The United States Health Care System

COMBINING BUSINESS, HEALTH, AND DELIVERY

SECOND EDITION

Anne Austin, PhD, JD
Vice Chancellor of Research, Planning & Assessment
University of Arkansas
Community College at Batesville

Victoria Wetle, RN, EdD
Retired Program Chair
Health Services Management
Chemeketa Community College
Salem, Oregon

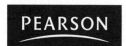

PEARSON

Boston   Columbus   Indianapolis   New York   San Francisco   Upper Saddle River
Amsterdam   Cape Town   Dubai   London   Madrid   Milan   Munich   Paris   Montreal   Toronto
Delhi   Mexico City   Sao Paulo   Sydney   Hong Kong   Seoul   Singapore   Taipei   Tokyo

Publisher: Julie Levin Alexander
Publisher's Assistant: Regina Bruno
Editor-in-Chief: Mark Cohen
Executive Editor: Joan Gill
Associate Editor: Bronwen Glowacki
Editorial Assistant: Mary Ellen Ruitenberg
Development Editor: Melisa Leong
Director of Marketing: David Gesell
Executive Marketing Manager: Katrin Beacom
Marketing Specialist: Michael Sirinides
Managing Production Editor: Patrick Walsh
Production Editor: Holly Shufeldt
Creative Director: Jayne Conte
Cover Designer: Karen Salzbach
Composition: Aptara®, Inc.
Printing and Binding: Edwards Brothers
Cover Printer: Lehigh-Phoenix Color

Chapter Opening Photo Credits: Getty Images, Inc.—Photodisc, pp. 2, 3, 52, 53, 68, 69, 116, 117, 148, 149; Centers for Disease Control and Prevention (CDC), pp. 132, 133, 166, 167; Victoria Wetle, pp. 184, 185, 200, 201

Library of Congress Cataloging-in-Publication Data

Austin, Anne
 The United States health care system : combining business, health, and delivery/Anne Austin,
Victoria Wetle.—2nd ed.
  p.; cm.
 Includes bibliographical references and index.
 ISBN-13: 978-0-13-139156-7
 ISBN-10: 0-13-139156-9
 1. Medical care--United States. 2. Medical economics—United States. I. Wetle, Victoria L. II. Title.
 [DNLM: 1. Delivery of Health Care—United States. 2. Health Care Sector—United States.
3. Health Services—United States. 4. Insurance, Health—United States. W 84 AA1]

 RA395.A3A955 2012
 362.10973—dc22

                                                                    2010043756

10 9 8 7 6 5 4 3 2 1

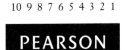

www.pearsonhighered.com

ISBN 13: 978-0-13-139156-7
ISBN 10:   0-13-139156-9

Contents

Preface

Over the last several decades, literally hundreds of books have been written about health care. Some are general introductions to the field; some are focused on specific narrow issues. We decided to add our book, *The United States Health Care System: Combining Business, Health, and Delivery*, to meet what we believed was an unfulfilled need.

Of all those books, there didn't seem to be one specifically designed for community college students and lower-division four-year students enrolled in allied health programs. What these students needed was a book that introduced them to the breadth of the field of health care without overwhelming them with detail. And it had to be written in an engaging, easy-to-follow style.

In any introduction to a field of study, a choice must be made between breadth and depth of coverage. Health care is a complex subject; for example, whole books can and have been written solely on Medicare eligibility, to pick just one topic. As authors and community college instructors, we have chosen to err on the side of breadth. We have intentionally introduced many topics with sufficient detail to identify them and have eliminated nonessential details that merely confuse or bog down the beginning student. Our hope is that students will leave the class with a broad overview of health care and all its components, thus establishing the building blocks for further learning in subsequent classes and in their careers. We're delighted to offer a second edition that encompasses the many changes that have occurred in both health care and in the United States since the first edition went to production.

Unique Perspective

Our book is unique in that it combines a health perspective with a business perspective. Health care is a major component in the U.S. economy and provides many employment opportunities. Students are attracted to the field not only because of a desire to help people but also because their studies pay off with jobs.

The first author provides the business perspective; her background is in management and marketing. Her view of health care is as an industry and business, facing the same challenges of all businesses to maintain a competitive advantage in the marketplace. The second author provides the delivery systems perspective; her background is in nursing, health care administration, and bioethics. Her view of health care focuses on the delivery system and addresses the perpetual tradeoffs among access, quality, and cost of services.

How This Text Is Organized

This book is organized around the pieces that make up health care. It addresses these questions: "What is this business called health care?" "How do we pay for health care?" "Who provides health care?" "Where and how is health care provided?" and "What else is included?" These questions are answered in the four parts of the book, in a total of 14 chapters, which permits the material to be presented in both quarter- and semester-long courses. The stand-alone nature of each part allows instructors to teach the material in the order that best suits their needs.

Part I introduces the world of health care. This section includes material on the size and scope of health care in the United States. The dual perspectives of business and delivery systems used in this text are presented as well as basic business and management concepts. The economic, government, and legal environments that impact health care are described. The payment process is presented as a framework for looking at health and money. The concepts of insurance and third-party payment are introduced, paving the way for subsequent discussion of managed care, Medicare, Medicaid, and other programs.

Part II introduces the people who provide care: those who the patient encounters first and those who work behind the scenes. Two chapters on clinical and non-clinical health care providers and professionals are included. We cover the roles of physicians and nurses in depth in one chapter and describe the roles of many other clinical and nonclinical providers in another.

Part III looks at where and how health care is delivered. It examines three health care delivery settings—the provider's office, clinics, and the hospital—to understand how primary and secondary care is delivered. This chapter describes the business organization, the roles played by managers and other business professionals, and the managerial decisions that are significant to these settings. Part III continues with chapter-length descriptions of long-term care, mental health, and public health. These are examined both as delivery systems and as specialty organizations.

Part IV expands the world of health care to include focused services and related industries. The industries of pharmaceuticals and medical technology are described to round out the student's understanding of the health care industry. Another chapter presents information about health care research and preventive care. Part IV goes on to discuss the important topics of cultural competency and ethical decision making. The text concludes with a chapter that provides an overview of the delivery systems in other countries as a counterpoint to the U.S. system that was the focus throughout the text.

How We Encourage Learning

Both the first and second editions of this textbook were intentionally written in a straightforward, student-friendly style to facilitate comprehension by college students, who field-tested a draft version. Based on our experience as instructors and the comments of students and reviewers, each chapter includes the following features to encourage student learning:

Learning Objectives

Each chapter begins with a preview of the material in a concise list of learning objectives. Students can use them to guide their reading and test their understanding of important points.

Profile

The text portion of the chapter begins with a real-life example that pertains to the topic of the chapter and is intended to increase students' interest in the material. One of the discussion questions in each chapter is related to the Profile scenario.

Exhibits

Each chapter includes exhibits. Diagrams or photos illustrate concepts or highlight the relationship between key points. Many aspects of health care are data based, and accompanying tables are presented to enhance students' understanding.

Glossaries

Like all fields of study, health care uses a specialized vocabulary that is often confusing and overwhelming to newcomers. To assist in learning vocabulary, key terms are boldfaced when they first appear in the text. Brief definitions are offered in the margin, and a complete glossary appears at the end of the book.

Chapter Summary and Questions

Each chapter closes with a summary of the key points that students should retain. Questions for Review test the students' comprehension of the chapter's learning objectives. In addition, Questions for Discussion allow students to expand their thinking beyond the facts presented in the chapter and provoke classroom discussion.

Chapter References and For Additional Information

Source materials are referenced in the text, and complete references are provided at the end of each chapter. The reference list allows students to explore topics of interest further and also models appropriate academic documentation for their own written work. Additional sources, including Web sites, are available for both faculty and student research.

Acknowledgments

We would like to thank Mark Cohen, our editor at Pearson Health Science, for his continued support of this book. We're proud of the final product his team at Pearson Health Science has produced.

We would also like to thank the reviewers who gave generously of their time and expertise. We particularly want to acknowledge the students in the Chemeketa Community College "Introduction to Health Care Services" classes of 2005 and 2006 for their thoughtful review of this material.

Anne—All my thanks to Frank, Frances, and Kathryn for their ongoing love, support, and patience.

Vikki—As always I am grateful for the love, support, and encouragement of my husband, Myron, and for the joy given to me by Jonathan, Shannon, Clara, and Luna.

Reviewers

The United States Health Care System

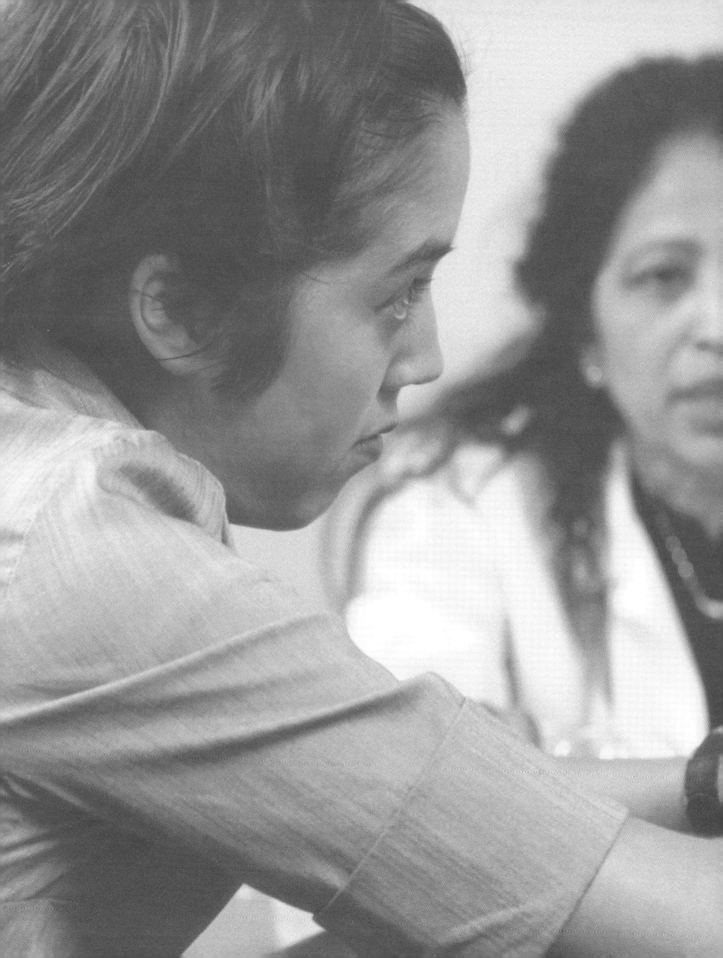

1

Health and Health Care in America

An Introduction

Learning Objectives

After reading this chapter, you should be able to:

1. Define health and health care.
2. Compare the medical and wellness models of health.
3. Identify major demographic categories of the American population.
4. Describe key indicators of the health of the American population.
5. Describe the size and scope of the health care industry in the United States.
6. Describe recent health reform efforts.

Sally Meets Health Care Providers

Sally, a college student majoring in health sciences, woke up with a very sore throat and an earache. Because the college does not have an urgent clinic or any student health program, Sally called her primary care physician's office. After a phone assessment by the triage nurse, Sally was directed to come into the clinic for a throat culture because of the possibility of a streptococcal infection.

Sally raced to the clinic between classes, thinking it would only take a moment to get a throat swab. The receptionist had Sally fill out a patient record visit, used her computer to determine which phlebotomist had an opening, and asked her to take a seat. After a 30-minute wait, Sally was taken back to the laboratory area, had her throat swabbed, and was told to give the receptionist her cell phone number so they could contact her if she needed an urgent appointment.

She had missed one class but went back to school for her next class. A public health epidemiologist would have told her to stay home because she was exposing everyone in the class to her germs.

Sally got a message to call her physician. When she returned the call after class, Sally scheduled an appointment for that evening with a nurse practitioner. The nurse practitioner explained Sally had a streptococcal infection, which had to be treated with antibiotics; without treatment, there might be a danger of kidney complications. Sally went to a nearby pharmacy; her prescription was taken by a pharmacy technician and filled by a licensed pharmacist who explained how to take the medication and what to do if certain side effects occurred. She took her medication as directed for the full 10 days. Sally was just fine at this point, but as predicted by our public health official, there were seven other cases of streptococcal throat infection in the class that term.

A simple throat swab generated a lot of activity that Sally never saw. Her chart was put together, notes written, and the laboratory results posted to the chart. Then a medical coder found the correct code to insert on the form that would be sent to the Sally's insurance company. This involved analyzing the information on the chart—called abstracting—and then posting the code. At this point, the chart notes went to the medical biller who actually put in the charges allowed and sent the electronic form

Introduction

Discussions of health care bring to mind images of doctors and nurses, hospitals, and nursing homes. The nightly news gives us stories about the latest government initiative to improve our nation's health, the outcome of a big malpractice case, or the impact of rising costs on access to care. In this chapter, you will learn about health care in the United States. You'll explore demographic data that provide a picture of health in the American population. You'll also look at data such as how many health care workers are employed, who the major employers are, and how much is spent for health care services to understand the impact of health care on the economy. The latest efforts to reform health care are presented, raising questions that you'll revisit throughout the semester. Finally, the chapter concludes with a brief overview of the topics covered in this textbook.

Health and Health Care in the United States

medical model
A viewpoint about health that focuses on the diagnosis and treatment of disease.

Any examination of health care needs to begin with an understanding of health and how health occurs in the population. You would think that defining health would be a simple matter, but it actually generates a great deal of controversy. Traditionally, health has been defined using a **medical model**. This model assumes that illness and disease require treatment; therefore, health care focuses on the diagnosis and treatment of disease. In the medical model, Western medicine is the answer to health.

into the insurance company where another medical coder verified the information, batched the file, and sent it on to the payer. The insurance company sent an electronic notification back to the physician's office verifying it paid the bill, the accounts receivable clerk posted the notice, and a record was also sent to Sally.

The state epidemiologist was given the report filled out by the nurse practitioner on an infectious disease and checked for other cases in the area. A public health specialist interviewed Sally and others in the class. The vector, or cause of the outbreak, was not Sally, but another student in a different class whose children all had come down with streptococcal throat infection from their grade school.

Meanwhile, Sally's ears had gotten worse, and she had an appointment with an otolaryngologist. After examining Sally, the otolaryngologist ordered more antibiotic followed by an audiometric examination to be done by an audiometric technologist 10 days after she finished her medication. The examination turned out to be within normal ranges, so no further treatment was necessary.

A few weeks later, Sally had a dental appointment for a routine check and cleaning: the dental hygienist did the preliminary exam, and then the dentist checked her X-rays and physically examined her mouth. The hygienist cleaned her teeth and prescribed a flossing routine. While she was in the office, Sally met a medical equipment salesperson who was demonstrating a new computer program that allowed the dental surgeon and orthodontist to take digital pictures rather than X-rays, which were then projected on a screen in the exam room, saving X-ray exposure for everyone.

During Christmas break, Sally had an appointment to check her eyes. At the ophthalmologist's office, the certified ophthalmology technician measured the refraction with a computer instead of the old-fashioned eye chart. The optometrist used this data to determine the strength of the glasses Sally would now need. She took this prescription to the optometrist who fitted her with glasses.

Sally had to give the same medical and insurance information to each office. She looked forward to something she had heard about in class: a single electronic record that all her caregivers could access.

In recent decades, there has been a shift of interest from illness to wellness. The **wellness model** of health care focuses on the prevention of disease and the maintenance of well-being. From the perspective of the wellness model, health is defined as the optimal functioning of each human being in his or her mind, body, and spirit.

wellness model
A viewpoint about health that focuses on the prevention of disease.

Which perspective you use to study health care will influence what data you select to examine whether a population exhibits health or not. It will also drive your decisions about how health should be achieved, including what resources should be allocated where.

A Snapshot of the American Population

A good place to begin the study of the American health care system is to look at some **demographic** data about the United States. Demographic data include innate personal characteristics of individuals, such as age, race, and gender. A key source of demographic data is the U.S. Census Bureau. The Census Bureau conducts a census every 10 years; the last census was in 2000. Data have been collected for the 2010 Census, although that data won't be fully available until 2012. According to Census 2000, there were 281.4 million residents in the United States. The bureau collects additional data in the intervening years using the American Community Survey. According to data released in 2010, the population had grown to 301.2 million residents in 2008 (There is always a lag between when the data are collected and when they are available to the public). Table 1.1 illustrates some characteristics of these residents and the changes between 2000 and 2008.

demographic
The data from human populations that describe vital statistics, size, and distribution.

Table 1.1	*Demographic Characteristics of United States Residents*	
	2000	**2008**
Total population:	281.4 million	301.2 million
Age of population:		
Under 18	72.3 million (26%)	73.5 million (24.4%)
Age 18–64	174.1 million (62%)	189.8 million (63.0%)
Over 65	35 million (12%)	37.9 million (12.5%)
Gender of population:		
Male	138.1 million (49.1%)	148.4 million (49.3%)
Female	143.4 million (50.9%)	152.8 million (50.7%)
Ethnicity of population:		
White	216.9 million (77.1%)	223.9 million (74.3%)
Black	36.4 million (12.9%)	37.1 million (12.3%)
Hispanic	35.3 million (12.5%)	45.5 million (15.1%)

Source: U.S. Census Bureau, *Census 2000* and *2008 American Community Survey*.
Note: Numbers do not add to 100% because of rounding error and method of questioning.

Age, gender, and ethnicity alone do not tell the whole story. In later chapters, we consider the impact of culture on health and health care delivery decisions. As these population figures are further subdivided and trends are considered, a more detailed picture emerges. This data can be used to predict what might happen in the future.

Consider two trends that emerge from the demographic data about age and their impact on health care. First, Americans as a whole are living longer. Life expectancy is now 77.9 years from birth, the highest it has ever been. Men and women who reach age 65 can expect to live to ages 82 and 85, respectively (Centers for Disease Control and Prevention, Chartbook 2008). The second trend is the impact of the baby boomers. Record numbers of babies were born in the years 1946 to 1964. Between 2010 and 2030, the 76 million baby boomers will reach age 65.

Both of these trends impact health care. An aging population increases demand for home health care and geriatric care. As longevity increases, an interest in the quality of that life becomes a major factor. As a result, preventive health care, including well visits and diagnostic screenings, becomes more important. Individuals seek information on exercise, diet, and alternative treatments such as acupuncture and hypnosis.

Gender also impacts the demand for health care. Women have a need for reproductive health care in addition to their general health care. Women are more often single heads of households, and they more often live in poverty. Women tend to live longer than men. Because of these gender-related needs, women require more access to health care over their lifetime.

Census data also indicate that the United States has increased its ethnic diversity. The Census 2000 was the first time respondents could identify themselves as more than one race. Of those who reported themselves as "white," 1.9 percent (about 5.5 million people) reported themselves as both "white" and one or more other races. The black population has increased faster than the total population; the Hispanic population has nearly doubled since 1990. The Hispanic population is also younger than the total population. When demographic data are combined with health status data, you will see that different populations experience health and illness differently. In later chapters, you will explore the issues of how diverse populations can best be served.

How Healthy Are Americans?

Epidemiology is the study of the nature, cause, control, and determinants of the frequency of disease, disability, and death in human populations (Timmreck 1994). In the United States, the **Centers for Disease Control and Prevention (CDC)** is responsible for collecting and interpreting volumes of health care statistics that present a picture of illness among Americans. Combined with Census-type data, health statistics can be used to design strategies to either prevent illness or encourage wellness.

Based on responses to the *2009 National Health Interview Survey*, America's health is good. Over 65 percent of respondents rated their health as "very good" or "excellent." Level of education and family income are closely related to good health. College graduates were more than twice as likely to be in excellent health as people who have not graduated from high school. Those with incomes above $75,000 were also twice as likely to be in good health as those with incomes of $20,000. Since 1998 there has been a steadily increasing number of Americans, now 7 percent, who report that they did not receive health care due to cost.

In addition to surveying Americans, the CDC also collects and reviews all the health statistics that are required to be reported. For example, the cause of death must be reported, which enables the CDC to track that outcome in the population. Table 1.2 reports the leading causes of death.

In the last century, huge strides have been made in terms of health outcomes. Over the last 30 years, the morbidity and mortality of the leading cause of disease has steadily declined by almost 50 percent. Healthier lifestyles account for much of that decrease. New vaccines have also improved health outcomes. Disease such as measles, mumps, chicken pox, whooping cough, tetanus, and diphtheria, which 30 years ago killed young children, have virtually been eradicated. However, widespread immunization policies must be continued in order to maintain such outcomes. Hospital discharges for children younger than 15 years have dropped over 50 percent in the last 30 years. In the last 10 years, new vaccines against hepatitis B, *Haemophilus influenzae*, and pneumonia have saved countless lives.

A road map of the preventive activities to improve American's health is presented in *Healthy People 2020*. The focus areas indicate major concerns of Congress, the **National Institutes of Health**, and the CDC. These focus areas are discussed in detail in a later chapter; however, access to health care remains one of the major goals of the country. The healthy outcomes are directly related to being able to get medical

epidemiology The study of the nature, cause, control, and determinants of the frequency of disease, disability, and death in human populations. Also the study of the history of a disease and its distribution throughout a society (public health).

Centers for Disease Control and Prevention (CDC) A group of federal governmental agencies responsible for collecting and interpreting health care statistics.

National Institutes of Health (NIH) A group of federal governmental agencies responsible for the health of the nation.

Table 1.2	*Leading Causes of Death 2007*
Total number of deaths	2,424,059
Heart disease	615,651
Cancer	560,187
Stroke	133,990
Chronic lower respiratory disease	129,311
Accidents	117,075
Alzheimer's disease	74,944
Diabetes	70,905
Pneumonia/flu	52,847
Septicemia	34,851
Suicide	33,185
Homicide	17,520

Source: Xu, J., Kochanek, K. and B. Tejada-Vera 2009.

care when needed. National legislation signed in 2010 addresses some of the issues related to improving access.

The focus areas and patterns of disease in the population also direct research efforts. Research can be directed at cure, control, or prevention with the ultimate aim of minimizing the impact of disease on a population. Curative research gets most of the headlines, but prevention has the widest impact on the daily lives of the population.

The Health Care Industry

The health care needs of the American population are met by the health care industry. Used broadly, this term includes all the workers and business settings involved in health. The health care industry encompasses all types of workers who provide health care services directly or who provide support or business services. The industry also includes all the different facilities and systems in which health care services are provided, such as physicians' offices, hospitals, long-term-care facilities, and laboratories. Health insurance providers, pharmaceutical companies, medical equipment and technology companies, and government agencies play important roles in the health care industry.

Health care is both one of the largest and one of the fastest growing industries in the United States. In 2009, the United States spent $2.5 trillion on health expenditures, or 17.6 percent of the country's gross domestic product (GDP). By 2018, the Centers for Medicare and Medicaid Services estimate spending will reach $4.3 trillion, or 20.3 percent of GDP (Kaiser 2009). **GDP** (or **Gross Domestic Product**) is the dollar value of all the final goods and services produced by businesses within a country's borders. Table 1.3 presents some figures from the most recent *Economic Census* that indicate the economic impact of health care businesses.

Health Care Employment

The U.S. Department of Labor forecasts that almost 22 percent of the new jobs created between 2008 and 2018 will be in health services. Employment of home care aides is expected to increase by 50 percent by 2018, medical assistants by 34 percent, physician assistants by 39 percent, and physical therapy assistants by 33 percent.

As identified by the Bureau of Labor Statistics, the four categories of health care occupations are (1) professional and related occupations; (2) service occupations; (3) office and administrative support occupations; and (4) management, business, and financial occupations. Professional and related occupations account for 43.8 percent of employees. This category includes doctors, nurses, and other health care professionals who provide health care services directly to patients. Service occupations represent

Gross Domestic Product (GDP) The dollar value of all the final goods and services produced by businesses within a country's borders.

Table 1.3	*Economic Impact of Health Care Businesses*		
	1997	**2007**	**% increase**
Number of establishments	645,853	779,519	20.7
Revenues	$885 million	$1,697 million	91.8
Annual payroll	$378 million	$665.8 million	76.1
Paid employees	13.6 million	16.9 million	24.3

Source: U.S. Census Bureau, *2007 Economic Census*.

another 34.2 percent of those employed. Dental and medical assistants, nursing and home health aides, medical transcriptionists, and food service and housekeeping are included here. Office and administrative support represents 17.7 percent of those employed. This category includes medical secretaries, billing and accounting clerks, and receptionists. Management, business, and financial occupations represent just under 5 percent of those employed (Bureau of Labor Statistics 2010–11).

The health care industry will continue to expand. The Department of Labor has identified three reasons for the continuing growth in health care employment. First, as already discussed, the aging of the population increases demand for health services. Second, advances in medical technology, covered later in this text, have changed both the way patient care is delivered and the way health care businesses are managed. Finally, continued interest to manage costs will also impact employment.

Health Care Delivery Systems

The three major places of employment are hospitals, nursing and residential care facilities, and practitioners' offices. More than 40 percent of health care jobs are in hospitals, 21 percent are in nursing or residential care facilities, and about 27.9 percent are in practitioners' offices (Bureau of Labor Statistics 2010–11). However, these are not just places of employment, but complex systems that deliver various types of services to specific groups of patients. Each delivery system combines the business side and a service model to address the needs not only of the individual patient, but the institutional and global nature of health. Some of the delivery systems discussed in this book are described below.

Long-term Care Long-term care (LTC) is and will continue to be one of the fastest growing sectors of health care. The term LTC means providing health care services to an individual for more than 90 days. A wide range of care facilities and professionals are involved in LTC. Most of the recipients (80%) of LTC assistance receive it in the community. Nursing homes account for a small percentage (4.1%) of the total. LTC also includes hospitals, assisted living and community-based residential facilities, adult day care, respite care, hospice care, rehabilitation centers, mental health facilities, adult foster homes, children's chronic care facilities, and care provided by family and friends (http://www.aoa.gov/AoARoot/Aging_Statistics/Profile/2009/6.aspx).

Mental Health The availability and quality of mental health services affect every family and employer in the United States. Most mental illness is a chronic lifetime disease that interferes with an individual's ability to participate fully in family life, work, and school. Mental illness strikes one out of every five adults, or about 26 percent of the population. This figure includes both mental illness diagnosis and substance abuse. It is further estimated that only about half the people who have mental illness get adequate treatment. Part of this inadequacy is because of economic and insurance status, cultural barriers, and the stigma of mental illness, and part is related to the inadequacy of the system itself (U.S. Department of Health and Human Services 1999, 405–7).

Public Health Public health can be seen in our everyday lives in things as simple as the crosswalk lines on a street that allow us to cross a roadway without getting hit by a car or the laws requiring construction workers to wear hard hats so that they are not injured by falling construction debris. It is also recognizable in state and nationwide campaigns to reduce smoking, heart disease, and cancer. Public health is seen every day by such activities such as nurses providing free immunizations to low-income children and police officers enforcing laws around seat belt and helmet use.

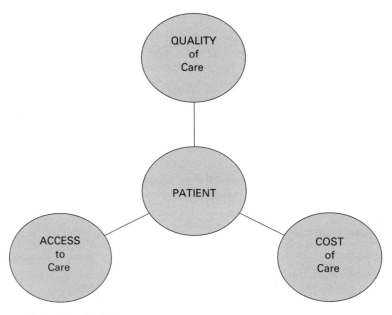

Figure 1.1   Policy Trade-Offs

Health Care Policy

Health care policy attempts to address the issues of access, quality, and costs, as indicated in Figure 1.1. It is difficult to design a policy, however, that will accomplish more than two of these goals simultaneously. What typically happens is that legislators identify a problem and then focus legislation on a solution to that problem.

The most recent federal legislation attempted to address all three goals. As signed into law by President Obama in March 2010, the Patient Protection and Affordable Care Act intends to improve health care for Americans in three ways (Kaiser 2010b). First, the act includes provisions to expand access to care by increasing access to insurance. For example, individuals are required to have coverage, employers are required to provide coverage, and benefits under public programs such as Medicaid and CHIP are expanded. Second, the act makes provisions to control health care costs. The Medicare and Medicaid programs will see significant changes over the next several years. Third, the law seeks to improve the health care delivery system's performance and quality through numerous specifically targeted mandates. Many of the provisions will be described in more detail later in this book.

Any time there are sweeping policy changes at the federal level, it takes time for these to take effect and for people to adjust. Survey data indicate that a slight majority of Americans (46%) view the law favorably, although 55 percent of respondents said they were confused about the law (Kaiser 2010a).

How we pay for health care in the United States Our system is a complicated process. While the specifics are covered in later chapters, patients may pay directly or through insurance coverage. Patients who meet the eligibility requirements of age, income, military service, or some other status receive health care as a benefit. By mandating insurance coverage, the Patient Protection and Affordable Care Act attempts to reduce the number of people who are uninsured, and thus not receiving care at all.

The idea that something needs to be done to control the costs of health care is not new. A major shift in the health care industry over the last 25 years has been the shift to **managed care**. Managed care combines health care delivery with health care services.

managed care
Describes the combination of payments for health care and delivery of services into one system.

Two things are managed: one is the patient's utilization of services and the other is the price paid for those services. The objective of managed care is to provide only those services that are necessary to contain costs. Although no one disagrees that health care has become increasingly more expensive, the shift to managed care as part of the effort to control costs has created considerable debate. A primary concern is that patients may not receive the care they really need.

Part of the focus on costs is because in the United States all industries operate in a market economy—they provide the goods and services that consumers indicate they want by paying for them. Business managers approach policy, or strategic decisions about the direction their business should take, from a **sustainable competitive advantage** approach. A business with a competitive advantage is able to maintain its position in the marketplace. Unless that advantage is sustainable, however, it will soon lose its position to its competitors.

sustainable competitive advantage Anything about a business that allows it to outperform other businesses and maintain its position over time.

What constitutes a sustainable competitive advantage varies from business to business and depends on the objectives the firm is trying to achieve. For example, a business could have an advantage because of cost: its product is low priced because its labor or materials don't cost it very much. This is why certain services are provided by a nurse practitioner instead of a physician. It could also have an advantage related to quality, either in its products or in its employees. Hospitals, for example, cultivate their reputation for providing the best care. A business could be competitive through speed: it's the first to offer a new product or service. Pharmaceutical companies try to be the first to market a patent-protected drug so that they will receive all the revenues from its sales.

Like health care policy makers, health care business managers must make trade-offs because all sources of advantage cannot occur simultaneously. And health care business must also try to meet the national policy objectives of quality, cost, and access.

Health care policy makers look to the major ethical theories of equality and justice for help in making health care allocation decisions. Most people will agree that there should be fairness and equality in the distribution of health care benefits across all parts of society. However, it will be clear as we study the health care system in the United States; and when we briefly consider health care systems in other countries, that fairness and equality are not easy to achieve. We will review some major ethical theories that provide a systematic way to allocate scarce and expensive resources.

This Book's Approach

This book presents an overview of health care in the United States, considering health care from two viewpoints. First, health care is a set of delivery systems that provides health care services to those who need them. At the same time, health care is a set of related businesses, all of which must operate as profitable entities. Figure 1.2 presents an overview of all the topics covered in this text

The book begins by exploring how health care services are paid for. It is rare for patients to pay from their own pocket, so the systems and businesses that are in place to pay must be understood. The impact of the health reform act is discussed.

At the heart of health care is an encounter between a patient and a provider. This book describes the various health care providers and professionals the patient may encounter. The encounter takes place in various settings depending on what types of services the patient needs. These settings, ranging from the simplest office visit to the complexity of LTC, are presented next. Each setting is described both in terms of a delivery system and as a type of business.

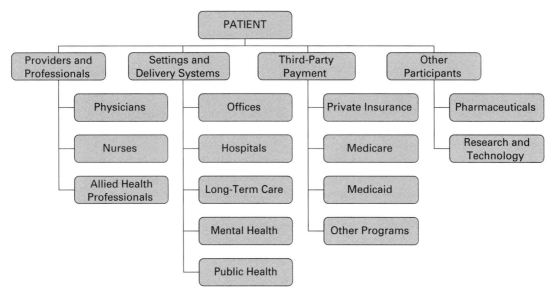

Figure 1.2   Organization of this Book

Finally, other entities that influence health care are considered. In some texts, these are not considered to be part of the health care system because they do not deliver services directly to patients. They are included in this text because we believe that the business and policy decisions made by and about pharmaceutical companies and medical research and technology have an enormous impact on the patient. The U.S. system is compared with other systems in terms of form, costs, and outcomes.

Summary

This chapter presents a picture of health and health care in the United States. Demographic data, such as age, gender, and ethnicity, were presented to understand some of the major characteristics of the American population. Health statistics, such as the major causes of death, were described, and the impact on the health needs and priorities of the country was discussed. The size and scope of the healthcare industry that meets these needs was presented. The criteria for making effective policy were discussed and compared to the criteria for effective decision making in business. Health care reform is expected to have a major impact on the industry.

Questions for Review

1. Define health. What is the difference between the medical and wellness models of health?
2. List two of the leading causes of death in 2007.
3. List two health care occupations that are expected to grow by 2018.
4. Describe one provision in the new health reform act.

Questions for Discussion

1. This chapter presented a list of the most common causes of death in the United States. How do these vary by demographic categories?
2. Why is health care such a large percentage of GDP? How does this compare to other segments of the economy, such as education, housing, or military spending?
3. Conduct a survey among your friends and family. What do they know about the newest health reform act? Is their opinion generally favorable? Why or why not?
4. How could the provisions in the new health reform bill improve Sally's access to health care (see the chapter profile)?

Chapter References

Bureau of Labor Statistics, U.S. Department of Labor. 2010–11. *Career guide to industries, Healthcare.* Available at www.bls.gov/oco/cg/cgs035.htm.

Centers for Disease Control and Prevention. 2008. *Chartbook, Health. United States 2008.*

Department of Health and Human Services, Administration on Aging. 2009. www.aoa.gov/AoARoot/Aging_Statistics/Profile/2009/6.aspx.

Henry J. Kaiser Family Foundation. 2009. *Trends in health care costs and spending.* March. Pub #7692-02, available at www.kff.org.

_____. 2010a. *American remain divided on health reform bill but are confused about the law and how and when it will affect them.* April 22. Available at www.kff.org.

_____. 2010b. *Summary of new health reform law.* April 21. Pub #8061, available at www.kff.org.

Timmreck, T. C. 1994. *An introduction to epidemiology.* Boston: Jones & Bartlett.

U.S. Census Bureau. 2002. *Statistical abstract of the United States.*

_____. *2007 Economic Census, Industry Series Reports.*

_____. *2008 American Community Survey.*

U.S. Department of Health and Human Services. 1999. *Mental health: A report of the surgeon general.* Rockville, MD: U.S. Department of Health and Human Services, Substance Abuse and Mental Health Services Administration, Center for Mental Health Services, National Institutes of Health, National Institute of Mental Health.

Xu, J., Kochanek, K., and B. Tejada-Vera. 2009. Death: Preliminary data for 2007. *National Vital Statistics Reports*, Centers for Disease Control and Prevention, August 19.

For Additional Information

Griffith, J. R., and K. R. White. 2002. *The well-managed healthcare organization.* 5th ed. Chicago: Health Administration Press.

Lee, R. H. 2000. *Economics for healthcare managers.* Chicago: Health Administration Press.

Shi, L., and D. A. Singh. 2001. *Delivering health care in America: A systems approach.* 2d ed. Gaithersburg, MD: Aspen.

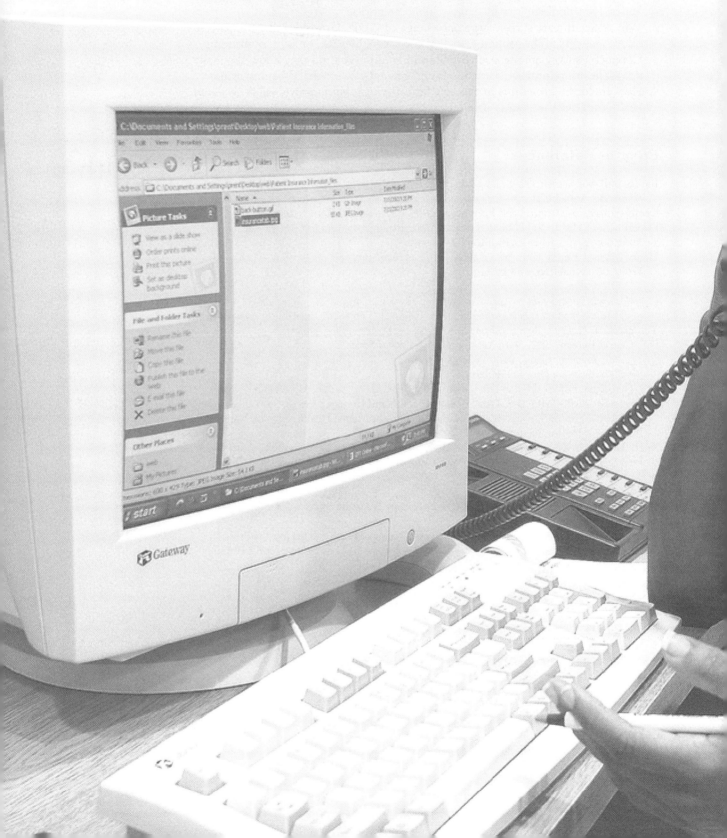

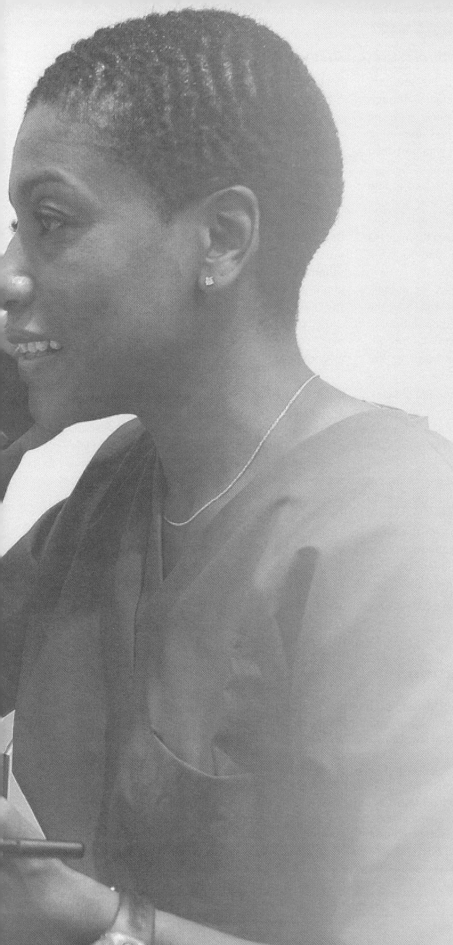

The Business Side of Health Care

Learning Objectives

After reading this chapter, you should be able to:

1. Identify legal forms of business ownership.
2. Describe key business functions.
3. Identify the major components of the health care industry.
4. Describe the ways economic activity is defined and measured.
5. Identify key laws that influence the health care industry.
6. Describe how health care businesses can monitor and evaluate the external environment.

Competition Comes to Town

Dr. Anderson put down a copy of the industry newsletter and leaned back in her chair. Although her ophthalmology practice was doing well, the first discount eye care chain had just opened in town, and she was concerned about what impact it might have on her business.

Like most ophthalmologists, she had a solo practice. She employed an office manager and one technician. She also had a retail operation that sold frames and contact lenses. The glasses themselves were manufactured offsite. Two people were employed on the retail side.

Before the discount chain opened, her competition was the one other ophthalmologist and the three optometrists in town. The population of 14,000 had seemed to support them all comfortably. On the plus side, a large portion of her patients were elderly: they needed the specialized care she gave, not just prescriptions for glasses. On the negative side, the town's largest employer, a manufacturing plant, was talking about layoffs, so those people would want the cheapest glasses they could get.

There weren't too many places she could cut expenses. One big expense was salaries, but all four employees were needed to take care of the patients. She had a long-term lease for the office and retail space at a good rate for the town. She had been considering some new patient-tracking software and a new piece of equipment. She could delay both purchases, but both were intended to make the office more efficient and modernize eye care.

Maybe she could increase revenues. About 35 percent of her revenues came from the retail business; the other 65 percent was from patient visits. If she was open on Saturdays and in the evenings, she could see more patients. But she'd have to have extra help to cover the extra hours. She already gave a discount to a patient who provided a referral, but maybe she could explore other ways to get more patients. At one meeting she'd attended, one doctor had given discounts for family members and for regular visits. She didn't know what the others charged for an office visit; maybe they needed to get together and discuss their fees.

On the retail side, maybe she needed to offer some less expensive frames in addition to the brands she already carried. Perhaps she could find a less expensive fabricator, although she was very pleased with the quality of the lenses they received. She wasn't sure if they had any customers from the other ophthalmologists; maybe she needed to advertise or offer second-pair discounts.

Tomorrow morning, Dr. Anderson decided, she'd meet with her employees and see what ideas they had for how to deal with this competitive threat.

Introduction

Businesses make decisions about the products they offer, the customers they try to attract, and how they organize and manage their employees and operations. As they develop plans and strategies, businesses must monitor and assess the potential impact of other businesses in their industry and changes in the external environment. Figure 2.1 presents these relationships visually.

In this chapter, you are introduced to basic business concepts, including organizational forms and key business functions. Key components of the health care industry are presented. This chapter describes two external environments that impact the design and operation of health care businesses: economic and political-legal. These environments are the frame of reference in which business decisions are made. The chapter concludes with an example of one strategic tool businesses use to integrate their decision-making process with the external environment.

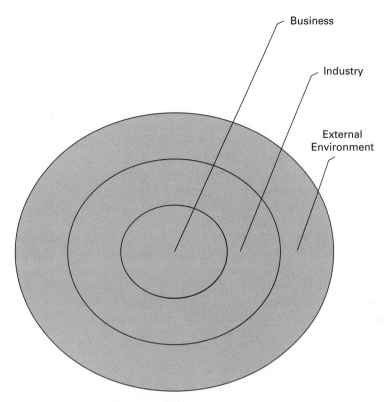

Figure 2.1   Business and Its Environment

What Is Business?

Broadly defined, **business** involves providing a product or service to customers for a **profit**. When a business provides a product or service, it generates revenues by selling the product or service to customers. However, it costs the business something to create that product or service because the business has to pay for materials and labor and equipment. When these costs are subtracted from revenue, what is left is profit.

All businesses, regardless of industry type, must make a profit, or else they will be unable to remain in business. However, a distinction is made between a **for-profit** business and a **not-for-profit** business. In a for-profit business, such as pharmaceutical giant Abbott Laboratories, profit is the primary reason for the business to exist. A not-for-profit business has something other than profit as its main objective. A not-for-profit hospital, for example, may focus on serving the poor in its community. The hospital will actually lose money on many of its poor patients, but as long as the hospital can generate enough revenue from operations or through donations to cover its expenses, that is okay.

If you look at a business that sells potato chips, it's easy to understand what the product is and who the customer is. In health care, those questions are a little tougher. Just what product or service does the industry provide? A physician's office could define its service as diagnosing illness or as preventing illness. Who exactly is the customer? The customer could be the patient, the individual who receives the service. It also could be the insurance company that pays for the service. How a business answers these questions helps the business organize and manage itself.

business The activity of providing goods and services to customers for profit.

profit The amount left when a business subtracts its expenses from its revenues. If the amount is a negative number, it is a loss.

for profit Making a profit is identified as the primary reason for the business to exist.

not-for-profit The primary reason for the business to exist is some reason other than profit.

Forms of Business Ownership

In the United States, there are only three legal structures for operating a business: sole proprietorship, partnership, and corporation. Each has advantages and disadvantages, depending on the needs of the business. As you can see in Table 2.1, the forms vary in terms of ownership, personal liability, income taxation, and ease of formation.

Solo practices, most common among dentists and ophthalmologists like the Profile's Dr. Anderson, are typical examples of sole proprietorships in health care. In a **sole proprietorship**, one person owns the business. The owner makes all the decisions, takes all the risks, and reaps all the rewards.

A medical group practice is frequently organized as a partnership. In a **partnership**, two or more people work together to achieve the objectives of the business. Decision making, risks, and rewards are shared among the partners.

Nursing homes and hospitals are often owned as corporations. A **corporation** separates ownership and management. The shareholders own the business, but they give their right to make decisions to managers. Their risk is then limited to their investment, as is their right to receive part of the rewards.

Although in a free enterprise system a business can chose which form of ownership best suits its needs, state law may determine the form of ownership for physicians and hospitals. These restrictions were enacted by legislators who wanted to promote public safety and quality of services. These forms are discussed in more detail in later chapters.

Business Functions

Regardless of the business's legal form, providing products and services to its customers requires a number of activities. These are known as business functions and are presented in Figure 2.2.

Management is the broadest function because it involves people at all levels of the business. Management is the process of planning, organizing, directing, and controlling the business's resources to achieve the objectives of the business. In the planning part of the process, managers define their objectives and develop strategies and plans to achieve the objectives. In the organizing part, managers develop an organizational structure that helps the business operate efficiently. The organizational structure also indicates who is responsible for what. The directing part focuses on the business's human resources—how can they be motivated effectively. Finally, the control part of the process is a feedback loop. Managers must monitor to see if the business is meeting its goals and make adjustments if necessary.

sole proprietorship A legal form of business ownership that has only one owner.

partnership A legal form of business ownership that involves at least two people called partners.

corporation A legal form of business ownership that can have many owners. The percentage of the business owned is determined by the number of shares held by the owner, also known as a shareholder.

management The business function of planning, organizing, directing, and controlling the business's resources.

Table 2.1	*Characteristics of Business Forms*		
	Sole Proprietorship	**Partnership**	**Corporation**
Ownership	One owner	At least two partners	Infinite
Legal Liability	Personally liable	Personally liable	Loss limited to initial investment
Taxation		Owner pays income tax on business profits as part of individual income; entity is a pass-through	Corporation pays tax on its income; shareholder pays tax on dividends
Formation	Simple	More complex	Difficult

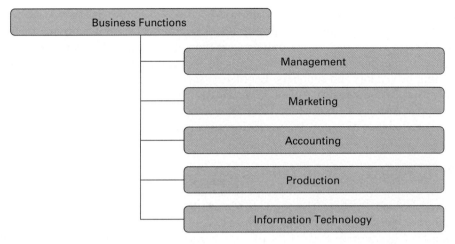

Figure 2.2 Business Functions

At the top of the organizational chart is the board of directors, the president or chief executive officer (CEO), and top management. These managers have responsibility for the whole organization. For example, the person in charge of a hospital is the CEO. Middle management refers to managers who have responsibility over a particular part of the business. The vice president of patient care, for example, is responsible for most of the nurses employed by the hospital. Line or supervisory management is responsible for a group of employees performing a specific task. An office manager supervises clerks, data processors, and receptionists. All the levels of management must work together.

Marketing focuses on the exchange process between a business and its customers. Marketing develops a plan that includes the product, its price, promotion, and distribution to the consumer. Marketers do research to help them understand what products and services their customers want. A pharmaceutical company, for instance, develops a new product: a drug to control allergies. The company lets its customers know about the product by advertising on TV and in magazines. It sets a price for the product. Its sales representatives visit doctors to tell them about the benefits of the new drug and provide free samples to encourage physicians to prescribe it for their patients.

Accounting keeps track of the money. Accountants track the flows of money in and out of a business. Money comes in when customers pay for the goods and services (called accounts receivable), and money goes out when the firm pays its employees and bills for raw materials and supplies (called accounts payable). Managers can use accounting data to make better decisions. For example, by analyzing cost data, a manager can decide whether the medical practice could save money by hiring an independent medical transcriptionist instead of using a full-time employee to do this job.

Production refers to the process of physically creating the product or service. Managers analyze the process to see if they can improve efficiency without sacrificing quality. When manufacturing a product, managers improve productivity by considering factors such as how the machines are laid out. Similar issues are considered when analyzing services. A manager might look at the process of admitting a patient to the hospital to see where steps could be saved so that waiting time could be reduced.

Information technology (IT) refers to the use of technology to manage information. Primarily this involves computers and computer networks. Health care organizations collect huge amounts of data that they store, retrieve, and process. IT helps

marketing
The business function that focuses on the exchange process between the business and its customers.

accounting
The business function that tracks flows of payments in and out of a business.

production
The business function that designs and manages the process that manufactures the business's products.

information technology
The business function that manages all the technology used to run the business and collects information for decision making.

design the systems to do this as efficiently as possible. The move to electronic storage of patient data has created a new profession—health information management. However, patient health records are only one example of the data collected by health care providers. The business also has data about its own employees and other records concerning its vendors and suppliers. Legislation such as the **Health Insurance Portability and Accountability Act of 1996 (HIPAA)** impacted how this function is performed in health care businesses. The American Recovery and Reinvestment Act of 2009 created incentives for the use of electronic health records technology.

The Health Care Industry

As you learned in Chapter 1, the U.S. Census Bureau considers more than 700,000 businesses part of the health care industry. Under code 62 of the North American Industry Classification System (NAICS), the government tracks the activities of the sector of the economy it calls health and social assistance. The businesses in code 62 are divided into four categories: ambulatory health care services, hospitals, nursing and residential care facilities, and social assistance. Each category is further divided. Every 5 years, the Census Bureau tracks the economic activity by measuring number of employees, size of payroll, and revenues. Revenues are broken out by what types of products are being sold (U.S. Bureau of the Census 2007).

The Impact of the Economy

Businesses in the US operate in a **market economy** (also called a private or free enterprise system). Competition is the central feature of a market economy. Anyone can open a business and offer whatever product he or she chooses. The business will succeed if it can provide a product that the market (customers) wants. The business must provide value—measured by the quality of the product and the level of customer satisfaction—to make itself different from its competitors. Dr. Anderson, the ophthalmologist described in the chapter Profile, is facing the question of how to remain competitive.

Some parts of the health care industry do not operate in a true market economy. In some geographic regions, there may be only one or two hospitals or only three dentists. A market where there are only a few sellers is called an **oligopoly**. If a pharmaceutical company holds a patent and sells the only drug for heartburn, then it is a **monopoly**. In markets where there is very little competition, sellers can raise prices and do not have to be as sensitive to their customers.

The allocation of resources in a market economy can be understood by understanding the demand and supply of goods. From the customers' side, the lower the price of a product falls, the more of it they are willing to buy. For example, if the price of cough syrup is $3.59, I might buy two bottles. If the price was $2.79, I might be willing to buy three bottles, and so on. This is the **demand** for the product.

From the producers' side, the higher the price goes, the more they are willing to produce for the market. At $2.79 per bottle, the manufacturer might be willing to produce one bottle; at $3.59, the manufacturer might be willing to produce two bottles. This is the supply for the product. As shown in Figure 2.3, the two sides meet at a point called the equilibrium price or the price at which the amount consumers demand and the amount that the producers supply are equal. In our example, the equilibrium price is $3.59.

Health Insurance Portability and Accountability Act of 1996 (HIPAA) A federal law that mandates insurance portability and sets up procedures for electronic data exchange.

market economy An economy in which many sellers compete for customers.

oligopoly An economy with only a few sellers.

monopoly An economy with only one seller. The one seller is able to set whatever price it chooses.

demand The amount of a good a buyer is willing to purchase at a given price.

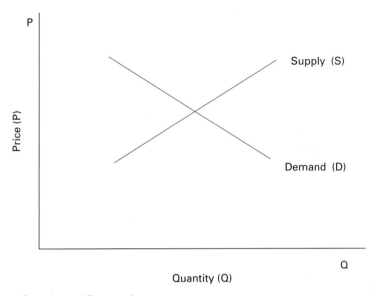

Figure 2.3   Supply and Demand

This basic economic model helps us understand the behavior of consumers and producers. The model can be used to understand why the price of generic drugs is less than brand-name drugs or why a nurse will change jobs to obtain a raise.

The health of the overall economy can be analyzed by studying data known as **economic indicators**. Among the key indicators that tell us how the economy is doing are the interest rate, the inflation rate, and the unemployment rate. Studying changes in these indicators helps health care managers plan for the future (Lee 2009).

Interest is the price paid when an individual or business borrows money. The price is quoted as an annual percentage rate. The lower the interest rate, the cheaper it is to borrow money. This encourages businesses and individuals to borrow, which allows them to spend more.

Inflation is an increase in the general price level, or average of prices at a given time. Inflation occurs when total spending in the economy increases in relation to the supply of goods, often during the expansion phase of the business cycle. Inflation has a variety of causes, such as a high demand for bank loans, heavy spending by the government, and a continuing demand for wage increases. Because prices tend to rise faster than incomes, consumers become afraid their savings will lose value as purchasing power declines. Often this leads consumers to spend their savings.

Unemployment is the lack of jobs for those who are willing and able to work at the going wage rate. Although some unemployment is considered normal in an economy, economists become concerned when the number of unemployed rises above the normal level (called full employment). The health care sector generally has a lower unemployment rate than the overall economy.

These economic pieces can be put together by considering the **business cycle**, the regular cycles of growth and decline. There are four possible scenarios: prosperity, recession, depression, and recovery. Each is measured by the change in the GDP per quarter. Figure 2.4 presents the relationship between the key economic indicators and the stage of the business cycle.

In the prosperity phase of the business cycle, times are good—GDP is increasing, and the interest rates, inflation, and unemployment are all low. Because individuals have jobs, they have extra money in their pockets. This is money they can spend on

economic indicators Key measurements that provide information about the health of the economy.

interest The amount, stated as a percentage, paid to borrow money.

inflation An increase in the price level.

unemployment A lack of jobs in an economy for those willing and able to work.

business cycle Regular cycles of decline and growth in an economy over a time period.

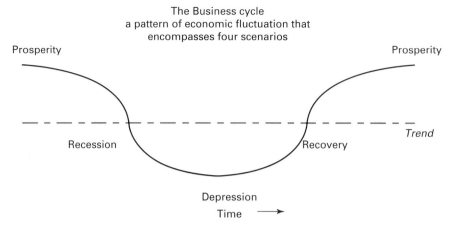

Figure 2.4 The Business Cycle

items beyond necessities. For instance, an individual might decide to have elective surgery, get braces, or buy a pair of prescription sunglasses. Health care providers also spend money: they add additional employees, buy new equipment, and expand the office building. Businesses that are doing well might decide to add additional health care benefits for their employees, which in turn improves the health care provider's business.

In the recession phase, the economy slows down. Inflation and interest rates begin to increase. This causes businesses and individuals to spend less and to borrow less because these activities are more expensive. Individuals may only seek the health care services they must have. Businesses may lay off employees and cut health care benefits as they try to save money. Health care providers might also have to cut staff and postpone purchases of new equipment. All of these have been seen during 2007–2010, when the United States has been in a period of recession. The unemployment rate has exceeded 10 percent in most areas of the country, and the number of uninsured increased.

If a recession persists, it is called a depression. Economic activity comes to a near standstill. Individuals buy only the necessities, and they may not be able to afford all of those. Unemployed individuals turn to the government for health care or do without.

The government may intervene in the free market economy to move the economy into the recovery phase. The government can lower interest rates and cut taxes to stimulate spending. In the recovery phase, things begin to improve. Businesses hire back employees, and business and individuals are able to purchase the items they need.

Economic cycles appear inevitable. The difficult part of a manager's job is to predict how often a cycle will occur and how long any of the phases will last. Like other businesses, the health care industry must monitor and assess economic conditions to make appropriate decisions.

The Role of Government

Even though the United States does not have a national health system, the government's involvement in health care is significant. Government actually plays three roles: as a provider of health care services, as a payer for services provided by others, and as a regulator of health care providers. The first two roles are discussed in other chapters of this book; government's role as a regulator is discussed here.

Government regulates health care by using the political process to make laws. The idea for a law can come from anywhere. Doctors and hospitals might want the level of Medicaid reimbursement increased. Older individuals on fixed incomes might want a law that sets prices for prescription drugs. A professional organization might want to change the licensure standards for its members. Each group would contact its legislator to make its ideas and needs known.

Industry representatives work with legislators to influence the political process. The American Medical Association and the American Hospital Association, as well as medical associations at the state level, lobby legislators to protect the interests of their membership.

Industries also create their own regulatory groups so that government will decide no additional regulation is needed. The **Joint Commission** (formerly JCAHO) is a case in point. TJC evaluates and accredits nearly 17,000 health care organizations in the United States to improve the quality and safety of health care services. Their standards are considered so good that TJC accreditation often substitutes for federal certification surveys for Medicare and Medicaid (www.jointcommission.org).

Joint Commission (TJC) National organization that evaluates and accredits health care organizations.

Traditionally the laws that the government uses to regulate health care have had two broad objectives. One objective has been to ensure fair competition in the marketplace. Another objective has been to protect the public.

The **antitrust** laws are an example of how the government regulates competition. These laws are presented in Table 2.2. Basically, antitrust law prohibits businesses from taking actions that lessen competition. This can include mergers, attempts to create monopolies, and price fixing and price discrimination (www.usdoj.gov/atr/). Health care organizations must make decisions within the boundaries of antitrust laws. For example, a hospital that limits the number of physicians admitted to its medical staff may be accused of conspiring to limit competition from other physicians and medical groups. A health maintenance organization (HMO) or participating provider option (PPO) might be accused of price fixing and price discrimination when it negotiates fees and contracts. Dr. Anderson, the Profile's ophthalmologist, could be in violation if she discussed fees with other similar physicians in her region. Although potentially more efficient for the business, a merger of two hospitals or medical groups has the potential to lessen competition because patients would have fewer choices of health care providers.

antitrust An area of federal law that prohibits monopolization and other activities that lessen competition in the marketplace.

Legislatures also pass laws that are expected to protect the public. Table 2.3 presents some examples of laws that are broadly related to the public's health. Some legislation designed to protect the public specifically regulates how health care

Table 2.2	*Antitrust Laws*	
1890	Sherman Antitrust Act	Prohibits restraint of trade and monopolization
1914	Clayton Act	Restricts practices such as price discrimination, exclusive dealing, and tying contracts where the effect "may be to substantially lessen competition or tend to create a monopoly"
1914	Federal Trade Commission Act	Establishes Federal Trade Commission to investigate business practices that are unfair methods of competition
1936	Robinson-Patman Act	Prohibits price discrimination; prohibits selling at unreasonably low prices to eliminate competition

Table 2.3	*Consumer Protection Laws*	
1906	Pure Food and Drug Act	Establishes Food and Drug Administration; prohibits misbranding and adulteration of food and drugs
1938	Federal Food, Drug, and Cosmetic Act	FDA given authority to regulate cosmetics and therapeutic products
1962	Kefauver-Harris Drug Amendment	Manufacturers required to test safety and effectiveness of drugs; generic or common drug name must be on label
1983	Orphan Drug Act	Sets incentives and grants exclusive marketing rights to promote development of drugs for rare diseases
1984	Drug Price Competition	Shortens application process for approval of Patent Term Restoration Act generic versions of certain drugs
1990	Americans with Disabilities Act	Protects rights of people with disabilities

providers must behave. Examples are presented in Table 2.4. Some legislation, like the Social Security Act of 1965 that created both Medicare and Medicaid, has been in existence for almost 40 years but continues to be important to health care businesses because of the influence reimbursement policies and amounts have on patients and providers alike.

Other legislation, such as the Hill-Burton Act, appeared to have been deactivated but have now made a comeback. When originally passed, the legislation

Table 2.4	*Health Care Laws*	
1965	Medicare/Medicaid	Part of the Social Security Act; Medicare provides health care insurance (including hospitalization) for elderly and patients with disabilities; Medicaid provides health care for the indigent
1946	Hill-Burton Act	Also called the Hospital Survey and Construction Act; federal government funded construction of private facilities pursuant to a Certificate of Need; facility required to provide care to underserved populations; enforcement regulation passed in 1979
1989	"Stark I"	Amendment to the Social Security Act, which prohibits referrals to clinical lab service where provider has a financial interest.
1993	"Stark II"	Expands Stark I to include referrals to "designated health services"
1996	HIPAA	Provides for health insurance portability and protects the privacy of health records
2009	ARRA	Special provisions to protect laid-off workers and to encourage electronic records technology
2010	Affordable Care Act	Patient Protection and Affordable Care Act; Requires U.S. citizens to have health insurance. Expands government programs. Specifies insurers' ability to deny coverage and raise premiums.

required Certificate of Need (CON) approval before new hospitals could be built; the rationale was to ensure that facilities were built in rural areas. A few state legislatures have debated whether to revive their certificate of need laws (Wysocki 2002). The current rationale is a debate over how to provide sufficient care at reasonable costs.

A major piece of legislation that directly regulates health care is HIPAA, cited earlier. Although the law was passed in 1996, some provisions did not go into final effect until April 2003. Part of the delay was caused by continuing debate about how the health care industry would comply with the law's provisions and whether the law would actually achieve its intent. The legislation has five parts, or titles. Title I provides for insurance portability. Title II includes two major components. The first deals with fraud and abuse and reform of medical liability. The second mandates administrative simplification, which includes privacy and security provision for health data and requires electronic data interchange (EDI). Title II involves taxes; Title IV, the requirements for group health plans; and Title V, revenue offsets.

The American Recovery and Reinvestment Act of 2009 (ARRA) includes the "HITECH Act" (Health Information Technology for Economic and Clinical Health Act), which adds programs under Medicare and Medicaid related to electronic health records technology. In another section, ARRA provides temporary COBRA subsidies to recently laid-off workers to cover 65 percent of the insurance premium.

The Patient Protection and Affordable Care Act was signed into law by President Obama in March 2010, although some of the provisions do not take effect until 2014 and beyond. Many refer to it as the "health reform act," because it addresses many of the access, cost, and quality issues that are addressed throughout this text. The primary purpose of the legislation was to expand access to insurance coverage, whether through private employer or government plans. The plan provides mechanisms for uninsured individuals to obtain private insurance, mandates employers provide basic plans, and expands government programs such as Medicare and Medicaid. Some of the specifics are described in later chapters. The law also creates a number of programs to improve the quality and effectiveness of health care as well as programs aimed at prevention (Kaiser 2010).

Integrating Business and Its Environment

As you have seen, the state of the economy as well as changes in federal and state laws can dramatically affect a health care business. Although managers can't change the environment, they can change the business's activities to meet the demands of the environment. As part of the process of developing business plans and strategies, managers assess the environment. This involves collecting data to understand what the environment is like at the present moment. It also involves making predictions or forecasts of what the environment will be like in the future. Managers can use a number of techniques to integrate the business activity with what is occurring in the environment around it.

Many managers use a technique called **SWOT analysis** to determine where the business is in relation to its environment (Thompson and Strickland 2003). SWOT stands for *S*trengths, *W*eaknesses, *O*pportunities, and *T*hreats. As illustrated in Figure 2.5, managers analyze the strengths and weaknesses of their business and try to identify opportunities and threats in the environment. Managers then try to match strengths with opportunities to plan for the future.

SWOT analysis
A method used by businesses to analyze the external environment.

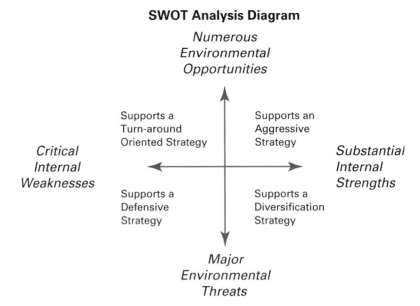

Figure 2.5   SWOT Analysis

Summary

Health care is a business as well as a delivery system. Business involves providing a product or service to customers for a profit. Health care businesses must define what their product or service is and who their customers are. The business may be legally organized as a sole proprietorship, a partnership, or a corporation. Regardless of form, the business will perform the key business functions of management, marketing, accounting, production, and information technology. Two external environments impact the operation and design of health care businesses: economic and political-legal. These environments are the frame of reference in which health care businesses make decisions. SWOT analysis can be used to integrate the decision-making process with conditions in the external environment.

Questions for Review

1. Define partnership and corporation.
2. Define the four areas of management.
3. What items are included in a marketing plan?
4. Define interest, inflation, unemployment, and supply and demand.
5. What are the key provisions of the 2010 Patient Protection and Affordable Care Act?

Questions for Discussion

1. If a manager cannot control changes in the external environment, why should the manager be concerned about those changes?
2. Do some research. What are the current interest, inflation, and unemployment rates in your region? Have those rates been improving or declining?

3. What activities could a health care business begin during an economic decline to improve the profitability of the business? (Hint: Review this chapter's Profile and assess the probability of success of each of Dr. Anderson's ideas.)
4. Interview your employer or other health care businesses to discover what changes they have made in their procedures to be in compliance with HIPAA, ARRA, and the new health reform law.
5. In addition to TJC and federal laws, what other means exist to ensure patients receive quality health care?

Chapter References

Department of Justice, Antitrust Division (www.usdoj.gov/atr/).

The Joint Commission (www.jointcommission.org).

Kaiser Family Foundation. 2010. *Summary of new health reform law*. Publication #8061 available at www.kff.org.

Lee, R. H. 2009. *Economics for healthcare managers*. 2nd ed. Chicago: Health Administration Press.

Thompson, A. A., and A. J. Strickland. 2003. *Strategic management*. 13th ed. New York: Irwin/McGraw-Hill.

U.S. Bureau of the Census. 2007. *Economic Census. Industry Series Reports. Health Care and Social Assistance*.

Wysocki, B. 2002. Regulation or competition? States battle over how to get reasonable, quality health care. *Wall Street Journal*, May 7, p. A4.

For Additional Information

Federal Trade Commission (www.ftc.gov).

Fremgen, B. F. 2008. *Medical law and ethics*. 3rd ed. Upper Saddle River, NJ: Prentice Hall.

Mescon, M. H., C. L. Bovee, and J. V. Thill. 2001. *Business today*. 10th ed. Upper Saddle River, NJ: Prentice Hall.

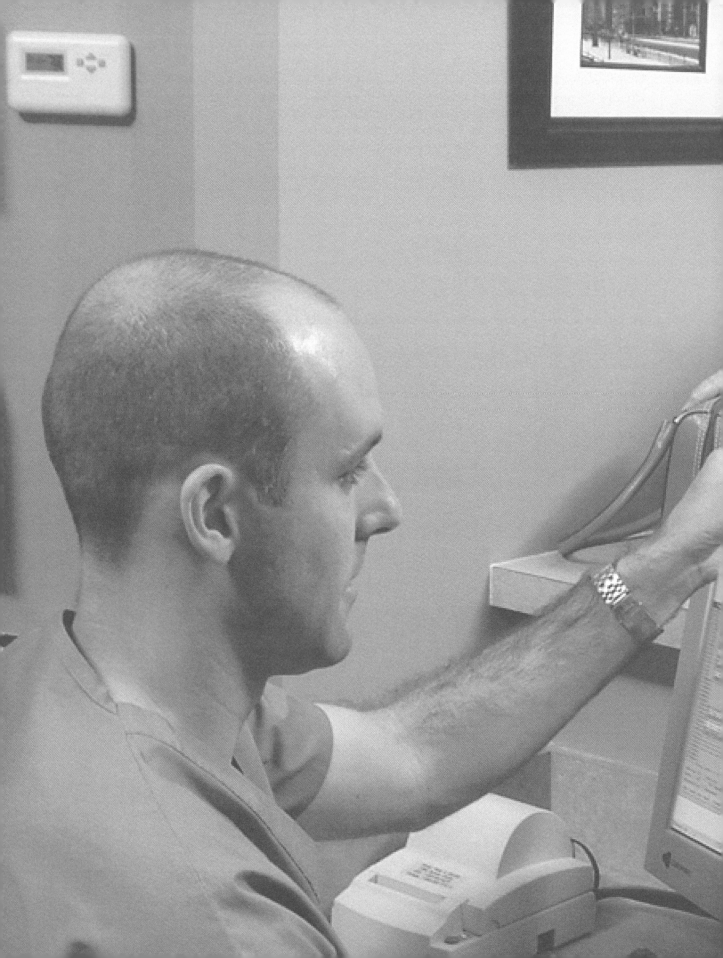

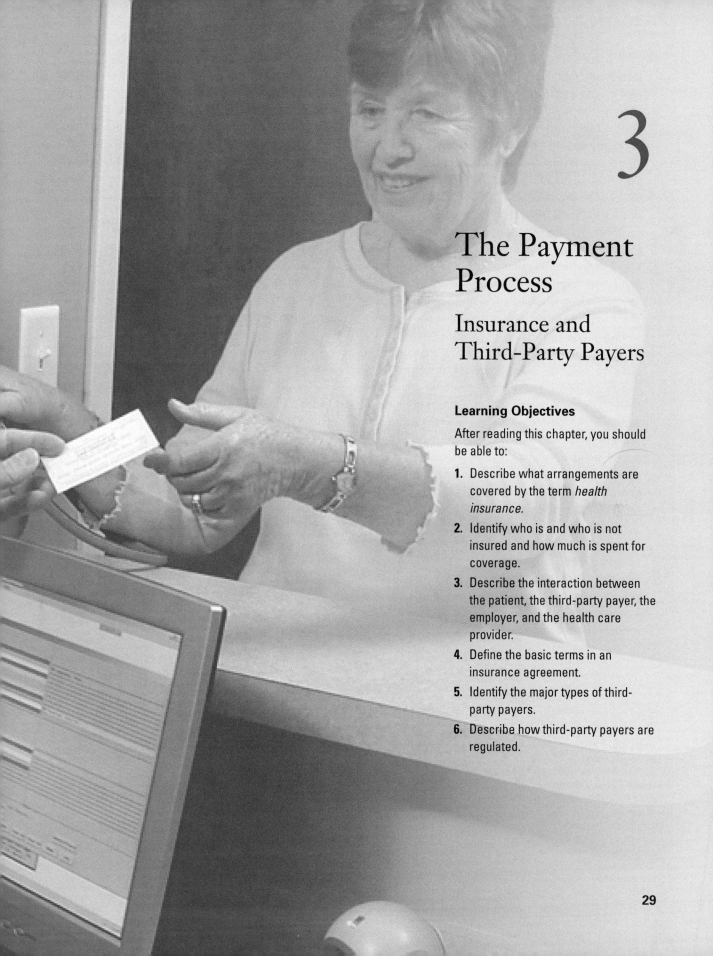

3

The Payment Process

Insurance and Third-Party Payers

Learning Objectives

After reading this chapter, you should be able to:

1. Describe what arrangements are covered by the term *health insurance.*
2. Identify who is and who is not insured and how much is spent for coverage.
3. Describe the interaction between the patient, the third-party payer, the employer, and the health care provider.
4. Define the basic terms in an insurance agreement.
5. Identify the major types of third-party payers.
6. Describe how third-party payers are regulated.

Consumers embrace Health Savings Accounts

Health savings accounts (HSAs) were developed as a way to engage consumers in their own health care, while lowering premiums and promoting tax-free savings. Instead of the managed care company saying "no" to the consumer, the consumer says no, because they bear the cost directly. The HSA is a savings account linked to a high-deductible health plan (HDHP). In 2009 the deductible is $1,150 for an individual and $2,300 for a family. Out-of-pocket costs can be no more than $5,800 for individuals and $11,600 for families. The individual must not be covered by other insurance, including Medicare and Medicaid. The savings account is similar to an **individual retirement account (IRA),** which provides tax-deferred savings. The individual deposits pretax dollars into the HSA account. The money in the account is used to pay for health services until the high deductible is reached. At that point, the insurance plan takes over, paying 100 percent of the cost of services. An employer can also make contributions to the HSA. There is a maximum that can be deposited each year. If the money in the HSA is not used by the end of the year, it rolls over to the next year. Even better, if the individual leaves the employer, the HSA goes with him or her.

HSAs got a lot of positive press because of their potential to lower insurance costs. The premiums on a HDHP are usually 45 percent to 55 percent less than a traditional copayment-type plan. Some people indicated they switched recently specifically in order to lower premium costs. The number of employers offering HDHP doubled between 2006 and 2008 as did number of employees enrolling. Surveys indicate that HDHPs are achieving the aim of engaging consumers: 72 percent agree that individuals should be responsible for managing their own health care costs; 64 percent ask about generics; 48 percent read bills closely; and 47 percent indicate they ask providers about health care charges. HSAs are an attractive product for financial services companies to offer. Fifth Third Bancorp, one of the early providers of HSAs, indicates that the number of its accounts rose 94 percent in last 2 years, and balances increased by 170 percent. But providers find it's a challenging marketplace. Customers want easy-to-use, no-fee products similar to IRAs. One company offers a tool for prospective individuals to determine eligibility, calculate contribution maximums, and estimate potential savings. Other banks link customers HSAs with their money markets and other accounts. The proposed changes/health reform has caused uncertainty.

Sources: By the numbers: Health savings accounts, *Best's Review* (November 2009), p. 24; S. Garmhausen, Fifth Third reaps benefits of push for HSA business, *American Banker* (October 27, 2009), np; W. Johnson, HSAs: Six insights for employees leaving or losing a job, *Benefits & Compensation Digest* (November 2009), pp. 24–29; K. Klug and L. Chianese, Health savings accounts: Back to the future, *Benefits Quarterly* (First quarter 2010), pp. 21–23; Lo Sasso, A., Helmchen, L. and R. Kaestner, The effects of consumer-directed health plans on health care spending, *Journal of Risk and Insurance* (January 2010), pp. 85–103; www.Optumhealth.com; Priebe, J. and K. Dunkelberger, Employees embrace health savings accounts, *National Underwriter* (November 16, 2009) pp. 18, 30; Principal Financial Group (www.principal.com/hsacalculator); U.S. Department of the Treasury (www.ustreas.gov/offices/public-affairs/hsa/).

individual retirement account (IRA)
Individuals may deposit money into an IRA to save for retirement. These accounts have certain tax benefits, and there are penalties for withdrawing the money prior to retirement.

Introduction

How services are to be paid for is one of the critical components of the health care industry. Most people use the term *health insurance* when they describe how they will pay for the services they have received. As you will learn in this chapter, health insurance covers a very wide range of payment arrangements. This chapter helps clarify what insurance really is, how individuals obtain coverage, and the categories of insurers and how they differ. A behind-the-scenes look at the process of paying for services is explored by following a claim from submission to payment.

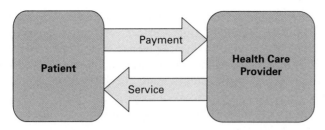

Figure 3.1 The Simple Payment Process

What Is Health Insurance?

Before health insurance became the primary method of payment, if you were sick you paid for health care services directly. You paid the doctor, you paid for a nurse, you paid the pharmacist for medicines, and so on. If you couldn't pay, you depended on charity or you did without.

As the cost of health care services increased, people began to develop creative ways to pay for those services. Plans that allowed prepayment of services, either on an individual basis or connected to an employer, have existed since the beginning of the 20th century. However, there was always the concern that you didn't know who would get sick or how sick they would be. Before health insurance, the family had to figure out how much to save for unexpected health care costs. But the family was never sure if they'd saved the right amount. A serious illness, then as now, could financially devastate a family.

Purchasing insurance is a way to handle that uncertainty and chance of financial loss. Insurance is the business of shifting the **risk of loss** from the individual to a third party. For example, if you own a house, there is some risk, or probability, that your house might catch fire and burn. If this loss occurs, like most of us, you will probably not be able to afford to replace the house and its contents.

risk of loss
The probability that the insured-against event will occur.

This is where the insurance companies step in. You purchase insurance from them. If the house then burns, they replace the house. By purchasing insurance, you have shifted the risk of the possible loss to the insurance companies. The house burning is now their problem.

The insurance company is willing to take the risk because it can make money by doing so. Most people are obligated to purchase insurance to protect their homes. However, the chance is that only a few of those houses will burn. So the insurance company is predicting it will make a profit by taking in more money than it will have to pay out. The process is known as **risk pooling**.

risk pooling
The process of combining all the insureds into one group so the group's overall risk of loss is reduced.

Health insurance is a similar process of shifting the cost of illness from the sick person to the insurance company. Based on what it knows about your health and the probability that you will get sick, the insurance company charges you a price. As with the house example, it is predicting it will come out ahead because you'll stay healthy and not need the services it has agreed to pay for.

The concept of shifting the risk of loss to another party is very straightforward. Health insurance gets complicated in the details.

Who Is Insured?

We protect our houses and vehicles from loss by purchasing our own casualty insurance. But only 5 percent of Americans under age 65 purchase private individual health care insurance. How do the other 95 percent pay for health care services?

For most Americans and their families, health insurance coverage is an employment benefit. Of the 262.8 million Americans who are under age 65, 60 percent have insurance as part of an employer-sponsored plan (Kaiser 2009b). Eighteen percent of those under 65 are covered by Medicaid and other public forms of insurance (Medicaid, Medicare, and other government programs are covered in Chapter 4). This leaves 45.7 million people, or about 17 percent of those under age 65, without health insurance. These numbers add to more than 100 percent because some people have insurance coverage from more than one source.

Among large employers (those with more than 200 employees), almost all offer health care benefits. In smaller companies, the number drops to about 59 percent of companies. Only a few states require employers of more than 25 people to offer health insurance. However, insurance is a benefit that attracts better qualified employees and encourages them to remain with the company.

Employees can opt not to participate in their employer's plan. Even in the companies that offer benefits, only about 81 percent of employees choose to be covered (Kaiser 2009b). Although some have coverage elsewhere (for example, through their spouse's employer), some are unable to afford the employee share of the premiums.

Health care is an expensive benefit for an employer to offer to its employees. In 2009, the average premium for single coverage was $4,824 and for family coverage was $13,375. In the past decade, premiums have risen about 130 percent (Kaiser/HRET 2009).

As premiums have increased, employers have passed the increases on to their employees. Although employees currently pay a similar percentage of the premium as they did a decade ago, the total amount in dollars has increased significantly. The 2009 average contribution for single coverage was $779, or 17 percent, and for family coverage the average was $3,515, or 27 percent. In addition to contributing to premiums, employees share costs for office visits, prescriptions, and deductibles (Kaiser/HRET 2009). Actual amounts can vary considerably depending on the type of plan and the size of the employer.

Many insurance companies have realized that it is cheaper to provide services to people who aren't very sick or before they get sick. Most plans now cover common areas of preventive care, including prenatal care, annual visits to the gynecologist, and well-baby care. Some also include mental health care and prescription drug coverage.

There is a strong correlation between having insurance and being able to access the health care system. Most studies indicate that those with insurance are generally healthier than those without. The uninsured are twice as likely to postpone or go without care due to cost than those with insurance. If they do seek care, they are more likely to do without prescription drugs, again due to cost (Kaiser 2009a).

More than 18 percent of the American population under the age of 65, about 46 million people, is uninsured. Most of the uninsured (63%) are from low-income families, and most (66%) are from families with at least one full-time worker (Kaiser 2009a). Low-wage workers and blue-collar workers are less likely to have employer-sponsored health plans and less likely to participate if a plan is available (largely due to cost). The 2007-2009 period saw an increase in the number of uninsured as unemployment rose above 10 percent. Expanded Medicaid and SCHIP coverage was able to absorb some of the newly unemployed.

The reforms encompassed in the 2010 Patient Protection and Affordable Care Act seek to change this picture (Kaiser 2010). As the provisions of the law take effect, most U.S. citizens and legal residents will have health insurance. The law mandates that all Americans obtain insurance. Effective immediately, a temporary high-risk program is available for those uninsured who have pre-existing conditions. Once the state insurance exchanges become available in 2014, this program will be phased out. Each of the plans available in a state exchange must include basic care and prescription coverage, with

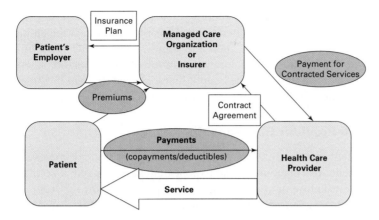

Figure 3.2   The Third-Party Payer Process

limits on deductible and copays. Plans will not be able to refuse coverage. As described in the next chapter, the new law also expands Medicare and Medicaid coverage.

How Does "Insurance" Work?

When you compare the process in Figure 3.2 to the process in Figure 3.1, once the employer and the insurer are involved, the process of obtaining and paying for health care services becomes more complex than when the patient paid the provider directly. The insurance company, government agency, or managed care organization (MCO) is known as the third-party payer (sometimes just "payer") because it is the third part of the transaction between the patient and the service provider. This section of the chapter explores each relationship in the process.

The Patient/Employer–Third-Party Payer Relationship

When the individual patient or his employer considers which insurance company to do business with, they decide which company's plan offers the best combination of benefits at the most acceptable price. **Benefits**, or coverage, and price, or **premiums**, are a tradeoff. The patient and the employer would like to obtain a long list of benefits—office visits, immunizations, hospital stays, mammograms, and so on—and would like to do so at a low price. But the more benefits that are covered in the plan, the more the benefits are going to cost.

The third-party payer will set a price for the benefit package. In addition to the benefits that will be included in the insurance plan, the price is determined by the number of people being insured and the general state of their health. As an outcome of risk pooling, the more people who are insured and the better their health, the more likely it is that the insurance company will not actually have to provide any of the benefits it has agreed to pay for. An **actuary** at the insurance company calculates this risk and helps the insurance company set a premium that will make the insurance company profitable.

Once the employer has negotiated an agreement with the insurer, the employer can offer health care benefits to its employees. The employer is not limited to just one plan: it can negotiate with several insurers and managed care companies to provide employees with options. Larger firms are more likely to offer a choice of plans to their employees. The employer decides what portion of the premium it will pay on behalf of its employees and what portion, if any, the employee will pay for the coverage. If the workforce is unionized, this is often negotiated as part of the union contract.

benefits The items that are covered under an insurance plan. Also referred to as coverage.

premium The price paid by the insured for insurance coverage.

actuary A professional who calculates insurance and annuity risks, premiums, and dividends.

policy The agreement, or contract, that describes all of the terms and conditions of an insurance policy.

the insured The person who will receive benefits under the terms of an insurance policy.

enrollment period The time period during which people, usually employees, can sign up for or change their insurance coverage.

enrollees The employees who sign up for insurance coverage from the employer.

deductible An amount specified in the insurance policy that must be paid by the insured before the insurance company will pay.

copayment (coinsurance) A payment made by the insured at the time services are received.

coordination of benefits If a service is covered under more than one policy, then the insurance companies determine which policy pays.

ICD-9-CM The abbreviation for the International Classification of Diseases, 9th revision, Clinical Modification. This classification is used to code office visits to process an insurance claim.

Healthcare Common Procedure Coding System (HCPCS) A classification system used to code and process an insurance claim.

The insurance plan is a legally binding contract known as a **policy**. If an individual purchases insurance directly, then he or she is the **insured**. If the employer is providing a plan to its employers, then the employer is actually the insured. The employer will have a time period, known as an **enrollment period**, when employees may decide to take advantage of the benefit being offered to them by the employers. If they take the benefit, they are known as **enrollees**.

The Patient–Provider Relationship

Once the patient receives services from a provider, the payment process begins. Even though a patient "has insurance," the patient may have to make a number of out-of-pocket payments before or after the third-party payer pays for services.

The first of these out-of-pocket payments is the **deductible**. A deductible is a dollar amount of services that must be paid by the patient or the person responsible for the bill as in the case of minors or dependents before the third party will begin to pay. Usually the higher the amount of the deductible, the lower the cost of the policy.

Most agreements now require a **copayment (coinsurance)** at the time that services are rendered. This means that the patient pays for a portion of the services up front. For example, that patient must pay $30 for an office visit to the primary care provider.

A patient may be insured under more than one policy. For example, a woman might have an individual policy through her employer and be covered under a family policy through her husband's employers. The policies will have a **coordination of benefits** clause that will determine which third party pays for services.

The Provider–Third-Party Payer Relationship

After the doctor or hospital has provided services, the provider now files a claim with the insurance company. A health insurance claim is simply a request for reimbursement for the services that have been provided. Accurate coding and billing are essential to this process.

Coding The initial stage of filing an insurance claim is the process of correctly coding what diagnoses, procedures, and services were provided to the patient. The provider selects the appropriate description of the service, and the coder assigns the number. The health care industry has moved toward standardizing the coding system by using two systems: ICD-9-CM and HCPCS. **ICD-9-CM** (the abbreviation for the *International Classification of Diseases, 9th Revision, Clinical Modification*) is used for physician office claims and reports diagnoses and reasons for the encounter. The other coding system is HCPCS (pronounced "hick picks"), which is the abbreviation for **Healthcare Common Procedure Coding System**. The HCPCS consists of two levels: **current procedural terminology (CPT)** is for procedures and services performed by providers and **national codes (HCPCS level II codes)** are for procedures, services, and supplies not found in CPT. (The third level, local codes, was phased out at the end of 2003.)

Billing Charges for services must be posted to client accounts. Claims are then transmitted to the third-party payer electronically. The claims are submitted on forms that are standardized for all payers. The payer replies with a transmittal notice and then begins to process the claim. An **explanation of benefits (EOB)** is sent to the patient to explain the results of the process. Payment is sent electronically to the provider. The amount of the payment will depend on what type of payment process is used by the payer, as described in the next section. If the payer does not completely reimburse the provider for that service, the provider may or may not be able to bill the patient for the difference.

Payment can be denied for a number of reasons. If there was an error in the process, then the provider can file an appeal. Other reasons for denial include such incomplete documentation, noncovered benefits, termination of coverage, failure to obtain **preauthorization**, and out-of-network provider (Green and Rowell 2010).

Types of Third-Party Payers

Patients and providers alike use the term *insurance* to cover any and all third-party payment arrangements. Unfortunately, the term simply isn't comprehensive enough to cover all the variations of third-party payers that can occur. There are significant differences in the types of payers.

Indemnity Insurers

Indemnification is a legal term that means someone else takes the place of the person at risk. Indemnity insurance is the classic form of insurance. In a traditional **indemnity** insurance agreement, the insurance carrier has agreed to indemnify, or pay for, the loss to the insured. With health insurance, the loss is the need to obtain health care services. In its purest form, once the patient has paid the provider for those services, the insurance company reimburses the patient (usually at a preset amount).

The insurance company may also reimburse the provider directly, usually on a fee-for-service basis. Payment is not made to the provider of services until covered services are used. Generally, indemnity insurance has no restrictions on the patient's choice of provider.

Self-Insurers

Many employers have shifted from traditional indemnity plans to self-insurance. From the employee's perspective, a self-insured plan seems no different than traditional insurance. In a **self-insured plan**, the employer assumes the risk of loss for medical costs instead of a commercial insurance company or a managed care organization. The employer must use its own revenues to pay for the health care costs of the employees as they arise. Often a **third-party administrator (TPA)** is hired by the employer to administer the health care benefits and process claims.

Self-insured plans are exempt from state insurance regulation. Instead, they are regulated by the **Employee Retirement Income Security Act of 1974 (ERISA)**. That statute provides rules for how employer-funded benefit plans, including health insurance, must be administered.

Blue Cross/Blue Shield

Most members of the public would be able to identify Blue Cross/Blue Shield as a health insurance company, but they probably would not be able to say what makes a Blue plan different from some other plan. Blue Cross was originally a group of teachers who paid Baylor University Hospital a small monthly sum in return for 21 days yearly of hospitalization. Many other hospitals adopted the idea. Blue Shield developed as a similar method to prepay physician expenses.

Today the Blue Cross and Blue Shield Association is a national federation of 39 local plans. In 2009, more than 100 million Americans were enrolled in some form of Blue plan (BlueCross BlueShield Association). What the plans have in common is the idea of prepaying medical expenses. Although most plans are nonprofit organizations, in 1996,

Current Procedural Terminology (CPT) A part of the HCPCS used to code procedures and services performed by providers.

national codes (HCPCS level II codes) The part of HCPCS used to code procedures and services not found in CPT.

explanation of benefits (EOB) A form sent to the patient that explains which claims were paid at what level.

preauthorization Many insurers require that certain procedures be authorized by the insurer before they are performed. Failure to obtain preauthorization may result in denial of the claim.

indemnity One party is exempted from incurred liabilities by the other party.

self-insured plan A plan where an employer pays for employees' health care.

third-party administrator (TPA) A company that manages the paperwork for an employer who establishes a self-insured plan.

Employee Retirement Income Security Act of 1974 (ERISA) Federal legislation that mandates how employer-funded benefit plans must be administered.

some converted to for-profit status by establishing publicly traded subsidiaries. An individual subscribes to a plan, so they are known as subscribers rather than policyholders. Local plans can develop HMOs and PPOs, and many serve as Medicare contractors.

Although the plans are a type of prepaid service, the subscriber is still responsible for deductibles, copayments, and any noncovered services. The typical way to reimburse providers is through a **usual**, **customary**, **and reasonable payment program (UCR)**. The usual fee is determined by what the provider normally charges for that service. The customary fee is based on the fee charged by similar providers within that geographic area. Finally, the reasonable fee considers any special circumstances of this particular incident. Determining the amount of payment can be a complicated process.

Managed Care Models

Thus far, the types of third-party payers described in this chapter are organizations whose primary business is insurance. These organizations do not deliver health care services; they only pay for the services.

Managed care describes both a system for paying health care providers and a system for delivering health care services. A managed care organization does both. Managed care has become the dominant mode of delivery because of its potential to reduce costs and increase efficiency. One of the key functions in a managed care model is **gatekeeping**. The patient can only access certain services from the primary care provider and can only obtain specialist and rehabilitative services if referred by the primary provider. This provides cost savings because only patients who are judged to need them have access to more expensive care.

Ninety-five percent of workers covered by an employer plan were enrolled in managed care in 2009, up from 27 percent in 1988. Table 3.1 lists the largest managed care firms. As indicated by the revenue and enrollment figures, managed care is the dominant feature of the health insurance industry.

Managed Care Structures

A number of organizational structures are classified as managed care, including health maintenance organizations (HMOs), preferred provider organizations (PPOs), and exclusive provider organizations (EPOs). Each is described in more detail in the following sections. Sometimes one company will offer several types of plans, which add to the confusion. In 2009, the majority of employees were enrolled in PPOs

usual, customary, and reasonable payment program (UCR) A method of reimbursing providers by examining what other providers are paid for that service.

managed care Describes the combination of payments for health care and delivery of services into one system.

gatekeeping A process of restricting access to services.

Health Maintenance Act of 1973 Federal legislation that provided incentives for the formation of Health Maintenance Organizations.

Health Maintenance Organization (HMO) Employer prepays a flat fee to the HMO; employees receive services as they need them.

Table 3.1	*Largest Publicly Traded National Managed Care Firms By premium revenue, 2008*	
Company	Revenue*	Total Enrollment**
United Health Group	$20.2 billion	30.3 million
WellPoint	15.3 billion	35.3 million
Aetna	7.8 billion	17.7 million
Humana	7.1 billion	8.4 million
CIGNA	4.1 billion	11.9 million
Health Net	3.8 billion	6.7 million
Coventry Health Care	3.0 billion	3.7 million
AMERIGROUP	1.1 billion	1.7 million

*Revenue for third quarter, 2008, from health premiums and fees
**As of Sept. 30, 2008
Source: Adapted from Atlantic Information Services, Inc. November 2008. Available at www.aishealth.com/ManagedCare/CompanyIntel/TenLargest.html.

(60%), followed by HMOs (20%) and POS plans (10%). High deductible health plans account for 8 percent and conventional plans 1 percent (Kaiser/HRET 2009).

The **Health Maintenance Act of 1973** was a strong incentive for the growth of HMOs. The act gave the federal government the authority to provide financial incentives to new HMOs and required employers to offer HMOs as an alternative to indemnity insurance. An HMO could be formed under the new law if the organization could prove its ability to provide comprehensive health care. The act specified basic health services the HMO had to provide and supplemental services it could choose to provide. The HMO must document to the government its ongoing ability to provide services in order to continue as an HMO.

Health Maintenance Organizations **Health maintenance organizations (HMOs)** are a form of **prepaid health plan (PHP)**. Payments are made in advance of the services being provided. The **capitation** payment entitles the patient to a certain dollar amount of services over a time period, either monthly or yearly. Usually the payments are made by the employer, on behalf of its employees and their families. Whether the employee uses fewer services or more services, the employer has prepaid a flat fee to the HMO. If the employee uses fewer services, the provider keeps the difference. If the employee uses more services, the provider has to absorb that cost. This creates a financial incentive to provide fewer services to the patient, whereas the fee-for-service model such as Blue Cross provides an incentive for providers to give more services.

HMOs have evolved from the simplest prepaid models of the 1970s. There are currently several ways the providers of the services can be organized. In the **staff model HMO**, the physicians are employees of the HMO and compensated by the payment of a salary. This organizational structure is different from the traditional structure for a primary care provider (described elsewhere in the text). In the **prepaid group practice model**, the physicians are employees of an independent group that contracts with the health plan to provide services. In a **network HMO**, the HMO contracts with at least two group practices to provide services. Finally, in the **independent practice association (IPA) model**, physicians contract independently with the IPA to treat the members of the HMO. The physician is reimbursed on a **fee-for-service** or capitation basis as treatment is provided. The IPA is basically the organization that markets the health plan.

Prepaid health plans are attractive to employers because they know in advance what the cost of providing health care will be. They are also attractive to the service provider because the number of patients is fixed and a certain revenue level is guaranteed. Service providers are given financial incentives to control costs by a withholding amount. A percentage of the payment from the employer is withheld until the end of the year. If services have been over utilized, then the HMO keeps that money. But if services are under the stated utilization rate, then the withheld amount is paid to the provider.

Preferred Provider Organizations A **preferred provider organization (PPO)** is a delivery network. The PPO does not receive premiums or assume financial risk. Instead it acts as the go-between, negotiating and managing contracts on the part of providers. The patient may choose his or her physician or hospital. If the patient chooses to uses a preferred provider, services are provided at a lower cost. If the patient chooses a provider who is not preferred, those services are provided at a higher rate. The patient gets more benefits by using the preferred provider.

Exclusive Provider Organizations **Exclusive provider organizations (EPOs)** have features that are similar to both HMOs and PPOs. A patient must select his or her care providers from those in the network. This is what makes the organization exclusive. If

prepaid health plan (PHP) Refers to all types of health plans in which fixed payments are made before services are rendered.

capitation A payment method under which each patient is entitled to receive a set dollar amount of services in each time period.

staff model HMO Physicians are employees of the HMO and paid a salary.

prepaid group practice model Physicians are employees of an independent group that contracts with the health plan to provide services.

network HMO The HMO contracts with at least two group medical practices, described as "in network" to provide services.

independent practice association (IPA) model The IPA markets the health plan. Physicians contract with the IPA to treat members of the HMO.

fee-for-service A method of reimbursement that pre-sets the fee that will be paid for the service that is provided.

Preferred Provider Organization (PPO) A delivery network that manages and negotiates contracts on behalf of the providers, who provide services at lower cost.

Exclusive Provider Organizations (EPOs) Delivery networks in which patients must use the services of those providers.

the patient chooses to go outside the network, then those services are not covered by the EPO. Unlike HMOs and PPOs, EPOs are regulated by state insurance law.

Regulation of Third-Party Payers

Insurance is a regulated industry. State governments have the authority to regulate the insurance companies that operate with their boundaries and sell products to their citizens. The agency charged with regulatory authority is usually called the insurance commission. The agency regulates all insurers, not just those who sell health insurance products.

Insurance companies must be licensed. As part of the process of issuing a license, the state reviews the company's financial health, its business practices, the policy forms it uses, who it insures, and the premiums it charges. The intent of this review is to make sure that the policyholders receive the coverage they were promised and that they paid for.

Because HMOs and other managed care organizations are not technically insurance companies but are classified as health care providers, they are regulated differently. Most states regulate HMOs by separate statute. However, the intent is similar to the regulation of insurance. In addition, HMO statutes also set standards for the provider side of the HMO. Thus, they set out processes for consumer complaints, quality review, and utilization review.

Many states have added additional consumer protection statutes. All 50 states now mandate breast cancer screening as a benefit that must be provided. Twenty-two states insist on mental health parity. External review of health plan decisions is required in 44 states.

At the federal level, HIPAA regulates portability, access, and mandated benefits. Congress also recognized the close relationship between employment and coverage by passing COBRA (Consolidated Omnibus Budget Reconciliation Act). COBRA provides that the employee may continue to be insured through the employer's plan even after the employment relationship has terminated. The catch is that now the employee picks up the total cost. Because obtaining coverage as an individual is prohibitively expensive, COBRA provides a way of staying insured. Under the American Recovery and Reinvestment Act of 2009 (ARRA), recently laid-off employees are eligible for a 9-month federal subsidy that covers 65 percent of those premiums. This is a temporary expansion of COBRA as a mechanism to maintain insurance during a recessionary period.

The 2010 Patient Protection and Affordable Care Act has numerous provisions that regulate the actions of insurers. For example, insurers cannot deny coverage for pre-existing medical conditions and can no longer place limits on the amount they will pay. All new plans must include preventive care and screenings, many for free. Adult children can now be carried on a family plan until they reach age 26. Older enrollees can be charged no more than three times the rate of younger adults (Kaiser 2010).

The law requires that states establish American Health Benefit Exchanges and Small Business Health Options Program Exchanges so that the uninsured and small businesses can obtain coverage. States may also create their own Basic Health Plans. In order to advocate for individuals with private coverage, states must establish an office of health insurance consumer assistance (Kaiser 2010).

Summary

Health insurance is a way to shift the possibility of financial loss caused by illness from the patient to the insurance company. Most Americans obtain health insurance through their employer as a benefit. The cost of the premiums is usually shared between the employer and the employee. Rising premiums are an ever-present concern to both employers and patients. Some costs have already been passed to the employee, such as higher deductibles and copayments for office visits and prescription drugs. Although all forms of third-party payment are called insurance by the public, only a few are traditional indemnity insurance plans. Various prepaid options also exist. Managed care organizations combine paying for and providing services in one business. These organizations can be structured as HMOs (health maintenance organizations), PPOs (preferred provider organizations), and EPOs (exclusive provider organizations). Whatever the form, health insurance is regulated at both the state and the federal level.

Questions for Review

1. What is risk of loss? How does insurance address this problem?
2. Provide a profile of insurance coverage for Americans.
3. Define the following terms: *policy, deductible, coinsurance, premium, claim.*
4. Define self-insured plan, HMO, PPO, EPO.
5. Who licenses insurance companies?

Questions for Discussion

1. Why is insurance so complicated? Can the process be simplified?
2. Review a health insurance policy. What's covered? What's not covered? Do you understand the terms and conditions of the policy?
3. Refer to the profile at the beginning of the chapter. What are the pros and cons of using a health savings account for yourself? Would you save money on health insurance? In what ways would you be motivated to reduce your health care costs?
4. Does the requirement of referral from the primary care physician keep costs down?
5. Some people feel that quality of care is compromised in the third-party payment system. What do you think?
6. Federal law now requires that almost all Americans have health insurance. How has this new law impacted you, your family, and/or your employer?

Chapter References

BlueCross BlueShield Association (www.bcbs.com).

Green, M. A., and J. C. Rowell. 2010. *Understanding health insurance: A guide to billing and reimbursement.* 10th ed. New York: Delmar Cengage Learning.

Kaiser Family Foundation and Health Research and Educational Trust. 2009. *Employer health benefits. 2009 Summary of findings.*

Kaiser Family Foundation. 2010. *Summary of new health reform law* (Publication #8061).

Kaiser Family Foundation. 2009a. *Five basic facts on the uninsured* (Publication #7806-02).

Kaiser Family Foundation. 2009b. *The uninsured: A primer. Key facts about Americans without health insurance* (Publication #7451-05).

U.S. Census Bureau. *Statistical Abstract of the United States: 2007.*

For Additional Information

Claxton, G., and J. Lundy. 2008. *How private health coverage works: A primer. 2008 update (Publication #7766).* Kaiser Family Foundation.

Henry J. Kaiser Family Foundation (www.kff.org).

Finkelman, A. W. 2001. *Managed care: A nursing perspective.* Upper Saddle River, NJ: Prentice Hall.

Kongstvedt, P. R. 2008. *Managed care: What it is and how it works.* 3rd ed. Sudbury, MA: Jones and Bartlett.

Skipper, H. D., and K. Black. 1999. *Life and health insurance.* 13th ed. Upper Saddle River, NJ: Prentice Hall.

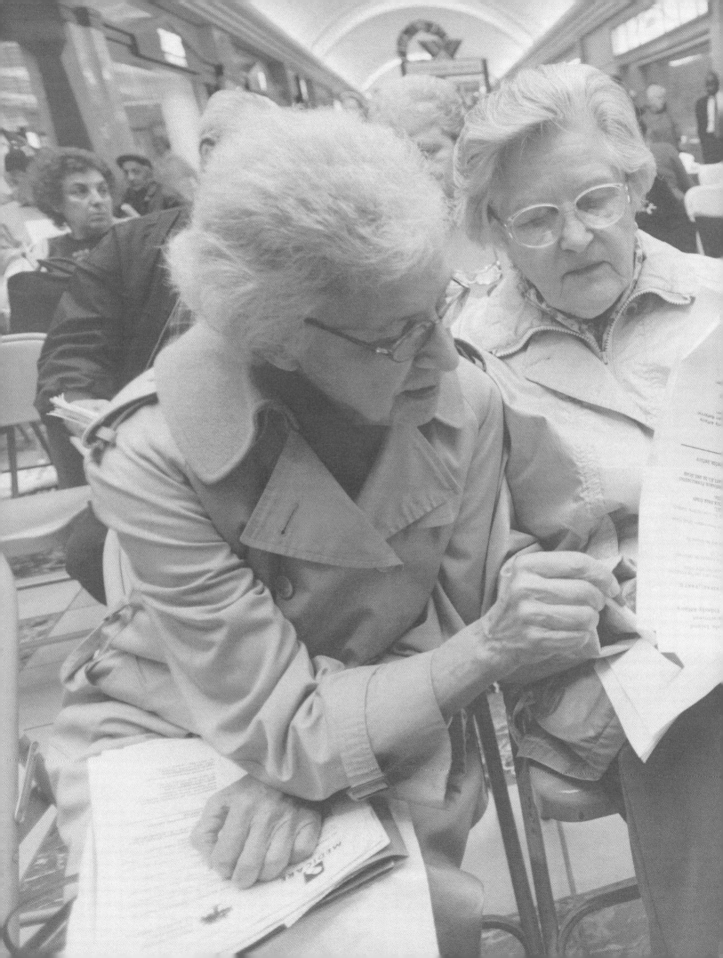

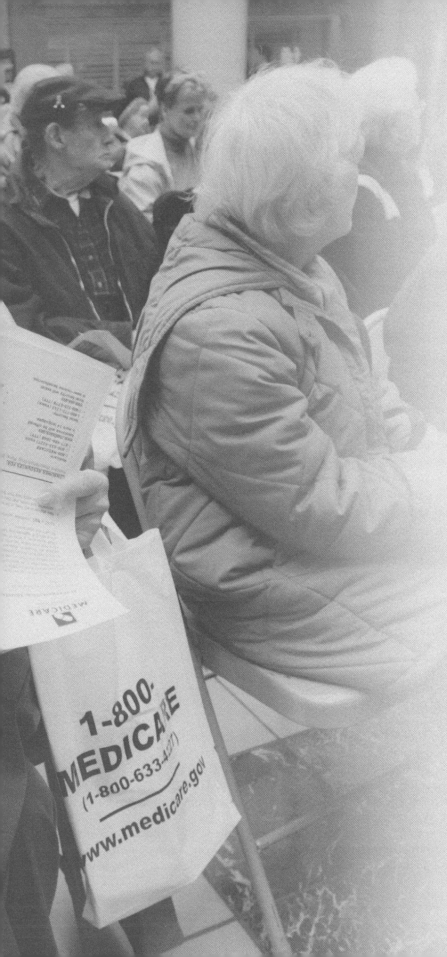

4

The Payment Process

Government Payment Programs

Learning Objectives

After reading this chapter, you should be able to:

1. Identify when a person is eligible for Medicare and what benefits are covered.

2. Describe how providers are reimbursed for Medicare services.

3. Identify when a person is eligible for Medicaid and what benefits are covered.

4. Describe how providers are reimbursed for Medicaid services.

5. Define SCHIP and identify who is eligible under this program.

6. Describe how fraud and abuse occur, and what penalties are imposed.

7. Describe health insurance programs for government workers and military personnel.

8. Identify when a person is eligible for workers' compensation.

9. Describe how workers' compensation is funded.

Medicare Offers Prescription Drug Coverage

On January 1, 2006, Medicare offered a new benefit: prescription drug coverage. This new benefit, Medicare Part D, was part of the Medicare Prescription Drug, Improvement, and Modernization Act of 2003 (MMA). Prior to this legislation, Medicare did not cover outpatient prescription drugs; consequently, 40 percent of the 40 million Medicare beneficiaries had no drug coverage. The others had coverage through a combination of employer plans, Medicaid, HMOs, Medigap, and other state assistance. Those without coverage paid considerably more for their prescriptions than the people did who had coverage. The legislation was primarily designed to help the low-income elderly. Health outcomes are often compromised in this group because prescriptions are unfilled or are taken at below optimal doses to extend the prescription.

Five years later, more than 27 million people are enrolled in Medicare Part D. Currently, the annual deductible is $310. Medicare pays about 75 percent until expenses reach $2,830. Then Medicare pays nothing until expenses reach $6,440, the so-called "doughnut hole," after which Medicare again pays about 95 percent. Since plan premiums, deductibles, co-pays, and formularies vary widely and change, enrollees are encouraged to review their plans and prescriptions during the fall open enrollment period to see if their current plan remains optimal for their needs. Medicare now provides an online comparison tool to assist decision making.

Analysts are just now beginning to assess the impact of the legislation, and so far results are mixed. Enrollment has been strong, yet one study indicated that there was no strong evidence that Medicare Part D had dramatically altered access to four categories of widely used medications (antidepressants, antipsychotics, lipid-lowering medications, and antihypertensive agents). An ongoing concern is the long-term cost of the plan. New benefits create new users. Congress initially pledged more than $400 billion over the next 10 years to pay for the benefit, but program costs may exceed $700 billion in that time span. Physicians face two challenges. One is identifying the period when a patient is in the "doughnut hole" and will have to pay all drug costs out-of-pocket, and the other is keeping track of patients' plans, since some drugs may not be covered at all.

The Medicare Improvements for Patients and Providers Act of 2008 made some improvements to Part D. Changes under the Patient Protection and Affordable Care Act phase in coverage of the "doughnut hole." By 2020, patients will pay only 25 percent of their prescription costs during that period.

Source: R. Alonso-Zaldivar, Medicare's drug benefit plan unveiled, *Los Angeles Times* (January 22, 2005), p. A16; M. Domino and J. Farley, Economic grand rounds: Did Medicare part D improve access to medications? *Psychiatric Services* (February 2010); G. Jacobson and G. Anderson, Medicare part D: Ongoing challenges for doctors and patients, *Annual Review of Medicine* (2010); G. Riley, J. Levy, and M. Montgomery, Adverse selection in the Medicare prescription drug program, *Health Affairs* (November/December 2009); M. Walberg and R. Patel, Potential opportunity cost of neglecting to annually reassess Medicare Part D standalone prescription drug plan offerings, *Journal of the American Pharmacists Association* (November–December 2009); What happens next—the drug benefit rollout, *AARP Bulletin* (June 2005), p. 18; W. Wolfe, Medicare lets people compare drug costs, *Star Tribune (Minneapolis)* (November 14, 2009)

Introduction

In addition to payments for services through the private health insurance plans you learned about in Chapter 3, health care costs can be paid by several government programs. The two dominant programs are Medicare and Medicaid. Medicare provides health care services for the elderly; Medicaid provides services for the poor of all ages. In addition, there are special programs for children, government workers, and military personnel. Workers' compensation pays for work-related injuries. Although workers' compensation is administered by the government, it is funded by payments by employers. In this chapter, you will learn the details of each of these programs and consider the issues facing federal and state government as health care costs continue to rise.

Medicare

The **Medicare** program was created in 1965 as part of the Social Security Act. At this time, it is administered by the **Centers for Medicare & Medicaid Services (CMS)**, formerly known as the Health Care Financing Administration (HCFA). CMS is part of the Department of Health and Human Services (HHS). Because Medicare is a purely federal program, the federal government establishes the rules for who is eligible, what benefits are covered, and how health care providers are reimbursed. Medicare is financed by payroll taxes, government revenues, and premiums paid by the beneficiaries.

Not only have overall health expenditures grown dramatically since the 1960s, but Medicare's share has more than quadrupled. In 2007, national health expenditures were $2.24 trillion; Medicare accounted for 19 percent of these. In 1966, the number was only 4.1 percent of $45.1 billion (Centers for Medicare & Medicaid Services 2009).

medicare A federal program that pays health care costs for the elderly, the permanently disabled, and those with end-stage renal disease.

Centers for Medicare & Medicaid Services (CMS) The federal agency that administers the Medicare and Medicaid programs; previously known as the Health Care Financing Administration (HCFA).

Eligibility

An individual qualifies for Medicare in three ways: if he or she is over 65 and is eligible for Social Security retirement benefits, is permanently disabled, or has end-stage renal disease. Eighty-four percent of those enrolled in Medicare are eligible because of their age; almost 12 percent of the total U.S. population is over age 65. Table 4.1 provides information about the number of people enrolled in the Medicare program.

Covered Benefits

Similar to a private health insurance plan, Medicare benefits include hospital care and physician services (Centers for Medicare & Medicaid Services, Medicare & You 2010). **Part A** of Medicare is hospital insurance. Part A covers inpatient hospital services, critical access hospitals, skilled nursing facilities (not custodial or long term), limited and medically necessary home health care services, and hospice. An individual does not have to pay premiums to have Part A coverage if he or she paid Medicare taxes while working. Like other insurance, Medicare requires a deductible and coinsurance or copayment. The deductible varies depending on the service and the enrollee's plan.

Part B covers physician services, outpatient hospital care, and some services and supplies. An individual who chooses to have Part B coverage pays monthly premiums. In 2010, the premium was $110.50 per month if the individual's income was less than $85,000. When care is received, the individual pays the deductible and a copayment for the service. In 2010, the deductible was $155.

Medicare Part A This part of the Medicare program pays for inpatient hospital services, critical access to hospitals, and skilled nursing facilities.

Medicare Part B This part of the Medicare program pays for physician services, outpatient hospital care, and some services and supplies.

Table 4.1	*Medicare Enrollees (in millions of people)*			
	1980	**1990**	**2000**	**2008**
Total	28.5	34.2	39.6	45.2
Over 65	25.5	30.9	34.2	37.8
Disabled	3.0	3.3	5.4	7.4

Source: U.S. Census Bureau, *Statistical Abstract of the United States: 2010,* Table 139.

Except for a limited time period following inpatient hospital care, Medicare does not cover long-term nursing care or home health care, both important issues for the elderly. Table 4.2 presents data on Medicare expenditures.

A number of modifications have been made to the Medicare program in an attempt to control costs. As part of the Balanced Budget Act of 1997, **Part C**, known as Medicare+Choice, was added to Medicare. Medicare+Choice offered individuals a variety of managed care–type options to provide the services covered under Parts A and B. The **Medicare Prescription Drug, Improvement, and Modernization Act of 2003 (MMA)** added new coverage for prescriptions and preventive care (Part D), replaced Medicare+Choice with **Medicare Advantage** and adds new Medigap plans, and made changes to fee-for-service payments. The 2009 American Recovery and Reinvestment Act added additional services such as cardiac rehab and HIV screening to enhance preventive care and wellness. The 2010 Patient Protection and Affordable Care Act made numerous specific changes, including closing the coverage gap in Medicare Part D and improving coverage of prevention benefits (Kaiser Family Foundation 2010).

As of 2010, an individual has two main choices about the Medicare coverage he or she can receive. An individual can select Original Medicare (Parts A and B), and then decide if he wants to add prescription drug coverage through Part D and a Medigap policy to cover services not provided under Parts A and B. The other choice is a Medicare Advantage Plan (Part C) to deliver the services of Parts A and B. An individual can add Part D, but does not need a Medigap policy (Centers for Medicare & Medicaid Services 2010). Through their Web sites and other information sources, the government attempts to assist individuals in making the best choice for their needs.

Medicare Part C This part of the Medicare program is an additional insurance plan intended to cover the gaps in Part A and Part B coverage.

Medicare Prescription Drug, Improvement, and Modernization Act of 2003 The most recent modification of the federal legislation. In particular, it added coverage for prescription drugs.

medicare advantage A revision of the Medicare+Choice offered under Part C of Medicare.

Reimbursement for Health Care Services

To process payments, the federal government contracts with private insurance carriers to act as intermediaries or carriers on behalf of the government. However, it is still the federal government that determines the level of reimbursement. Medicare was one of the earliest to begin adopting managed care strategies to control its costs.

Medicare uses a **prospective payment system (PPS)** to reimburse providers. The amount of the payment is determined prospectively, that is, before the patient receives services, and it is based on the patient's classification into a diagnostic-related group (DRG). Hospitals, skilled nursing facilities, and home health agencies are reimbursed on an "episode of care basis" using a PPS formula. Physicians are reimbursed on a fee-for-service basis. The fee schedule is based on the Resource-Based Relative

prospective payment system (PPS) A payment system in which the amount of reimbursement is determined prior to the patient receiving services and is based on the patient's classification into a diagnostic-related group (DRG).

Table 4.2	*Medicare Disbursements (in millions of dollars)*			
	1980	**1990**	**2000**	**2008**
Total	35,025	109,709	219,275	455,076
Part A hospital	24,288	66,687	130,284	230,240
Over 65	20,951	58,503	110,142	184,267
Disabled	2,825	7,218	15,850	33,524
Part B medical	10,737	43,022	88,991	177,709
Over 65	8,497	36,837	76,507	151,298
Disabled	1,256	3,758	10,750	31,991

Source: U.S. Census Bureau, *Statistical Abstract of the United States: 2010,* Table 137.

Table 4.3	Medicare Benefits by Provider Type (in millions of dollars)			
	1980	**1990**	**2000**	**2008**
Type of Provider				
Part A hospital	23,776	65,721	125,992	226,275
Inpatient hospital	22,860	57,012	86,566	128,754
Skilled nursing facility	392	2,761	10,593	23,919
Home health agency	524	3,295	4,552	6,570
Hospice	NA	318	2,818	11,399
Managed care	NA	2,335	21,463	47,150
Part B medical	10,737	43,022	88,991	174,805

Source: U.S. Census Bureau, *Statistical Abstract of the United States: 2010,* Table 142.

Value schedule, which essentially pays more for specialty services. Medicare also sets limits on the total amount of payment.

The 2010 health reform law has numerous provisions regarding payments to physicians, hospitals, and other providers. The changes are intended to act as monetary incentives for productivity improvements and better primary care (Kaiser Family Foundation 2010). Table 4.3 provides data that illustrate which health care providers are receiving reimbursement from Medicare. Under Part A, hospitals receive the majority of payments. Skilled nursing homes and hospices are receiving more payments now than 20 years ago. These additional payments reflect the needs of an elderly population whose life expectancy has improved. Part D benefits have expanded from $216 million in 2004 to $46,734 million in 2008, again reflecting the needs of elderly people who are served by Medicare.

Medicaid

In 2007, Medicaid made up almost 15 percent of total national health expenditures; in 1966, the percentage was only 2.9 percent (Centers for Medicare & Medicaid Services 2009). By the end of 2008, Medicaid enrollment increased 4.8 percent due to the deepening recession (Ellis et al. 2010). **Medicaid** is a transfer program. It is funded by taxpayers' income tax payments to the government's general revenue. These revenues are then allocated by Congress to various national needs, such as health care. Like Medicare, Medicaid is also administered by the CMS. However, Medicaid is administered at the state level as well as at the federal level. This means that eligibility and coverage can and do differ from state to state.

medicaid A federal and state program that funds health care primarily on the basis of the recipient's income.

To receive federal funds, states must provide Medicaid coverage to certain individuals. The state's Medicaid spending is matched by the federal government using a formula called the federal medical assistance percentage rate (FMAP). This rate is based on a state's per capita income as compared to the national average. Almost 60 percent of Medicaid expenditures are financed by the federal government, with the rest coming from states' revenues (Kaiser 2008).

Eligibility

The two major eligibility groups for Medicaid are poverty related and medically needy (Centers for Medicare and Medicaid Services 2005). Poverty-related Medicaid eligibility is determined by income and resources; it is designed to provide health care for those who otherwise would be unable to afford services. When an individual applies for Medicaid, the state evaluates that person's needs based on his or her income. Usually, if a person is eligible for supplemental security income (SSI) or temporary assistance for needy families (TANF), he or she is also eligible for Medicaid.

Medicaid is also available if the state determines that the individual is "medically needy." People who would otherwise not meet the income limit can use unpaid medical bills to lower, or spend down, their income. This eligibility category allows groups with large medical bills such as the elderly, pregnant women, children, and persons with disabilities to receive Medicaid benefits.

As part of the effort to reduce the numbers of uninsured Americans, under the 2010 Patient Protection and Affordable Care Act states are required to expand their Medicaid programs to all non-Medicare eligible people under age 65 with incomes up to 133 percent of the federal poverty level. All newly eligible adults will receive a package that meets the "essential health benefits" that the states make available through their Exchange programs (Kaiser Family Foundation 2010).

According to census data, currently Medicaid recipients are predominantly white and mostly under the age of 18. Table 4.4 provides more complete information about the demographic characteristics of Medicaid recipients.

Covered Benefits

Federal law specifies three categories of benefits. The first are benefits that all states' Medicaid programs must cover. This includes hospital and physician services. The second category of benefits is those the state may cover. This can include pharmaceutical, dental, and eye care coverage. The third group is benefits the state may not provide. For example, federal law prohibits using Medicaid funds to pay for abortions.

Table 4.5 provides information about the utilization of Medicaid services. It reveals some interesting discrepancies. Although children are the largest group of Medicaid recipients, they do not receive the majority of Medicaid spending. The majority of spending is for the elderly and people with disabilities, even though they are only a quarter of the recipients.

Table 4.4	*Characteristics of Medicaid Recipients, 2000 and 2007 (in thousands)*	
Persons covered	**2000**	**2007**
Total	28,360 (100%)	39,327 (100%)
Ethnicity		
White	19,290 (68%)	27,046 (68.7%)
Black	7,164 (25%)	8,910 (22.6%)
Hispanic	6,226 (22%)	10,298 (26.2%)
Age		
Under 18	14,486 (51%)	20,673 (52.5%)
18–44	7,098 (25%)	9,827 (24.9%)
45–64	3,484 (12%)	5,565 (14.1%)
65+	3,293 (12%)	3,263 (8.3%)

Source: U.S. Census Bureau, *Statistical Abstract of the United States: 2002,* Table 129; *Statistical Abstract of the United States: 2010,* Table 141.

| Table 4.5 | *Medicaid Recipients and Payments, 2006* |

	Recipients	**Payments**
Total	57.7 million	$269.9 billion
Elderly	4.4 (7.6%)	$58.2 (21.6%)
Disabled	8.3 (14.4%)	$116.9 (43.3%)
Adults	12.6 (21.8%)	$33 (12.2%)
Children	26.8 (46.4%)	$45 (16.7%)

Source: U.S. Census Bureau, *Statistical Abstract of the United States: 2010,* Table 144.

States have used this type of data to determine what benefits they can provide. A tradeoff between the cost of some services and the number of people receiving benefits creates difficult decisions for state governments. The latest health reform law mandates states to reduce the numbers of their uninsured.

Reimbursement for Health Care Services

Medicaid reimburses providers on a fee-for-service/episode-of-care basis. Medicaid has managed care options in the same way Medicare has. In all but a few states, more than 50 percent of the Medicaid population is in managed care. These are primarily children and nondisabled, nonelderly adults (U.S. Census Bureau 2010).

States are required to use a public process to determine their Medicaid reimbursement rates. However, many providers feel the rates are too low to make their participation in the program financially worthwhile. Under the 2010 health reform law, reimbursements to physicians who provide primary care services will be increased to 100 percent of the Medicare rate (Kaiser Family Foundation 2010). Physicians and nursing homes are not required to accept Medicaid patients, which may limit a patient's ability to choose what provider they would prefer.

SCHIP

An additional federal health insurance program was created in 1997 as part of the Balanced Budget Act. The **State Children's Health Insurance Program (SCHIP)** covers targeted low-income children whose parents do not qualify for Medicaid yet are unable to afford private health insurance. Children under the age of 19, including the unborn, are eligible. Each state operates its own plan, with a combination of federal and state funding. States had three options to achieve the objective of the program: they could choose to expand Medicaid coverage, they could set up a separate child health program, or they could combine the two options (Centers for Medicare and Medicaid Services 2004). In 1999, all states had approved SCHIP plans in place to serve approximately 1.9 million eligible children. States have continued to expand eligibility, so that by 2008, total enrollment was close to 7.4 million children at a cost of $6.9 million (U.S. Census Bureau 2010).

The program was reauthorized in 2009 to preserve coverage through FY 2013. The reauthorization now permits states to utilize eligibility finds from other need-based programs in order to enroll the estimated 5 million eligible children who remain uninsured (Kaiser Commission 2010). The economic recession saw a dramatic increase in the number of uninsured adults, but a decrease in the number of uninsured

State Children's Health Insurance Program (SCHIP)
A federal program that targets low-income children whose parents do not qualify for Medicaid yet are unable to afford private health insurance.

children as states expanded Medicaid and SCHIP eligibility, conducted outreach efforts to families who had previously had private insurance, and simplified enrollment procedures (Kaiser 2009).

Waste, Fraud, and Abuse

Waste, fraud, and abuse of the Medicare and Medicaid programs are a serious concern. The 2010 Patient Protection and Affordable Care Act requires provider screening and enhanced oversight of new providers. A database to share information across states' and federal programs is being developed and penalties for false claims increased (Kaiser Family Foundation 2010). The 2010 Act is not the first time the government has addressed this problem. Provisions in the HIPAA legislation give the government greater authority to investigate and punish fraud. The Department of Health and Human Services and the Department of Justice developed joint fraud strike forces that have obtained indictments of more than 500 individuals and organizations for more than a billion dollars of billing fraud. Civil penalties include substantial fines; criminal penalties include imprisonment. Realistically, the most significant penalty is exclusion from the Medicare or Medicaid program.

Fraud occurs in a number of ways. Fraud may be committed intentionally to obtain payments the provider is not otherwise entitled to receive. For example, a provider might submit a claim for a service that was never provided or might submit the claim under a different code to receive a higher rate of reimbursement (called *upcoding*). Fraud is sometimes the result of good intentions. For example, when a sympathetic practitioner knows a service the patient needs is not covered, the practitioner may be tempted to code the service so it will be covered. Even with good intentions, this is still fraud.

self-referral arrangements Health care providers are prohibited under federal law from referring patients to laboratories or other health services in which they have a financial interest.

Federal legislation prohibits kickbacks and **self-referral arrangements**. The legislation prevents health care providers from making health care decisions based on the financial benefits they could receive, which include payments to induce referrals. Under Stark I, if a physician or his or her immediate family owns a clinical laboratory, the physician may not make referrals to that lab facility. Stark II is even broader and prohibits the physician from referrals to "designated health services" where there is a financial interest. "Designated health services" include clinical laboratories, physical and occupational therapy, radiology, equipment and supplies, and home health services. If the physician has made a prohibited referral, the health services may not bill Medicare for payment.

compliance programs A program that is implemented in a business to ensure the business stays in compliance with current legislation, especially changes in the Medicare or Medicaid programs.

Most health care organizations have chosen to meet this challenge by implementing **compliance programs**. A strong compliance program ensures that all claims submitted for payment have appropriate documentation. In addition, it is particularly important that providers receive regular training to stay current with Medicare and Medicaid regulations. Compliance programs are mandatory under the Patient Protection and Affordable Care Act.

Programs for Special Populations

In addition to the programs already described in this chapter, the federal government provides health insurance programs for two additional groups. One is government workers, and the other is military personnel.

Federal employees' health care needs are met by the **Federal Employees Health Benefits Program (FEHBP)**. The program is administered by the Office of Personnel Management (OPM), which is the human resources department of the federal government. The FEHBP is an employer-sponsored health insurance program. This makes it more similar to the insurance options described in Chapter 3 than the government programs such as Medicare and Medicaid described in this chapter.

Federal Employees Health Benefits Program (FEHBP) An employer-sponsored health insurance program available to employees of the federal government.

Federal employees, families, retirees, and survivors are covered under the FEHBP program, making it one of the largest employer-sponsored health insurance programs in the world. Enrollees can choose from a wide selection of plans, including fee-for-service, point-of-service, or HMOs. Because the federal government is a purchaser of insurance, it has the ability to influence what types of programs are offered and what level of premium is charged. The federal government began exploring managed care options in the 1970s, leading many other employer-sponsored health insurance programs to follow suit.

Health care coverage for military personnel is another government payment program. **TRICARE** is the Department of Defense's health insurance program for eligible beneficiaries in the uniformed services. The TRICARE program (formerly known as CHAMPUS) has a variety of managed care options such as HMOs, preferred providers, and fee-for-service. Care is provided by civilian health care providers who contract with TRICARE to become a preferred provider. Under certain circumstances, a military treatment facility may be the provider for TRICARE-covered services.

TRICARE A health insurance program offered by the Department of Defense to military personnel.

Retired military personnel may also be eligible for Medicare; there are regulations that cover which insurance program will pay for what services. However, neither Medicare nor TRICARE covers long-term care needs such as a nursing home.

As you'll read elsewhere, the federal government also takes the role of a health care provider through the Veterans Administration hospitals. The federal government's role in the TRICARE program is as a purchaser of insurance.

Workers' Compensation Insurance

Employees are another category of people who can receive health care benefits under a government-administered program called **workers' compensation**. Workers' compensation acts were designed to eliminate the need for an employee to sue the employer for negligence when the employee was injured in the workplace. In return for giving up the right to sue for damages, employees gain the certainty of compensation at a predetermined level.

workers' compensation A program that provides health care benefits to employees who are injured on the job.

The process is straightforward. When an employee is injured, he or she files a claim with the state government agency. In most states, this agency is called the workers' compensation commission or the workers' compensation board. The employee must prove that the injury was work related. The government agency determines if the claim is legitimate and what benefits the employee is entitled to receive. Benefits are predetermined based on the type of injury and the amount of time the employee will be unable to work. If the employee is denied benefits for some reason, he or she can appeal the decision. However, the employee cannot sue the employer unless the employer intentionally caused the injury.

Workers' compensation is funded by employers. Depending on state law, the employer either pays for workers' compensation insurance or self-insures by making payments into a contingency fund. An incentive to maintain a safe workplace is built into the system: employers' premium rates drop if they have a low numbers of accidents. New Jersey, South Carolina, and Texas have designed voluntary plans that allow the employer to decide if it will participate in the system or be open to negligence claims by the injured employee.

Like all insurance plans, workers' compensation is vulnerable to fraud and abuse. There are cases of employees claiming injuries that don't exist or were not work related. Back injuries, in particular, are prone to false claims. There are also cases of employees deliberately injuring themselves on the job in order to recover.

Issues for Government Payment Programs

The role of federal and state governments in providing health care services is controversial. Who should be eligible, what services should be provided, and how providers should be compensated are ongoing issues that governments must address. In these times of rising costs, the government must be both a good steward of taxpayers' money and at the same time provide health care as broadly as possible.

Eligibility and Benefits

As you've seen in this chapter, the eligibility and benefits issues go hand in hand. Especially at the state level, Medicaid programs have used different models to decide what services to provide. Decisions to expand access (prescription drugs) or limit access (abortions) are often based on political, rather than medical factors. Government programs continue to provide care for the elderly and the poor. The legislative changes in 2010 are intended to expand care, especially to those who were uninsured.

Payments

As one of the largest purchasers of health care services, the government has implemented strategies to manage costs. Through size alone, it can force providers to accept the payment program it offers. However, as seen with the Medicaid program, where providers feel that the financial incentives are inadequate, they will opt out of the program. Cost savings therefore translate into reduced access for certain categories of patients. The 2010 legislation requires a number of demonstration projects aimed at special populations and creates oversight boards to monitor costs.

Summary

Many people's health care costs are paid by government programs. Medicare provides benefits primarily to the elderly. Approximately 45 million people receive Medicare; the program costs the government $504 billion. Medicare pays for hospitalization, regular medical care, and, if elected, prescription drug coverage. Medicaid is a program primarily for the poor. Of the 50 million receiving Medicaid, almost half are children. However, the bulk of Medicaid spending is for the elderly, particularly for long-term care. Additional government programs address the needs of children and government/military employees. Workers' compensation is funded by employers, administered by the government, and covers work-related injuries.

Questions for Review

1. List three ways a person becomes eligible for Medicare benefits.
2. What is the difference in coverage between Part A and Part B of Medicare? What is covered under Part D?
3. How is a person eligible for Medicaid?
4. What is SCHIP?
5. Who pays for workers' compensation?

Questions for Discussion

1. What groups do you believe are not being served under the current system of government health care programs? How should they be served? What services should be provided? How will government pay for the services?
2. Should Medicare fund long-term care, regardless of income?
3. As discussed in the chapter profile, the "doughnut hole" was designed to keep the cost of Medicare Part D manageable. Has this objective been achieved? Are there better ways to manage costs?
4. Should the government require providers to accept Medicaid patients?
5. Do the mechanisms for preventing fraud and abuse seem adequate? How could they be improved?
6. Can an employer prevent fraudulent claims by employees of work-related injuries?

Chapter References

Centers for Medicare and Medicaid Services. 2004. *Program information on Medicaid & State Children's Health Insurance Program (SCHIP)*. Baltimore.

Centers for Medicare and Medicaid Services. 2005. *Medicaid at-a-glance 2005. A Medicaid information source*. Baltimore.

Centers for Medicare and Medicaid Services. 2009. *National health expenditure data, NHE tables*. Available at www.cms.hhs.gov/NationalHealthExpendData/25_NHE_Fact_Sheet. asp.

Centers for Medicare and Medicaid Services. 2010. *Medicare and you 2010*. Baltimore.

Ellis, E. et al. February 2010. *Medicaid enrollment in 50 states: December 2008 data update*. Washington, DC: The Kaiser Commission on Medicaid and the Uninsured.

Kaiser Commission on Medicaid and the Uninsured and the Children's Partnership. January 2010. *Building an express lane eligibility initiative: A roadmap of key decisions for states*. (Publication # 8043 available at www.kff.org).

Kaiser Commission on Medicaid and the Uninsured. December 2009. *Protecting children during the recession: Spotlight on state health coverage efforts*. (Publication #8027 available at www.kff.org).

Kaiser Family Foundation. April 2010. *Summary of new health reform law*.

____. November 2008. *The Medicaid Program at a glance*. (www.kff.org).

U.S. Census Bureau. *Statistical abstract of the United States: 2010*.

For Additional Information

Centers for Medicare and Medicaid Services (www.cms.hhs.gov).

Medicare, The Official U.S. Government Web Site for People with Medicare (www.medicare.gov).

Stop Medicare Fraud (www.stopmedicarefraud.gov).

TRICARE (www.tricare.osd.mil).

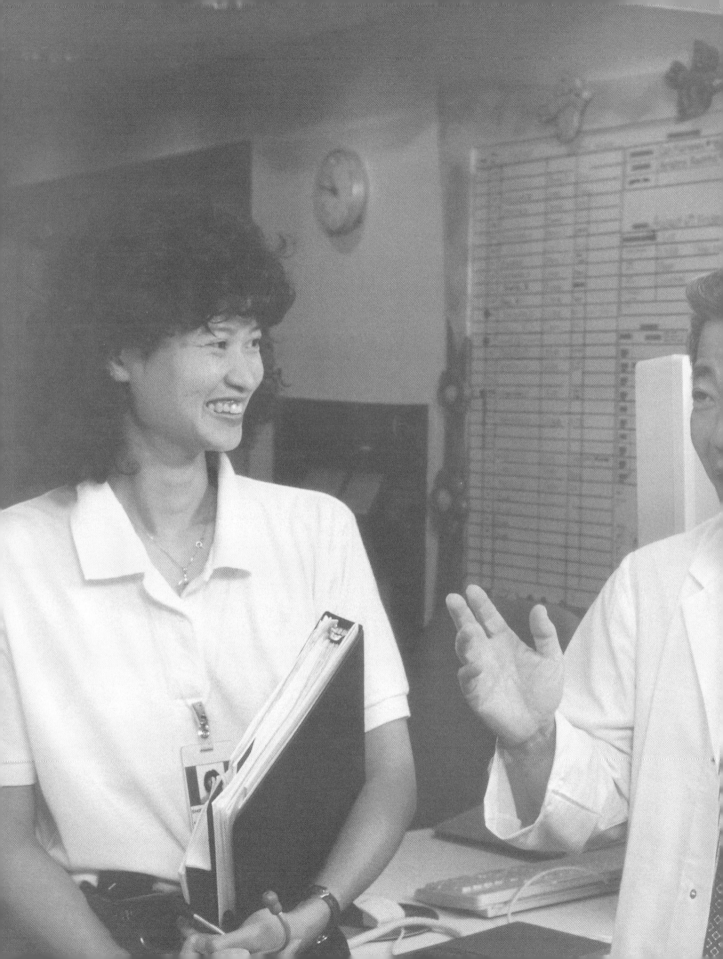

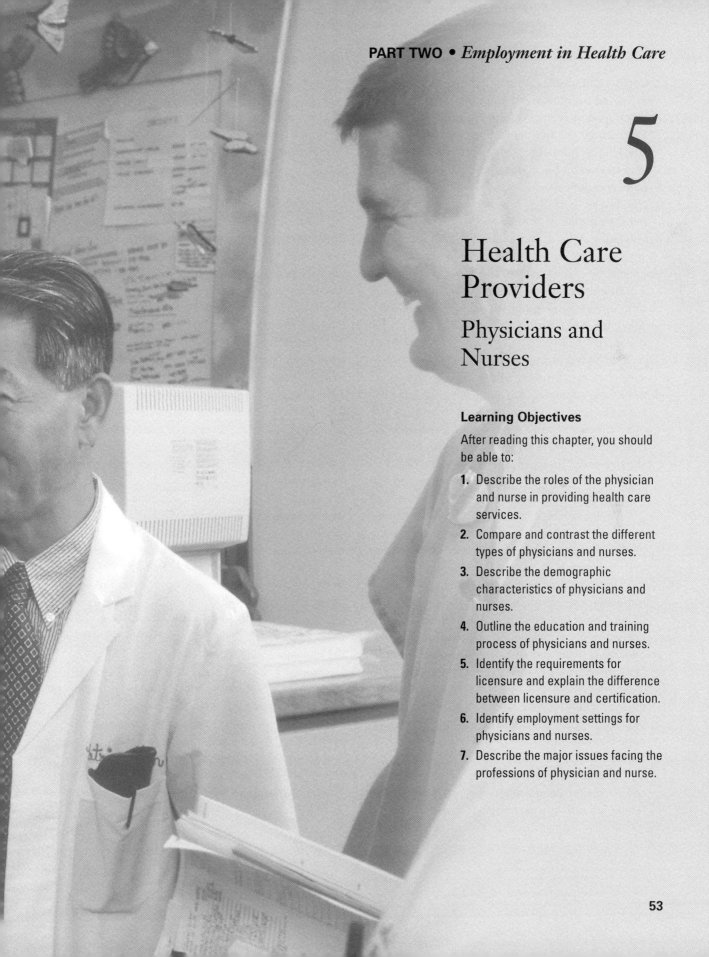

5

Health Care Providers

Physicians and Nurses

Learning Objectives

After reading this chapter, you should be able to:

1. Describe the roles of the physician and nurse in providing health care services.
2. Compare and contrast the different types of physicians and nurses.
3. Describe the demographic characteristics of physicians and nurses.
4. Outline the education and training process of physicians and nurses.
5. Identify the requirements for licensure and explain the difference between licensure and certification.
6. Identify employment settings for physicians and nurses.
7. Describe the major issues facing the professions of physician and nurse.

A Family Practitioner

Carrie Hunter, MD, advises that the best way for someone to understand what the life of a family practitioner is really like is to tag along for a week. They would see her interacting with patients and checking on her patients at the hospital, but they'd also see her on the phone, ordering tests and supplies and generally checking on things, or hitting the books and the Internet to investigate a patient's problem. "Even when you're not at work, you really still are. Sometimes you're the only one who can do what needs to be done for your patient."

Hunter is one of 18 family practitioners and four internists in group practice in Jonesboro, Arkansas. Her days start around 7:30 or 8 A.M. at the hospital. She usually has only two or three patients in the hospital, which is the way she likes it. "I want to treat them in the clinic so they don't have to be admitted." But if one of her patients has been admitted with pneumonia, for example, she'll order fluids and antibiotics. When she goes to the hospital, she checks on the blood work and X-rays she ordered. "Then I rely on the nurses to check on my patients." Sometimes she'll swing by again at lunch or in the evening.

By 9 A.M. she's at the clinic. She schedules patients every 15 minutes, preferring to have her mornings full and work through lunch rather than to stay late in the evenings. New patients or longer procedures such as Pap smears and lesion removals are scheduled for 30 minutes. Three times a week, she spends half her day in the practice's urgent care clinic. The clinic is open weekends and takes patients without appointments. They aren't necessarily even her patients. The clinic sees about 60 patients a day, and up to 100 during flu season. "We get overflow from the local pediatricians for colds and strep throat, and even people who should have probably gone directly to the ER."

"The best part about my job is really getting to see yourself making a difference," says Hunter. "In family practice you do routine illness and you follow patients with blood pressure, diabetes, and heart disease. You see them for a long time and get to know their whole family." One patient even brought a birthday gift for her daughter.

"Primary care is one-third psychiatry. It's counseling as well as technical knowledge." One of the frustrations is dealing with patients who aren't taking care of themselves. "Smoking and alcohol are big problems. Some patients just want you to fix them with a pill so they can keep doing what they're doing." Hunter notes that sometimes it's hard to be nice and supportive all day, every day when you see people who aren't at their best. Doctors internalize, she says: "Where do you go with all that bad stuff?"

Hunter recently took the exam to be board certified in family medicine. She considers it good review because she has to recertify every 7 years. Each year they get review modules, so she's up-to-date on the latest treatments for blood pressure or cholesterol. "Every day I see at least one thing I don't know about. I do research that day—either in my books or on the Internet. And I talk to my partners."

One of the challenges Hunter anticipates is the desire of female physicians to have a lifestyle where they can take care of both their patients and their families. All her female preceptors in medical school were career oriented and had never married or were divorced and childless. "All that has changed," Hunter notes. "Female physicians are like me. We're having children, and we want both—a life and a practice. If we can do both, then the men can back off too."

Hunter says, "I'm glad I do what I do. It's interesting work and I make a good living. The downside is there's no control over the hours." What she hopes to do in the next phase of her career is focus mostly on the clinic and women's health issues. "I'd like more of my patients to be the 18- to 45-year-old women. Sometimes they have trouble relating with a male physician. It's something I'd be good at."

Introduction

In the United States today, almost 16 million people are employed in the health care industry (Bureau of Labor Statistics, Healthcare 2010–11). Physicians and nurses make up about a quarter of all health care employees. Patient care is delivered by a team of professionals that includes physicians, nurses, and other clinical providers. The patient care team is supported by non-clinical staff and business professionals. Physicians play an important role in the delivery of health care services. In 2007 alone, American made more than 994 million office visits to physicians (U.S. Census Bureau 2010). Of all the health professions, nursing employs the largest number of people, with more than 3 million jobs in 2006 (Bureau of Labor Statistics, RNs 2010–11). In this chapter, you will learn about the roles of the physicians and nurse as part of a health care provider team, where they work, how they are trained and licensed, and the issues facing these providers as the health care environment continues to change. The following chapter addresses the other clinical and non-clinical providers.

The Physician's Role in Health Care Delivery

The role of physicians is to diagnose and treat the illnesses of their patients. When a physician sees a patient who has an injury or is ill, the physician must first identify the problem or diagnose the illness. The process begins with the physician obtaining the patient's **medical history** and performing a physical examination. To aid in the diagnosis, the physician may perform or order diagnostic tests and then interpret the results. Once the physician has made a diagnosis, treatment for the patient will be prescribed or administered. In addition, physicians give their patients advice about preventive health care and make suggestions about diet and hygiene that will help the patients live healthier lives (Bureau of Labor Statistics, Physicians 2010-11).

medical history The record of a patient's health, physicians' visits, symptoms, prescribed treatments, regular medications, and family medical history.

Types of Physicians and Medical Specialties

Physicians are either doctors of medicine (as indicated by the abbreviation MD after their name) or doctors of osteopathy (as indicated by the abbreviation DO). MDs practice **allopathic medicine**, which means they fight disease by using standard treatments, including surgery and drugs. Although the DO may use these same treatments, DOs practice **osteopathic medicine**, where a special emphasis is placed on understanding the body's musculoskeletal system and on providing preventive and holistic care that considers the relationship between the body, the mind, and the emotions of the patient (Bureau of Labor Statistics, Physicians 2010–11).

During medical school, students are exposed to the many medical specialties. In part, this exposure is designed to help them decide what area of medicine they would like to focus on. Physicians are usually described either as primary care providers or as specialists.

allopathic medicine A process of treating disease by using standard treatments, such as surgery and drugs.

osteopathic medicine A process of treating patients by providing preventive and holistic care.

Primary Care

More than half of DOs and a third of MDs are **primary care physicians**. A primary care physician sees the same patients regularly for preventive care and to treat a

primary care physicians The physician who sees a patient regularly for routine and preventive care.

internal medicine An area of medicine that focuses on the body's organs, such as the heart, eyes, ears, kidneys, and the digestive, respiratory, and vascular systems.

general and family practitioner Physician who focuses on providing comprehensive health care to patients of all ages.

pediatrician A physician who focuses on providing care to children.

surgeon A physician who performs operations.

variety of common health problems. The main areas of primary care are internal medicine, general and family practice, and pediatrics (Bureau of Labor Statistics, Physicians 2010–11).

Internal medicine focuses on problems associated with the body's organs. An internist is trained to diagnose and treat common problems and diseases of the heart, blood, eyes, ears, skin, kidneys, and the digestive, respiratory, and vascular systems. The patients an internist treats are usually adults, although internists often treat children with diabetes or chronic gastrointestinal diseases.

General and family practitioners diagnose and treat a wide variety of illnesses in patients of all ages. This requires a range of training that includes internal medicine, obstetrics and gynecology, and pediatrics. Special emphasis is placed on comprehensive health care of the family as a group.

Pediatricians focus their efforts on a particular group of patients: children. It is the norm for pediatricians to provide preventive health care for children through regular checkups and immunizations. However, they also diagnose and treat infections, injuries, and serious illnesses as needed by their patients.

Specialty Care

Health insurance coverage usually requires that the patient first see the primary care physician for diagnosis and treatment. If required, the primary care physician then refers the patient to a specialist, a physician who is an expert in that particular medical field. Table 5.1 lists some of the typical specialties and their definitions.

If the patient needs an operation to treat the injury or disease, the patient is referred to a **surgeon**. Most surgeons specialize in a particular type of surgery; these include orthopedics (skeletal system and associated organs), ophthalmology (eye), neurological (brain and nervous system), and plastic and reconstructive surgery (Bureau of Labor Statistics, Physicians 2010–11). During surgery, the patient will also need the services of an anesthesiologist.

Table 5.1	*Medical Specialties*
Allergy and immunology	Abnormal responses or acquired hypersensitivity to substances
Anesthesiology	Administration of medications to cause loss of feeling
Cardiovascular diseases	Diseases of the heart and blood vessels
Dermatology	Diseases of the skin
Emergency medicine	Acute illness or injury
Gastroenterology	Diseases and disorders of the stomach and intestine
Neurology	Diseases of the brain and nervous system
Obstetrics and gynecology	Pregnancy, childbirth, and diseases of the female reproductive organs
Pathology	Diagnosis of disease by studying changes in organs, tissues, and cells
Psychiatry	Diseases and disorders of the mind
Pulmonary diseases	Diseases of the lungs
Radiology	Use of X-rays and radiation to diagnose and treat illness
Urology	Diseases of the kidney, bladder, or urinary system

Characteristics of U.S. Physicians

The most recent U.S. Census data indicate that there are a total of 941,300 physicians (U.S. Census Bureau 2010). The demographic data indicate that the profession has slowly changed from one that only white men could enter to one with more opportunities for women and minorities. For example, in 1980 less than 12 percent of physicians were women; in 2007, almost 29 percent are women. Asians represent the largest group of minorities (about 9%), followed by Hispanics (about 4%) and African Americans (about 3%).

Because the population of the United States has become more diverse, it is important that the physician population also continue to diversify. Some studies show that patients report greater comfort and satisfaction with a physician whose ethnicity and gender mirror their own (Bertakis, Franks, and Azari 2003). A diversified physician population may also improve patient access. Minority and female physicians are more likely to practice in primary care and to serve disadvantaged populations. Data from the American Medical Association (AMA) indicate that 47 percent of women as compared to 30 percent of men are in general primary care.

Employment and Earnings of Physicians

Our image of a physician working as a solo practitioner is more a product of art and television than reality. According to the Department of Labor, 661,400 physicians were in active practice in 2008. Only 12 percent were self-employed in solo practice. About 53 percent were in office-based practice; almost 19 percent were employed by hospitals (Bureau of Labor Statistics, Physicians 2010–11). The others worked in the government, with the VA Hospital or the public health service of HHS, for example. The physicians who are not in active practice are teachers, administrators, and researchers. A small number are not involved in medicine at all.

The employment of physicians called **hospitalists** is a growing trend. The traditional model was for a primary care physician to admit patients to the hospital where she or he had staff privileges; in this model, the physician is not an employee of the hospitalist. In the hospitalist model, the hospitalist provides care for the admitted patient; the hospitalist is employed by the hospital. Close to 30,000 physicians are employed as hospitalists; 82 percent trained in internal medicine (Robeznieks 2009). The growth in the number of hospitalists is in part driven by physician practice factors such as declining revenues and desire for work-life balance and in part by hospital factors such as shortages of primary care physicians, emergency department coverage, and decreased physician involvement in hospital quality initiatives (Cors and Rohr 2010).

hospitalists
Physicians who focus on providing care to hospitalized patients.

It is typical for most physicians to work long, irregular hours. In 2008, 43 percent of physicians reported they worked more than 50 hours per week. One advantage of working in a group practice is that the heavy workload is shared by more physicians.

Because the health care industry is expected to continue expanding, the Department of Labor forecasts that the need for physicians will grow by more than 20 percent through 2018 (Bureau of Labor Statistics, Physicians 2010–11). Some specialties are oversupplied; due to the ageing of the American population, job prospects are better in specialties such as cardiology or radiology. Job prospects are also good for those willing to relocate to rural areas where there aren't as many physicians. Some states have tried to attract recent graduates to rural areas by offering to repay the student loans.

Although the workload is sometimes viewed as a disadvantage by those considering the profession, the salary is an advantage. Physicians have among the highest earnings of any profession. The median net income for physicians in primary care is $186,000 per year, according to the 2008 Medical Group Management Association's Physician Compensation and Production Survey. For many physicians, earnings are much higher. Income level varies by number of years in practice, geographic region, hours worked, and specialty. For example, median net income for specialty fields is $340,000.

Education and Training

The education and training required to become a physician has two components. The formal education component consists of an undergraduate degree from a university or college, followed by graduate medical education in medical school. The training component occurs on the job.

The first step toward becoming a physician is an undergraduate degree, usually with a pre-med or science major. The second part of a physician's formal education occurs in medical school. Medical school looks the way it does today thanks to the efforts of the AMA to move training from an apprenticeship style to a scientific university-based education. The Flexner Report in 1910 recommended what has become the current model of medical education: a 4-year program, with 2 years of basic science and 2 years of clinical experience (Beck 2004). Medical school curricula have continued to change as the medical field has changed. More students are exposed to complementary and alternative medicine. Students are also taught to care for culturally diverse populations. Today there are 154 medical schools in the United States— 129 teach allopathic medicine and award the MD; 25 teach osteopathic medicine and award the DO (Bureau of Labor Statistics, Department of Labor 2010–11). Admission to medical school is very competitive with less than half of the applicants being accepted. Of these, about 48 percent are women, 6.5 percent African-American, 21 percent Asian, and 7.5 percent Hispanic. Ninety-six per cent graduate (AAMC FACTS 2010).

residency The last stage of physician training. After medical school, the student completes on-the-job training in his or her specialty.

The final stage of a physician's preparation is **residency** now referred to as Graduate Medical Education (previously called internship and residency). It is paid on-the-job training. Depending on the specialty, residency can last from 1 to 7 years (www.acgme.org).

Medical school tuition and fees have increased by 50 percent for private schools and by 133 percent in public schools since 1984. Because medical school is so expensive, 80 percent of students borrow money so that they can attend. According to the Association of American Medical Colleges (AAMC), the average debt for a 2009 graduate is between $156,456; 79 percent of graduates carry more than $100,000 of debt (www.ama-assn.org).

The increased cost of medical school creates several concerns. The first is an increase in undesirable physician behaviors such as moonlighting and depression. A second concern is that the cost will disproportionately affect minority students, leading to a decrease in diversity. Finally, there is concern that students with high levels of debt may decide not to practice in the lower paying areas of primary care or to work in underserved areas.

Licensure and Certification

The final step is licensure. Every state sets its own requirements for licensure; however, the three standard requirements are graduating from medical school, completing 1 to 7 years of residency, and passing a licensing exam. The U.S. Medical Licensing

Examination (USMLE) is a three-step exam required for licensure in the United States (www.nbme.org). Only a handful of states require criminal background checks or fingerprinting of applicants. The state's specific requirements for licensure are set out in its **Medical Practice Act**, and the license is granted by the state's Board of Medical Examiners. Physicians may only practice medicine in a state where they have a license. To practice in another state, the physician must obtain a license in that state. The state may have a **reciprocity agreement**, which means it accepts the licensing requirements of the first state.

To stay licensed, the physician must pay an annual renewal fee. States also require that physicians stay current in the field by completing additional education, called **CME (Continuing Medical Education)**. Although state requirements may vary, the standard requirement is 75 hours of CME over a 3-year period. Physicians who do not meet these requirements can lose their licenses and hospital privileges.

The state's Medical Practice Act specifies the conditions when a state may suspend or revoke a physician's license. The conditions generally include unprofessional conduct, commission of a crime, or personal incapacity to perform one's duties. The licensing board provides notice to the physician and performs an investigation before a decision is made to revoke the license. The Board may choose to suspend the physician's license during this period if it believes that a dangerous situation exists.

Unlike licensure, **board certification** is voluntary and a way for the physician to indicate that he or she has additional training and skill in a particular area of medicine. To obtain board certification in any of 24 areas, physicians must complete the required years of residency in that specialty and then pass an exam. When these requirements are successfully completed, physician may refer to themselves as "board certified." Others refer to the physician as a "diplomat" of that particular board. The two organizations that control board certification are the American Board of Medical Specialists and the American Osteopathic Association.

The Nurse's Role in Health Care Delivery

As you can see from Table 5.2, there are a number of definitions of nursing; however, all include some aspect of caring for the patient as a whole. A brief definition of the nurse's role is that nurses "take care of people."

"Taking care of people" can include interviewing, examining, and evaluating patients when they first seek health care services. It may progress to providing treatment and care as the patient receives health care services. It may also include working with other health care professionals and referring the patient elsewhere for other services. It includes patient advocacy. The actual day-to-day tasks performed by a nurse are usually determined by the work setting. In addition to the traditional role of direct patient care, nurses' roles have expanded to include disease prevention and health promotion.

The **nursing process** is an organizing framework that provides a systematic method to deliver patient care (Harrington and Terry 2008). The five stages in the nursing process are assessment, diagnosis, care planning, implementation, and outcome evaluation. The process begins with assessment, or the gathering of information. Information can come directly from the patient or from friends, family, and other health care providers. The next step is a nursing diagnosis. The information that has been gathered is reviewed, the problem identified, and a nursing diagnosis made. The North American Nursing Diagnosis Association (NANDA) has developed a classification and formatting system for nursing diagnoses.

Medical Practice Act State legislation that sets out the requirements for physician licensure in that state.

reciprocity agreement An agreement between two states in which each accepts the professional licensing requirements of the other.

CME (continuing medical education) The state requirement that physicians receive a certain amount of additional training and education to remain licensed.

board certification A physician may become board certified by completing additional years of residency in the specialty and passing an exam.

nursing process An organizing framework that provides a systematic method to deliver patient care.

Table 5.2	*Definitions of Nursing*

The four essential features of contemporary nursing practice:
- Attention to the full range of human experiences and responses to health and illness without restriction to a problem-focused orientation
- Integration of objective data with knowledge gained from an understanding of the patient's or group's subjective experience
- Application of scientific knowledge to the process of diagnosis and treatment
- Provision of a caring relationship that facilitates health and healing

Source: American Nurses Association Social Policy Statement, 1995.

The "Practice of Nursing" means assisting individuals or groups to maintain or attain optimal health, implementing a strategy of care to accomplish defined goals, and evaluating responses to care and treatment.
Source: Model Practice Act, National Council of State Boards of Nursing, 1994.

The first level nurse is responsible for planning, providing, and evaluating nursing care in all settings for the promotion of health, prevention of illness, care of the sick, and rehabilitation; and functions as a member of the health team.
Source: International Council of Nursing, 1973.

Nursing is the diagnosis and treatment of human responses to actual or potential health problems.
Source: New York State Nurse Practice Act, 1972.

The essential components of professional nursing are care, cure, and coordination.
Source: ANA Position Paper, 1965.

<To have> charge of the personal health of somebody . . . and what nursing has to do . . . is to put the patient in the best condition for nature to act upon him.
Source: Florence Nightingale, 1859.

Source: Adapted from Joel and Kelly (2001), Exhibit 4.1.

Nursing Outcomes Classification (NOC)
A list of 385 identified outcomes that are responsive to nursing care.

Nursing Interventions Classification (NIC)
A list of 542 interventions that are the nursing treatments of choice for each nursing diagnosis.

Based on the nursing diagnosis, care is planned. Planning actually involves two steps: writing client goals and planning interventions to achieve the goals. There are 385 identified outcomes that are responsive to nursing care; these are classified on the **Nursing Outcomes Classification (NOC)** (Mooread, Johnson, Mass, and Swanson 2007). In the **Nursing Interventions Classification (NIC)**, 542 interventions are identified. These are the nursing treatments of choice for each nursing diagnosis (Bulechek, Butcher, and Dochteman 2007). Then the plan is implemented. Finally, the outcome is evaluated. In actuality, evaluation is ongoing so that modifications can be made to the care plan.

Characteristics of U.S. Nurses

Most of our images of the nursing profession come from the media, yet not all of these impressions are accurate. The media usually portrays nurses as young females. Of the more than 3 million people employed in nursing, it's estimated that 90 percent are women; however, men are increasingly choosing nursing as a profession. Less than 3 percent of nurses are under the age of 25; the average age of RNs is 46 (HRSA 2004).

Nursing continues to be a predominantly white profession. More than 80 percent of RNs are white, but, like other health occupations, the number of minority nurses has increased. African Americans represent about 4 percent of RNs, Asians about 3 percent, and Hispanics about 2 percent.

Types of Nurses

To the general public, a nurse is a nurse is a nurse. Contrary to this misperception, there are significant differences in the types of nurses. The differences include the tasks/responsibilities, the extent of training and education, and the requirements for professional licensing.

Nurses' Assistants and Aides

The nursing assistant or aide is not actually a nurse at all. In some health care settings, **nurses' aides** and home health aides are referred to as NAs and CNAs, depending on whether certification has been obtained. In 2008, there were about 1.5 million nurses' aides (Bureau of Labor Statistics, Nursing Aides 2010–11).

Under the supervision of an RN, NAs provide the most basic level of patient care. Basic care includes physical care of the patient, such as feeding and hygiene. An NA answers call bells, serves meals, and makes beds. The NA may help the patient get out of bed and walk and may escort the patient within the hospital or nursing facility. NAs also set up equipment and move supplies. In nursing homes, the NA is often the principal caregiver. In the home health setting, if they have taken advanced training, NAs may give oral medications to their patients (Sorrentino, Remmert, and Gorek 2010).

NAs are trained on the job or complete a short course of study offered by the hospital or nursing home or by a community/technical college. An NA may obtain the credential of **CNA (Certified Nursing Assistant)**; not all states require certification. NAs are not required to obtain a state license, but some states do require registration. Federal guidelines require that home health aides whose employers receive Medicare reimbursement pass a competency test (Bureau of Labor Statistics, Nursing Aides 2010–11).

> **nurse's aide** Health care worker who provides the most basic level of patient care, such as feeding and hygiene.

> **CNA (Certified Nursing Assistant)** A nurse's aide who has received the credential of CNA.

Licensed Practical or Licensed Vocational Nurse

The next level of care is provided by the **licensed practical nurse (LPN)** or the licensed vocational nurse (LVN). More than 753,000 LPNs were employed in 2008 (Bureau of Labor Statistics, LPNs 2010-11). The duties of the practical nurse include the basic bedside physical care of the patient. In addition to feeding patients and assisting with their personal hygiene, LPNs take vital signs, give medications and injections, and administer some IV medications.

Educational programs for LPNs last about a year. Ninety percent of programs are at technical/vocational schools or community colleges. The training includes both classroom and clinical experience. After completing their formal education program, LPNs must pass a national licensure exam to practice.

> **licensed practical nurse (LPN)** A nurse who has completed a state-approved program and passed a national exam. Generally, LPNs are supervised by RNs when providing patient care.

Registered Nurse

The majority (2.6 million in 2008) of nurses are **registered nurses (RNs)**. A higher level of care is provided by the RN. When performing direct patient care tasks, RNs observe, assess, and record symptoms, reactions, and progress. They may administer IV medication and blood. RNs perform patient assessments and plan care. As part of the nursing care plan developed and managed by the RN, the RN must instruct both the patient and the patient's family in proper care (Bureau of Labor Statistics, RNs 2010–11).

Some of the major differences between the LPN and the RN involve supervision, legal responsibilities, and IV therapy. The LPN and RN roles also vary in terms of the

> **registered nurse (RN)** A nurse who develops and manages a nursing care plan for a patient.

skill level required in communication, assessment, and client teaching (Harrington and Terry 2008). LPN training programs focus on the "how to" of patient care, whereas RN education emphasizes understanding "why" (Hill and Howlett 2008).

The educational program for RNs is more complex than that for LPNs. RNs complete additional coursework toward an associate's degree, which includes additional clinical hours. Many community college offer bridge programs, designed for LPNs who wish to move up. RNs are encouraged to complete the **BSN (bachelor of science in nursing)**. Like LPNs, to practice, RNs must pass a national licensure exam.

BSN (Bachelor of Science in Nursing) A bachelor's program usually takes 4 years to complete.

Additional promotions come from moving up a career ladder at a place of employment and assuming managerial responsibilities. RNs with the bachelor's or master's degree may choose a teaching career.

Advanced Practice Nurses

advanced practice nurse A nurse who has obtained a master's degree in a clinical specialty.

Advanced practice nurses provide their patients an even higher level of care. To become an advanced practice nurse, an RN must have a master's degree in a clinical specialty. A person can choose to become a **nurse practitioner (NP)**, a **clinical nurse specialist (CNS)**, a **certified nurse-midwife (CNM)**, or a **certified registered nurse anesthetist (CRNA)** (Blais and Hayes 2010).

nurse practitioner (NP) Advanced practice nurse who provides basic primary health care.

There are currently 135,000 nurse practitioners in the United States (www.aanp. org). NPs serve an important function in areas not adequately served by physicians such as rural communities and inner cities. They also are key health care providers for populations such as children in schools and the elderly. In these settings, NPs provide basic primary health care, including diagnosis and treatment of common acute illnesses. They can order and interpret X-rays and other laboratory tests. The nurse practitioner is able to prescribe medication, although state law may place restrictions on how this is done and limit the classes of drugs and may be able to practice independently without physician collaboration or supervision. Certification is available for NPs who wish to specialize in acute, adult, family, gerontological, or pediatric care (Blais and Hayes 2010).

clinical nurse specialist (CNS) An advanced practice nurse who specializes in a field such as oncology, neonatal care, or mental health.

Instead of focusing on primary care, nurse practitioners may choose the role of clinical nurse specialist (CNS). There are currently 54,000 clinical nurse specialists. Some of the specialties for practice include cardiac, oncology, neonatal, obstetrics/gynecology, pediatrics, neurological nursing, and psychiatric/mental health care.

certified nurse-midwife (CNM) An advanced practice nurse who provides prenatal and postpartum care and delivers infants.

Certified nurse-midwives (CNMs) and certified registered nurse anesthetists (CRNAs) are two additional areas of specialization. More than 18,500 CNMs in clinical practice provide prenatal care to healthy women, deliver babies, and provide postpartum care for their patients. Of all visits to CNMs, 90 percent are for primary preventive care including annual gynecological exams. Many of the patients (70%) whom CNMs serve are considered "vulnerable" because of their age, socioeconomic status, ethnicity, education, or location of residency (www.acnm.org).

certified registered nurse anesthetist (CRNA) An advanced practice nurse who specializes in anesthesia.

The more than 44,000 CRNAs in the United States play a central role in anesthesiology. According to the American Association of Nurse Anesthetists, nurse anesthetists administered approximately 32 million anesthetics in 2009. In nearly 100 percent of rural U.S. hospitals, the CRNA is the sole provider of anesthetics (www.aana.com). Unlike other areas of nursing, this is not a female-dominated specialty; 49 percent of nurse anesthetists are men.

supervised clinical experience Nursing students obtain hands-on experience with patients as part of their education.

Education and Training

At all levels, nursing education has two components: classroom instruction and **supervised clinical experience**. As nursing has evolved as a profession, the level of education and training has shifted from primarily on-the-job training to formal college-based education. Although there are a few **diploma programs** still offered by hospitals, the majority of RN programs are offered at the **ADN (associate degree in nursing)** level and the BSN level (Bureau of Labor Statistics, RN 2010–11). Either degree qualifies a licensed nurse for an entry-level staff position. However, advancement opportunities into management positions may require the bachelor's degree.

The profession is encouraging nurses to complete bachelor's, master's, and even doctoral degrees in nursing. Currently only 40 percent of nurses have bachelor's degrees or higher. Enrollment and graduation rates from BSN programs have continued to rise, but growth is constrained by lack of faculty and clinical sites. In 2009, almost 40,000 qualified applicants were not admitted (AACN 2009). Enrollment has increased 9 percent in master's programs and 20 percent in doctoral programs. Higher level degrees are required for teaching and research positions. Graduate training is required for management-level nursing positions and for advanced practitioner patient care.

Licensure

In each state, the **State Board of Nursing** (or its equivalent) specifies what educational, clinical, and licensure requirements are necessary to practice in that state. **Nurse Practice Acts** contain the states' requirements for practice. Although they vary from state to state in their details, practice acts generally define the scope of nursing practice, control who may use nursing titles, specify educational requirements, and identify causes for disciplinary action (Harrington and Terry 2008).

All 50 states require that nurses be and remain licensed in order to practice. Once a nurse has finished the educational program requirements, the next step is to take the national registry exam (NCLEX). At each level of practice, there is a separate licensure exam. If the exam is passed, then licensure by the state to practice follows, and the title LPN or RN can be used.

The continuing education requirements for nurses vary. Generally, the more specialized the practice, the more likely it is that continuing education is required to maintain licensure or certification. Like physicians, nurses are subject to disciplinary actions. They have to stay in good standing or risk having their license not renewed or even revoked.

Employment Options for Nurses

Everywhere health care services are provided, you'll find nurses. The work nurses do in hospitals, office, long-term care, home health, public health, and other settings is described in the following sections. The salaries earned by PNs and RNs and the percentage of each type of nurse working in different health care setting are presented in Table 5.3.

Hospitals

The entry-level position for an RN is **staff nurse**. Staff nurses provide bedside care and carry out medical regimes. They also supervise LPNs and NAs. A staff nurse is usually assigned to one area such as surgery, maternity, pediatrics, emergency department, or intensive care.

With more experience, an RN can be promoted to a **nurse supervisor** position. Nurse supervisors plan work schedules and assign duties for their area. They also provide training for other nurses. They visit patients to observe the patients' care. Maintaining records and ordering supplies are among the nurse supervisor's additional responsibilities.

diploma program
Hospitals used to provide on-the-job training programs for nurses and award a diploma upon completion. Very few diploma programs still exist.

ADN (associate degree in nursing)
An associate's program typically takes 2 years to complete and is usually offered by a community college.

State Board of Nursing Each state has an agency that oversees the profession and accredits educational programs.

Nurse Practice Act State legislation that sets out the requirements for nurse licensure in the state.

staff nurse An entry-level position for a nurse.

nurse supervisor A nursing position with more responsibilities and requiring more experience than a staff nurse.

Table 5.3	*Employment Settings and Salaries for Nurses*			
	LPNs		**RNs**	
Setting	**% employed**	**Avg Salary**	**% employed**	**Avg Salary**
Hospital	25	$38,080	60	$63,880
Office	12	35,020	8	59,210
LTC	28	40,580	5	57,060
Homehealth	5	39,500	5	58,740
Other	30	39,030	22	62,450

Source: Bureau of Labor Statistics, U.S. Department of Labor. 2010–11. *Occupational outlook handbook, Licensed practical nurses* and *Registered nurses.*

Medical Offices

Medical offices include all the physician offices and clinics where patients receive ambulatory primary care services. In those offices, nurses prepare patients for the health examination and assist with the exam. They also maintain patient records. Nurses perform many of the diagnostic tests once done by physicians and provide clinical care for monitoring patients with chronic disease.

Medical offices also include a number of services that used to be performed only in inpatient hospital settings. More sophisticated procedures, especially outpatient surgery, are now performed in medical offices and surgicenters. Here the nurse may also assist with the surgical procedure and administer medications and injections.

Long-Term Care and Home Health

Both long-term care and home health are providing increased opportunities for nurses. Because of the aging of the population, there is increased demand for long-term care services, especially to care for those with Alzheimer's or as a consequence of stroke or head injuries. Technological advances have made it possible for many complex procedures to be performed in the home, which has increased opportunities in that setting.

In the long-term care facility, the RN usually has an administrative or supervisory role. LPNs perform direct patient care tasks (Bureau of Labor Statistics, RNs and LPNs 2010–11). Home health care offers the opportunity to work independently. Both settings expect to see an increased demand for aides. Part of this is related to the growth in these settings, but part of it is because of high turnover among the aides. Their pay is low, with little opportunity to move up, and the job has high physical and emotional demands.

Public Health

As the health care industry shifts from an emphasis on treating disease to an emphasis on preventing disease, the industry has paid more attention to the public health setting. Nurses in this setting provide primary care services to the community, including immunizations, screenings, and pediatric care. They also play an important role as educators, instructing the community about health issues, disease prevention, and nutrition. Public health nurses must have at least a bachelor's degree.

Other Opportunities

Nurses who choose not to provide care directly to patients can find employment on the business side of health care. Many companies that provide home health and chronic care services employ nurses in management positions. In those positions, nurses perform the managerial roles of planning and development, marketing, and quality assurance. Their nursing experience provides the companies they work for with valuable insights. Nurses who decide to take this employment direction usually return to school for graduate-level management education.

Another area of employment is in education. Nursing faculty are in high demand. Those with a master's or a doctorate administer educational programs, as well as teach.

Issues in Health Care Delivery

As discussed earlier in this text, the health care industry faces challenges to improve access, maintain quality, and control costs. These are serious concerns for everyone employed in the healthcare industry. The same supply and demand concerns that affect the overall economy are present in the healthcare industry.

There is concern that there is an insufficient supply of health care providers of all types. Part of the problem lies in attracting applicants, but this chapter has demonstrated that both medical and nursing schools have more applicants than they can admit. To expand educational opportunities is a multi-year endeavor, requiring the construction and equipping of expensive facilities and an increase in the number of professional who are willing to become faculty, often at salaries less than what they can earn as practitioners. Rigorous educational and licensure requirements encourage quality, but restrict people from entering the profession.

To increase the supply of physicians, some states have developed incentive programs where they will pay for medical school if the physician promises to practice in an underserved area. As well as calling for medical schools to control costs, the AMA also supports an income tax deduction for the interest on medical school loans. States have also looked for ways to fund initiatives that would increase the number of nurses (AACN 2010).

Another part of the problem lies in retaining people in health care professions. **Burnout** is common in professions that demand a great deal of empathy from their practitioners. Burnout is generally caused by stress and overwork, both of which are common in health settings that are understaffed (Dunham and Smith 2005). Other serious concerns included back injuries, **needlestick injuries**, **latex allergies**, and physical and verbal abuse. The wide variance in compensation between various clinical providers can be another source of dissatisfaction that causes people to change professions.

Matching the supply of clinical providers to the demand for their services also causes gaps. Cost pressures in particular have led to staffing with less expensive professionals. The more expensive RN is replaced with the less expensive LPN or NA, or the patient is seen by a nurse practitioner instead of a primary care physician. Depending on the setting, this can raise questions about the quality of services provided to a patient.

The way services are billed and reimbursed also influences demand. Nursing care is not billed separately (it is part of the daily fee for hospitals, for example). Insurance may cover visits to one type of care provider, but not to another. Concerns about quality of care have influenced legislators and accrediting agencies to look closely at staffing levels, which then alter the demand for certain kinds of clinical providers.

burnout
A psychological condition in which a person loses the ability to care and becomes apathetic. Stress and overwork are thought to cause burnout.

needlestick injuries
Health practitioners can be injured and exposed to disease if they are inadvertently stuck by a needle.

latex allergies Many medical practitioners and patients are allergic to latex, which is the most commonly found material in gloves used in medical procedures.

Summary

The ways in which physicians and nurses deliver patient care are described. Physicians, whether MDs or DOs, see patients to diagnose and treat injuries and illness. Physicians are primary care providers or may choose an area of specialty. Most physicians work in some form of office-based practice. In addition to the required education and training, physicians must be licensed by the state to practice medicine. Physicians may describe themselves as "board certified" if they pass the residency and examination requirements of the American Board of Medical Specialties.

The nurses' role in the health care team is "taking care of people." The actual day-to-day tasks are determined by the nurse's employment setting and the licensure. Nursing care is provided by nursing aides, licensed practical nurses (LPNs), registered nurses (RNs), and advanced practice nurses. The State Board of Nursing specifies what educational and clinical requirements are necessary to obtain a license in that state; nurses must be licensed to practice. Nurses work in hospitals, medical offices, and long-term and home health care settings.

The supply of and demand for health care providers influence physicians and nurses. Access to care and quality while still controlling costs are concerns facing physicians and nurses.

Questions for Review

1. What tasks does the physician perform to provide health care services?
2. Describe the specialties of family practitioners, pediatricians, and surgeons.
3. Explain the difference between licensure and certification.
4. What are some of the differences between LPNs and RNs?
5. Describe one type of advanced practice nurse.
6. What is a Nurse Practice Act?

Questions for Discussion

1. As a patient, do the demographic characteristics of a health care provider (gender, race, age) make any difference to you? Should part of providers' education include more diversity training?
2. Many people believe that health care wouldn't be so expensive if doctors didn't get paid so much. What do you think about physicians' earnings and compensation?
3. Suggest ways that nurses can influence public opinion about the scope of the health care services they provide.
4. One argument used for allowing nurse practitioners more independent responsibility is that they are cost-effective providers of care. Do you believe this is a good strategy to improve access to care? Should advanced practice nurses be able to practice without supervision?
5. Interview a physician you know. Does he or she face any of the same concerns as Dr. Hunter (in the chapter profile) does?

Chapter References

AACN. 2009. Student enrollment expands at U.S. nursing colleges and universities for the 9th year despite financial challenges and capacity restraints. Available at www.aacn.nche.edu.

AAMC Facts: Applicants, matriculants, enrollment, graduates, MD/PhD, and residency applicants data. 2010. Available at www.aamc.org/data/facts/start.htm.

American Association of Nurse Anesthetists (www.aana.com).

American Association of Nurse Practitioners (www.aanp.org).

American Medical Association. 2008. *Physician characteristics and distribution in the U.S.* www.ama-assn.org.

____. *Medical school debt.* www.ama-assn.org. Accessed May 7, 2010.

Beck, A. 2004. The Flexner report and the standardization of American medical education. *Journal of the American Medical Association* 291: 2139–40.

Bertakis, K., Franks, P., and R. Azari. 2003. Effects of physician gender on patient satisfaction. *Journal of the American Medical Womens Association* 58(2): 69–75.

Blais, K., and J. Hayes. 2010. *Professional nursing practice.* 6th ed. Upper Saddle River, NJ: Prentice Hall.

Bulechek, G., H. Butcher, and J. Dochteman. 2007. *Nursing interventions classification (NIC).* 5th ed. St. Louis, MO: C.V. Mosby.

Bureau of Labor Statistics, Department of Labor. 2010–11. *Career guide to industries, Healthcare.* Available at www.bls.gov/oco/cg/cgs035.htm.

Bureau of Labor Statistics, Department of Labor. 2010–11. *Occupational outlook handbook, Licensed practical and licensed vocational nurses.* Available at www.bls.gov/oco/ocos074.htm.

____. *Nursing, psychiatric, and home health aides.*

____. *Physicians and surgeons.*

____. *Registered nurses.*

Cors, W., and R. Rohr. 2010. The 'ist' explosion: Driving forces, current trends and future directions for hospitalists. *Physician Executive Journal,* May–June. Retrieved from MEDLINE.

Dunham, K., and S. Smith. 2005. *How to survive & maybe even love your career as a nurse.* Philadelphia: F.A. Davis.

Harrington, N., and C. Terry. 2008. *LPN to RN transitions.* 3rd ed. Philadelphia: Lippincott, Williams & Wilkins.

Health Resources and Service Administration, U.S. Department of Health and Human Services. 2004. *The Registered nurse population: Findings from the 2004 national sample survey of registered nurses.* Available at hpr.hrsa.gov/healthworkforce/rnsurvey04/.

Hill, S., and H. Howlett. 2008. *Success in practical nursing: Personal and vocational issues.* 6th ed. Philadelphia: W.B. Saunders.

Joel, L., and L. Kelly. 2001. *The nursing experience: Trends, challenges, and transitions.* 4th ed. New York: McGraw-Hill.

Moorhead, S., M. Johnson, M. Maas, and E. Swanson. 2007. *Nursing outcomes classification (NOC).* 4th ed. St. Louis, MO: C.V. Mosby.

National Board of Medical Examiners (www.nbme.org).

Robeznieks, A. 2009. Hopitalists score. But program isn't exactly board certification. *Modern Healthcare.* 39/40. Retrieved on MEDLINE.

Sorrentino, S., L. Remmert, and B. Gorek. 2010. *Mosby's essentials for nursing assistants.* 4th ed. St. Louis, MO: C.V. Mosby.

U.S. Census Bureau. 2010. *Statistical abstract of the United States: 2010.*

For Additional Information

Accreditation Council for Graduate Medical Education (www.acgme.org).

American Association of Colleges of Nursing (www.aacn.nche.edu).

American Board of Medical Specialties (www.abms.org).

American Nurses Association (www.nursingworld.org).

Association of American Medical Colleges (www.aamc.org).

Buhler-Wilkerson, K. 2001. *No place like home: A history of nursing and home care in the United States.* Baltimore, MD: Johns Hopkins University Press.

Konefal, J. 2002. The challenge of educating physicians about complementary and alternative medicine. *Academic Medicine* 77: 847–50.

National Council of State Boards of Nursing (www.ncsbn.org).

National League for Nursing (www.nln.org).

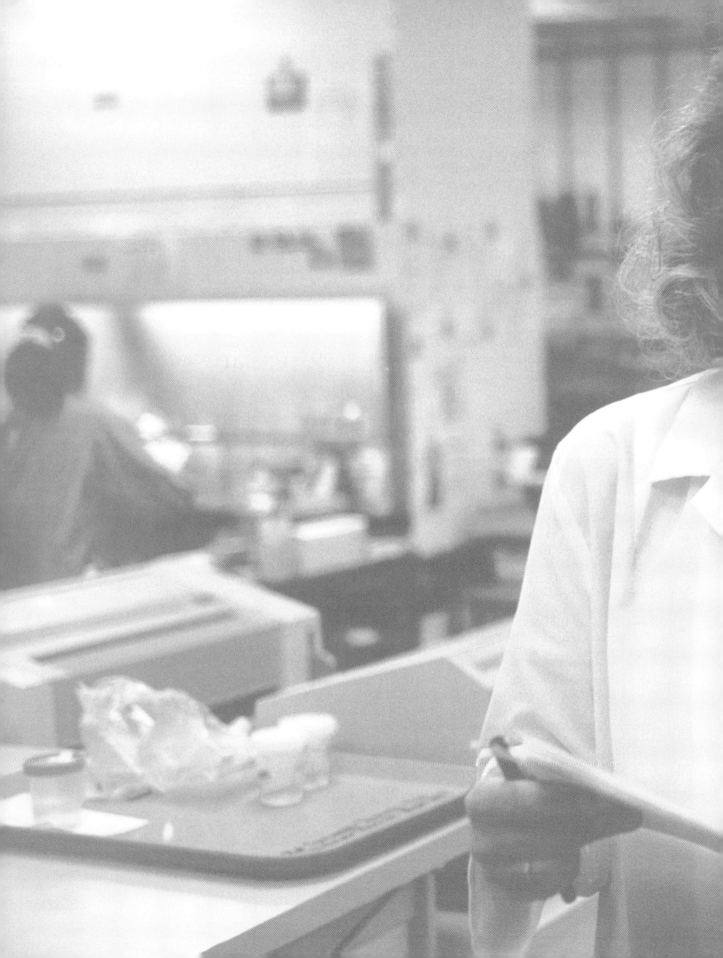

6

Other Clinical and Non-Clinical Health Care Providers

Learning Objectives

After reading this chapter, you should be able to:

1. Identify the role of physician assistants, medical assistants, and surgical technologists in hospital and office visits.
2. List the providers of diagnostic testing.
3. Identify the providers of therapeutic services.
4. Describe the role of health care professionals in emergency care situations.
5. Identify the role of dentists, optometrists, chiropractors, podiatrists, and dietitians/nutritionists in the health care system.
6. Define health administration.
7. Identify the role of health information managers and technicians.
8. Describe the role of professional billing and coding in the service delivery process.

Speech-Language Pathologist

Julie Pierce went to college thinking she wanted to be a nurse but she quickly discovered nursing wasn't her field. A friend in speech pathology urged her to talk to the professors in that department. Julie did, took the introductory courses, and fell in love with the field of speech-language pathology. She obtained her bachelor's degree in communication disorders and her master's in speech-language pathology. After a year of clinical practice under the direction of a licensed speech pathologist, Julie obtained her licensure. The rest, as they say, is history.

Julie is employed by the Midland School District in Arkansas as the speech-language pathologist. She sees 20 to 25 children each day, usually in groups of three to four. Her patients range in age from preschool to high school. In the morning, she works with the younger children. Most of what she does is articulation therapy, the actual producing of a specific sound. She starts with the sound, moves on to the word, the phrase, the sentence, and then conversation. When the child can successfully produce the sound in all of those settings, then the child graduates. Younger children are identified by their teachers and then tested by Julie to see if her services are needed. She also spends about an hour a day in the resource room doing overall lessons. Julie also does some language therapy, which focuses on the process of communication. She might work on speech or phrases or on the broader context of appropriate social behavior. Julie's services are free for the student; her salary is paid by the school district. An Individual Education Plan (IEP) is prepared for each student, and conferences are held regularly with parents to inform them of their child's progress.

Speech pathologists generally work with children or with adults. During their graduate training, students work with both groups of patients. They even experience many of the same tests their patients do. For example, to test a patient's ability to swallow, a moving video is taken of the patient swallowing a barium solution. "It was nasty," said Julie, "but now you know what it's like for the patient." Generally, there are more successes working with children. "Their bodies are amazing at regenerating," says Julie. Adult patients often need therapy as a result of traumatic brain injury or dementia. Although there are occasional gains, the work can be frustrating because the patient's overall condition is likely to deteriorate.

Julie says she prefers working with children because "I'd rather be thrown up on by a child than an adult!" She cautions that speech-language pathology is not a field for "the faint of heart. You're knee-deep in the mouth. I've been thrown up on, spat on, and even choked." What she loves, however, is helping people communicate. "It's wonderful when they grasp an idea. You can see the light come on."

Like many professional in health care, Julie finds the paperwork and bureaucracy the most difficult part of her job. "It's hard to see a child slip through the cracks because the funding isn't there." She notes that adults face some of the same funding challenges. Speech therapy and physical therapy are grouped together by Medicare without sufficient funding to obtain both. "A stroke victim in a nursing home has to make a choice between walking and talking. That's sad."

Introduction

If the physician's role focuses on diagnostics and the nurse's role focuses on caregiving, what roles are played by the other 200-plus health care occupations? This chapter cannot cover every health occupation, but it addresses some office-based occupations, diagnostic and laboratory services, and therapeutic services. In holistic patient care, the health care team encompasses many other clinical and non-clinical health care providers. Patients generally do not encounter many of these other health care professionals until they have seen their primary care physician, been admitted to the hospital, or had a medical emergency. Patients encounter many

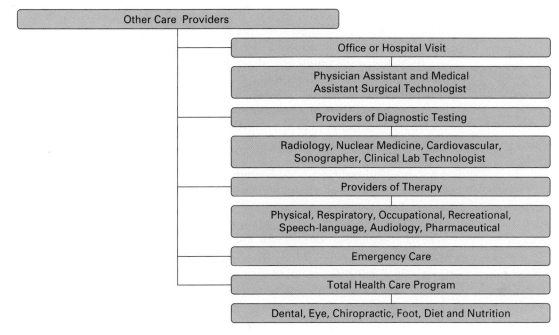

Figure 6.1 Other Care Providers

other health care professionals as part of a total health care program. This chapter also introduces the many non-clinical occupations available in the health care setting. Non-clinical employees use their skills and training to keep the businesses operating so that clinical employees can deliver patient care. Many of these forms of employment can be found in any business, but some, such as health information manager or coding specialist, are only found in health care. Figure 6.1 presents a list of all the other professionals covered in the chapter.

Office or Hospital Visit

In conjunction with an office or hospital visit, a patient comes into contact with other health care providers in addition to physicians and nurses. These include physician assistants and medical assistants in the office setting and surgical technologists in the surgical setting.

Physician Assistants

According to the American Academy of Physician Assistants, there were approximately 74,800 practicing physician assistants (PAs) as of 2009 (Bureau of Labor Statistics, Physician Assistant 2010–11). Working under the supervision of a physician, the PA provides health care services to patients; 90 percent of PAs are in clinical practice. This can include taking medical histories, examining patients, ordering tests and X-rays, diagnosing, and prescribing medications. In 2009, 37 percent of PAs worked in hospitals and another 35 percent worked with group practice physicians; 85 percent are employed full-time (www.aapa.org).

In all 50 states, the District of Columbia, Guam, and the Commonwealth of the Northern Mariana Islands, PAs are allowed to prescribe medications (www.aapa.org).

PAs are particularly in demand in rural and inner-city areas where it has been difficult to attract physicians. In these areas, the PA may be the principal care provider, reporting to the physician on the 1 or 2 days per week that the physician is present.

By state law, PAs must complete an accredited, formal education program; in 2008, 142 programs nationwide provided physician assistant programs (Bureau of Labor Statistics, Physician Assistant 2010–11). The majority of PAs hold a bachelor's degree, although PAs are employable with an associate's degree. Master's degrees in PA are available from 113 programs. With additional clinical hours, PAs can specialize in pediatrics, orthopedics, or surgery.

In addition to formal education, all states require that PAs pass the Physician Assistants National Certifying Examination (PANCE). Every 2 years, the PA must complete 100 hours of continuing medical education, and every 6 years, the PA must be recertified.

A 2009 salary survey conducted by the American Academy of Physician Assistants indicated that median earnings for PAs were about $93,500 (www.aapa.org). As with other health care professions, earnings vary considerably depending on location, specialty, and experience.

Because PAs represent a cost-effective way to provide routine health services, demand is expected to grow. Movements to restrict the number of hours physician residents may work and reduction in the number of residents in teaching hospitals will also increase the need for more PAs.

Medical Assistant

Although the name *medical assistant* sounds very similar to physician assistant, the role of the medical assistant (MA) is quite different. The MA provides administrative and clerical services to the physician. These can include working with patient records, scheduling appointments (including hospital admission and laboratory services), insurance forms, and billing. The MA may also provide limited clinical services to patients. Depending on state law and the size and type of medical practice, an MA's clinical duties might include taking medical histories and vital signs and assisting the physician during the examination of a patient. The MA may also collect and prepare laboratory specimens and perform lab tests (www.aama-ntl.org).

Most MAs have completed either a 1- or 2-year program of college study, resulting in a certificate or associate degree, respectively. Although there is no licensure requirement for MAs, employers prefer applicants who have passed a national certification examination.

Data from their professional association indicate that there were approximately 483,600 people employed as MAs in 2008. The majority (62%) work in physicians' offices, 13 percent in hospitals, and 11 percent in other practitioners' offices such as chiropractors and podiatrists. MA is one of the fastest growing occupations because of the increase in the number of health care facilities that rely on a high proportion of support personnel (Bureau of Labor Statistics, Medical Assistant 2010–11). The average earnings for a MA in 2009 were $30,834 (www.aama-ntl.org).

Surgical Technologists

The patient who requires a surgical procedure, whether performed on an inpatient basis in the hospital or on an outpatient basis in an office, will encounter surgical technologists. They assist the surgical team by preparing patients, preparing surgical instruments and equipment, passing instruments and supplies during surgery, transferring patients after surgery, and cleaning and restocking the operating room. Almost 71 percent of the 91,500 surgical technologists employed in 2008 worked in hospital operating and delivery rooms. The annual median earnings were $3,874, according to the Department of Labor (Bureau of Labor Statistics, Surgical Technologists 2010–11).

Formal education is acquired in programs lasting from 9 to 24 months. Depending on the length of the program, the surgical technologist earns a certificate or associate's degree. Licensure is not required, but most employers prefer professionally certified technologists. Depending on the certifying organization, certification is renewed through continuing education or reexamination.

Providers of Diagnostic Testing

Physicians frequently order a variety of **diagnostic tests** to provide them with the data to make a diagnosis. **Technologists** and **technicians** provide these services. The difference in the two titles represents the difference in amount of education and training. The most common form of training is a 2-year associate's degree, although some fields require a bachelor's degree. Many health care professionals cross-train by receiving a 1-year certificate. Growth is predicted in these fields because of the health care needs of an aging population. Technologists and technicians are found in hospitals, physicians' offices, and diagnostic imaging centers. Data concerning these career fields are presented in Table 6.1.

Medical Imaging Technologists and Technicians

Radiology is the field of medicine that utilizes X-ray and other **imaging technology** to diagnose medical problems. The technologists and technicians in this field (often called diagnostic imaging technicians or radiographers) work with the physician to take X-rays or other tests. A CT technologist uses tomography scanners to produce cross-sectional images of the patients' bodies. Magnetic resonance imaging (MRI) technologists use magnets and radio waves instead of radiation to produce images (www.asrt.org). More than half of all jobs are in the hospital setting. Since 1981 when Congress passed the Consumer-Patient Radiation Health and Safety Act, federal voluntary standards have protected both patients and practitioners from excessive exposure to radiation.

diagnostic tests tests ordered by a physician to provide information that assists in making a diagnosis.

technologist A professional who performs testing services. A technologist usually has more training than a technician.

technician A person who performs the routine tasks in a laboratory setting.

imaging technology a broad term referring to the many forms of technology that allow an image of the patient's body to be produced.

Table 6.1	Diagnostic Testing Careers 2008			
Position	**No. of Jobs**	**Annual Earnings**	**Education**	**License**
Radiology	214,700	$52,210	Associate's	Y (38 states)
Nuclear medicine	21,800	$66,660	Associate's	Y (25 states)
Cardiology	49,500	$47,010	Associate's	N
Sonography	50,300	$61,980	Associate's	N
Clinical lab	328,100	$53,500	Bachelor's	Varies

Source: Bureau of Labor Statistics, U.S. Department of Labor, *Occupational Outlook Handbook,* 2010–11.

Nuclear Medicine Technologists

Nuclear medicine uses radioactive drugs to diagnose and treat disease. The nuclear medicine technologist administers the radiopharmaceutical and operates the imaging equipment that traces the drug in the patient's body. Almost 66 percent of technologists work in hospitals (Bureau of Labor Statistics, Nuclear Medicine Technologists 2010–11). All technologists must comply with the federal standards regarding the administration of radioactive drugs and the operation of radiation detection equipment.

Cardiovascular Technologists and Technicians

As implied by the name *cardiovascular*, these technologists and technicians specialize in the heart and its peripheral blood vessels. Seventy-seven percent work in hospitals, most commonly in the cardiology department. Technologists specialize in invasive cardiology, echocardiography, or vascular technology (Bureau of Labor Statistics, Cardiovascular Technologists and Technicians 2010–11).

Cardiology technologists, those specializing in invasive cardiology, assist with cardiac catherizations and balloon angioplasty. They may also monitor patients during open-heart surgery. Noninvasive tests involve the use of ultrasound instrumentation. Vascular technologists or sonographers listen to the arteries to diagnose circulation disorders. Echocardiographers, or cardiac sonographers, use ultrasound to examine the chambers, valves, and vessels of the heart.

Cardiovascular technicians receive 8 to 16 weeks of on-the-job training to take basic electrocardiographs (EKGs). Those with advanced training can perform Holter monitoring and stress testing.

Diagnostic Medical Sonographer

Ultrasonography uses sound waves to generate an image to assess and diagnose various medical conditions. The best known use is in obstetrics where an ultrasound is used to examine the growth and health of the fetus. However, a number of other medical specialties utilize ultrasound technology. Abdominal sonographers scan the abdominal cavity to assess the gallbladder, bile ducts, kidneys, liver, pancreas, and spleen. Neurosonographers focus on the nervous system, including the brain. Ophthalmologic sonographers study the eyes (www.sdms.org). Approximately 59 percent of sonographers are employed by hospitals (Bureau of Labor Statistics, Diagnostic Medical Sonographer 2010–11).

Medical Laboratory Specialists

Laboratory testing of patients' body fluids, tissues, and cells plays an integral role in the diagnosis and treatment of disease. Medical laboratory specialists (formerly called clinical laboratory technologists or medical technologists) perform a variety of complex tests on the samples they receive. If they work for a larger lab, they may specialize in the type of testing they do. Clinical chemistry technologists analyze the chemical and hormonal contents of body fluids; microbiology technologists examine bacteria and other microorganisms; immunohematology technologists examine blood; immunology technologists focus on the human immune system; cytotechnologists examine cells for signs of cancer; and molecular biology technologists perform genetic tests (Bureau of Labor Statistics, Clinical Laboratory Technologists and Technicians 2010–11).

Medical technicians or clinical laboratory technicians perform less complex testing than technologists. Consequently the median annual salary is lower, about

$35,380 in 2008. Technicians also have less education, usually an associate's degree. Two areas of specialization for technicians include **histology** technicians, who prepare tissue samples for pathologists, and **phlebotomists**, who collect blood samples.

Some states require that lab personnel be licensed or registered. Advanced education is required to direct or manage a laboratory. Professional certification, although voluntary, is usually a job requirement.

histology the study of body tissues.

phlebotomist A health care professional who collects blood samples.

Therapy Providers

Part of the physician's treatment may be to order **therapy**. Depending on the patient's medical problems, the patient might need the services of a physical, respiratory, occupational, or recreational therapist. They might also need to work with a speech-language pathologist or audiologist. Therapists may work with assistants and aides. They must be properly supervised, and only a specific set of duties may be delegated to them. Table 6.2 presents data concerning these fields.

therapy Remedial treatment of a disorder.

Physical Therapy

Physical therapists (PTs) help patients restore mobility and manage pain by implementing a treatment plan that utilizes exercise, massage, and other therapies. About two thirds of PTs are employed by hospitals or in a PT practice. About 27 percent work part time. Nursing homes, rehabilitation centers, and home health agencies also employ PTs (www.apta.org).

Working under the supervision of the PT, the physical therapy assistant implements treatment plans and reports the outcomes to the PT. Physical therapy aides perform routine support tasks under the PT's supervision.

Respiratory Therapy

Respiratory therapists treat patients with breathing disorders. More than 80 percent work in hospitals in respiratory care, anesthesiology, or pulmonary medicine departments.

Table 6.2 *Therapy Careers 2008*

Position	No. of Jobs	Annual Earnings	Education	License
Physical therapist	185,500	$72,790	post-baccalaureate	Y
PT assistant	63,800	$46,140	Associate's	Y
PT aide	46,100	$23,760	OJT	N
Respiratory therapist	105,900	$52,200	Associate's	Y (48 states)
Occupational therapist	104,500	$66,780	Master's	Y
OT assistant	26,600	$48,230	Associate's	N
OT aide	7,800	$26,960	OJT	N
Recreational therapist	23,300	$38,370	Bachelor's	N
Speech-language pathologist	119,300	$62,930	Master's	Y (47 states)
Audiologist	12,800	$62,030	Doctorate	Y

OJT, on-the-job training.
Source: Bureau of Labor Statistics, U.S. Department of Labor, *Occupational Outlook Handbook,* 2010–11.

Entry-level positions often require that the therapist be certified (certified respiratory therapist); supervisory positions or therapists in intensive care are usually registered (registered respiratory therapist). Although certification or registration is voluntary, the exam is usually a required component of licensure (www.aarc.org).

Occupational Therapy

Occupational therapists (OTs) focus on improving patients' ability to perform daily living and work skills. Occupational therapists may work in hospitals, schools, mental health centers, or rehabilitation centers (www.aota.org).

OT assistants help with activities and exercises in the treatment plan developed by the occupational therapist. OT aides provide treatment support services and perform clerical tasks.

Recreational Therapy

Recreational therapy includes techniques such as arts and crafts, games, dance, drama, and music to improve the emotional and physical well-being of patients. Therapists work in hospitals and long-term care facilities. Many employers prefer to hire certified therapeutic recreation specialists (CTRS). This certification requires the bachelor's degree, an examination, and 480 hours of internship (Bureau of Labor Statistics, Recreational Therapist 2010–11). Four states require licensure.

Speech-Language Pathologist and Audiologist

Speech-language pathologists and audiologists are also therapists. Speech-language pathologists diagnose and treat a range of problems: speech, language, cognitive, communication, voice, and swallowing (www.asha.org). Audiologists work with patients with hearing, balance, and related problems (www.audiology.org). More than half of these pathologists and audiologists work school settings. Health care settings include hospitals, rehabilitation, and psychiatric facilities. A small number have independent practices where they do their own diagnostic work or see patients who have been referred by a primary care physician.

Eighteen states now require audiologists to obtain a doctorate. In addition to the appropriate degree, supervised clinical experience, professional clinical experience, and national examination are required for licensure. Continuing education is usually required to renew the license.

Pharmaceutical Care

Patients who have been to see their primary care physician often don't feel like the visit is complete unless they walk out of that office holding a prescription to be filled. The Food and Drug Administration regulates the pharmaceutical industry and specifies which drugs require a prescription and which can be purchased over-the-counter by the patient/consumer. The pharmacist is forbidden from dispensing any medication without the appropriate prescription. Depending on state law, only physicians, physician assistants, and nurse practitioners can prescribe. Table 6.3 presents the pharmacy career ladder.

Pharmacists dispense the drugs prescribed by the physician. They also provide information to patients about medications. The majority of pharmacists work in retail pharmacies (65%) and hospitals (22%) (Bureau of Labor Statistics, Pharmacists 2010–11).

Table 6.3	*Pharmacy Career Ladder*			
Position	**No. of Jobs**	**Earnings**	**Education**	**License**
Pharmacist	269,900	$106,410/yr	Pharm.D.	Y
Technician	326,300	$13.32/hr	High school/OTJ	N
Aide	54,900	$9.66/hr	OTJ	N

OJT, on-the-job training.
Source: Bureau of Labor Statistics, U.S. Department of Labor, *Occupational Outlook Handbook,* 2010–11.

While pharmacists hold an advanced degree (Pharm.D.) and must meet state licensing criteria, pharmacy technicians and aides usually have only a high school education and are trained on the job. Many states require certification. Their job duties include counting tablets and labeling bottles and other routine tasks. They also verify information, prepare insurance forms, and stock inventory. Questions concerning a prescription are referred to the pharmacist. Pharmacy aides usually perform clerk and cashier activities. Two thirds of technicians and 80 percent of aides work in retail pharmacies (Bureau of Labor Statistics, Pharmacy Technicians and Aides 2010–11).

Emergency Care Providers

Thus far we've seen encounters with health care professionals because the patient has initiated contact with the health care system by visiting the primary care physician. However, in an emergency situation, the patient may enter the system through encounters with a number of emergency care professionals. Emergency care services are locally designed to provide the best care for that community.

In an emergency, EMTs (emergency medical technicians) and paramedics are dispatched to the scene. They provide appropriate medical care on site and transport the patient to the hospital for further care. The precise nature of care depends on the level of training of the EMT.

The National Registry of Emergency Medical Technicians (NREMT) has four levels of service providers: first responder, EMT-basic, EMT-intermediate (85 and 99), and EMT-paramedic. First responders provide basic care. EMT-basic personnel care for patients at the accident scene and transport by ambulance. EMT-Intermediate personnel can administer intravenous fluids, use defibrillators, and advanced airway techniques and equipment. EMT-paramedics may also administer drugs, interpret EKGs, and use other complex equipment.

Department of Labor data indicate EMTs and paramedics held about 210,700 jobs in 2008 (Bureau of Labor Statistics, Emergency Medical Technicians and Paramedics 2010–11). Although earnings vary considerably as a function of training and geographic location, annual median earnings were about $28,200. Most work for hospitals and private ambulance services. Firefighters often have EMT or paramedic training; they are employed by the municipality.

Training and certification is required to become an EMT and paramedic. The training is a combination of college coursework and clinical and field experience. Paramedics usually obtain an associate's degree. Every state has an agency in charge of emergency services that issues licenses. Most states require that EMTs meet the certification requirements of the National Registry of Emergency Medical Technicians (www.nremt.org).

Total Health Care Program

There are some health care professionals whom patients encounter only if they specifically seek that type of care. No referral is necessary from the primary care physician.

Dental Care

As part of their total health care program, patients must decide who and how they will take care of their teeth. Table 6.4 presents data about the different professionals in dental care.

The dentist is the physician who provides oral health care. Like other physicians, dentists are licensed by the state and may prescribe medications for their patients. Dentists can be general practitioners or specialists. Common areas of specialization include orthodontia, the straightening of teeth; pediatrics, taking care of children's teeth; periodontics, gums and bones; oral surgery, operating on mouth and teeth; and endodontics, root canal. Dentistry has increasingly focused on preventive care, so dentists spend time educating their patients about the proper way to brush and floss their teeth (Bureau of Labor Statistics, Dentists 2010–11).

Most dentists are in private practice, usually as sole practitioners (75%); 15 percent work in a partnership. About 15 percent are specialists (www.ada.org).

However, the dentist employs a number of other professional to provide care. Chief among these are dental hygienists who do the bulk of health assessment, X-rays, and teeth cleaning. In some states, hygienists are permitted to perform additional duties related to fillings and surgery. Because many of the routine care tasks previously performed by dentists are now being done by hygienists, the field is expected to grow rapidly (Bureau of Labor Statistics, Dental Hygienists 2010–11).

The dentist's office also employs dental assistants who perform a combination of patient care, office, and laboratory tasks. Usually the assistant is in charge of the office's infection control procedures. If the assistant is permitted to perform radiological procedures, they must pass an exam offered by the Dental Assisting National Board (www.dentalassistant.org).

A large dentist office might have its own laboratory, but it is more common for dental laboratory technicians to work in a commercial dental laboratory. The technician creates all of the dental prosthetics such as crowns, bridges, and dentures, as prescribed by the dentist (www.nadl.org).

Eye Care

As part of their total health care program, patients must decide who and how they will take care of their eyes. More than half of all Americans need corrective eyewear.

Table 6.4	*Dental Care Professionals*			
Position	**No. of Jobs**	**Earnings**	**Education**	**License**
Dentist	141,900	$142,870	DDS	Y
Hygienist	174,100	$66,570	Associate's	Y
Assistant	295,300	$32,380	OTJ/college	Y
Lab technician	46,000	$34,170	OTJ/college	N

DDS, doctor of dental surgery; OJT, on-the-job training.
Source: Bureau of Labor Statistics, U.S. Department of Labor, *Occupational Outlook Handbook*, 2010–11.

Table 6.5	*Eye Care Professionals*			
Position	**No. of Jobs**	**Earnings**	**Education**	**License**
Optometrist	34,800	$96,320	Bachelor's + OD	Y
Optician	59,800	$32,810	Associate's	Y (22 states)
Lab technician	35,200	$27,210	OTJ/college	N

OD, doctor of optometry; OTJ, on-the-job training.
Source: Bureau of Labor Statistics, U.S. Department of Labor, *Occupational Outlook Handbook,* 2010–11.

Disorders such as diabetes or frequent headaches may require specialized vision treatment. Table 6.5 presents data about eye care professionals.

Ophthalmologists are physicians who treat diseases of the eye and perform eye surgery (see Chapter 5). They may also prescribe corrective lenses.

Optometrists provide primary care. Although this includes prescribing corrective lenses, it also includes treating and managing diseases of the visual system, such as cataracts and macular degeneration (www.aoanet.org). They are doctors of optometry (ODs). To earn this degree, the optometrist completes a 4-year optometry program, after completing a bachelor's degree or at least 3 years of a pre-optometry program. After passing written and clinical state board examinations, the optometrist is licensed to practice. Continuing education is required to renew the license. About two thirds of optometrists are in private practice; an increasing number are in group practice.

Dispensing opticians fill the prescriptions written by ophthalmologists and optometrists for the patient's corrective lenses. About 40 percent work directly for the optometrists, 13 percent for ophthalmologists, and another 33 percent work in retail optical stores (Bureau of Labor Statistics, Opticians 2010–11).

Ophthalmic laboratory technicians actually make the prescription eyeglasses. Contact lenses are usually produced by machine (Bureau of Labor Statistics, Ophthalmic Laboratory Technicians 2010–11).

Chiropractic Care

Chiropractic has become increasingly accepted as a form of health care, and usually treatment is covered by insurance. The chiropractor's approach to healthcare is holistic, but the focus is on the spine. Therefore, the primary intervention is manipulation of the spine.

Chiropractors are also known as chiropractic physicians or doctors of chiropractic (DCs). Usually a bachelor's degree and a 4-year chiropractic college course are required to obtain the doctor of chiropractic degree. All states require licensure, which requires formal education and examination, usually through the National Board of Chiropractic Examiners. Continuing education is required to maintain licensure. States vary widely in terms of what they permit chiropractors to do within the scope of their practice. However, all states prohibit chiropractors from prescribing medications and from performing major surgery.

Most chiropractors are in private, solo practice. According to the Department of Labor, in 2008, 49,100 chiropractors had median annual earnings of $66,490 (Bureau of Labor Statistics, Chiropractors 2010–11).

Foot Care

Podiatrists provide specialized care for the foot. There are relatively few podiatrists—about 12,200—and more than half are in solo practice. Average earnings are $113,560.

Podiatrists provide 39 percent of all foot care, according to the American Podiatric Medical Association (www.apma.org). That works out to about 60 million office visits per year. In addition, 81 percent of hospitals have a podiatrist on staff.

A license is required to practice podiatric medicine. The podiatrist must graduate from one of the seven accredited college of podiatric medicine. The program is similar to medical school, where students have clinical rotations in the third and fourth years, and complete hospital residency programs after receiving the doctor of podiatric medicine degree (DPM). Podiatrists can also become board certified in orthopedics, surgery, or primary medicine (Bureau of Labor Statistics, Podiatrists 2010–11).

Diet and Nutrition

medical nutrition therapy The use of nutrition to support health in a patient.

Dietitians are the food and nutrition experts. Health care practitioners recognize the link between food, fitness, and health. As part of the health care team, dietitians provide **medical nutrition therapy** to patients. In addition to direct patient care, dietitians are also employed in wellness programs and public health settings. They often find a role in teaching or research settings, or in food service, whether in a health care settings or in the food industry generally.

In health care, dietitians are frequently employed in hospitals, long-term care facilities, or physicians' clinics. The Department of Labor reports 60,300 people were employed as dietitians in 2008, with a median salary of $50,590 (Bureau of Labor Statistics, Dietitians 2010–11).

Most dietitians and nutritionists hold at least a bachelor's degree, and many obtain a master's degree to progress in the field. The dietetic technician holds an associate's degree. State laws vary regarding licensure and registration.

Health Care Employment in Non-Clinical Positions

In addition to the many clinical providers, patient care is supplemented by the non-clinical providers who keep the delivery systems functioning. These include administrators and managers, health information personnel, and support staff.

Health Administrators and Managers

Health administration is concerned about patient care, but also about profitability and other business issues. Professionals in this industry may be referred to as health administrators, health managers, or health executives, and they hold a variety of job titles. In 2008, there were approximately 284,000 positions in the health care industry, with an average salary of $80,240 (Bureau of Labor Statistics, Medical and Health Services Managers 2010–11). An administrator must understand the basics of management, marketing, and accounting and finance in order to effectively manage a health care business (Haddock, Chapman and McLean 2002). These functions were described in Chapter 2.

Health administration has grown more professional in recent decades. Administrators are often trained in business schools or health administration programs where they learn business concepts. Some administrators entered their professions as clinical providers and then moved into a management role. Other have a business background but have directed their interest to the health care industry.

While a bachelor's degree may be sufficient for an entry-level position, most managers have earned a master's degree (www.ache.org). There are three traditional paths: the Master of Business Administration (MBA), the Master of Public Administration (MPA), and the Master of Health Administration (MHA). While MBA and MPA programs might include health-related coursework, only the MHA is completely focused on the health care industry. The American College of Healthcare Executives offers board certifications, which are becoming an industry standard. Some administrators will go on and earn a doctorate, especially if they intend to teach in a university or administer a clinical research setting. There is some professional tension between the doctors who hold the MD and the doctors who hold the Ph.D.

Careers in Health Information

When used strategically, information technology can assist a health care business to achieve higher level of performance, both of personnel and financially. A variety of professionals manage the information technology needs of health offices. These include the areas of medical records management, privacy officer, risk management, medical coding, corporate compliance, and data analysis and reporting (www.ahima.org). The position of Medical Chief Information Officer has developed as physicians with advanced technical skills develop strategy and policy to meet the organization's IT needs.

Social media is another area of employment growth, as business and technology interact. Web sites, Facebook, RSS feeds, podcasts, blogs, and Twitter are not only ways to communicate, but also offer employment opportunities (Thielst 2010). While large companies can afford to have their own IT staff, many smaller offices outsource these functions.

Coding Specialist Increasing computerization of health care recording keeping and the HIPAA requirements for EDI are just two of the factors fueling the growth of coding specialists. The Bureau of Labor Statistics predicts that this field will grow faster than average in the next few years (Bureau of Labor Statistics, Medical Records and Health Information Technician 2010–11).

Based on the documentation provided by the patient's record, coding specialists assign codes, or numbers, to the diagnoses, services, and procedures. That data are used for reimbursement and also to support statistical research. Coding specialists may also be called health information specialists or health insurance specialists. Coders must have a strong background in medical terminology, anatomy, and physiology. Their communication and computer skills (Internet and software) must also be strong. A coder must be able to enter data with accuracy and have the ability to manage details. And of course, the coder must be thoroughly familiar with **CPT and ICD-9-CM codes**.

In a small practice, a coder may do many types of work tasks. In large practice, a coder's work may be more specialized. For example, one coder may process claims for a single payer such as Medicare. In addition to practice-based employment, a coder has opportunities in other settings. The coder could work for insurance companies, government agencies, private billing practices, or private educators who train medical office employees (Green and Rowell 2010). In 2008, there were 172,500 jobs in the field of medical records and health information technician, with an average salary of approximately $30,600 (Bureau of Labor Statistics, Medical Records and Health Information Technician 2010–11).

Coders can obtain professional credentials through two professional organizations: the American Health Information Management Association (AHIMA) and the

Current procedural terminology (CPT) A part of the HCPCS used to code procedures and services performed by providers.

ICD-9-CM The abbreviation for the International Classification of Diseases, 9th Revision, Clinical Modification. This classification is used to code office visits to process an insurance claim.

American Academy of Professional Coders (AAPC). AHIMA offers an entry-level coding credential, the Certified Coding Associate (CCA). When a student demonstrates competency in ICD-9-CM and CPT surgery coding, patient documentation, data integrity/quality, A&P, and pharmacology, he or she can achieve the title of certified coding specialist (CCS). Finally, by demonstrating expertise in multispecialty CPT, ICD-9-CM, and **HCPCS** national (level II) coding, the coder can become a certified coding specialist–physician-based (CCS-P) (www.ahima.org).

AAPC offers credentials that differentiate between patient care settings. For coders in physician practice and clinics, they offer the certified professional coder (CPC) and for coders in outpatient facilities, the certified professional coder–hospital (CPC-H). For those coders who have not yet completed the medical field experience required to obtain those credentials, AAPC also offers apprentice credentials for both settings: the certified professional coder–apprentice (CPC–A) and the certified professional coder–hospital apprentice (CPC-HA) (www.aapcnatl.org).

Healthcare Common Procedure Coding System (HCPCS) A classification system used to code and process an insurance claim.

Other Support Staff

Transcriptionists and secretaries are among the other support staff necessary to keep health care businesses running. There were about 105,200 jobs as medical transcriptionists in 2008, with an average hourly wage of $15 (Bureau of Labor Statistics, Medical Transcriptionist 2010–11). About 36 percent of transcriptionists work in hospitals and another 23 percent in physicians' offices, sometimes combining transcription duties with other tasks such as receptionist. A number of transcriptionists operate home businesses. The skill requirements for transcriptionists evolve as the technology changes (www.ahdionline.org). With the increased ability to send files electronically from anywhere in the globe, there has also been an increase in the use of off-shore transcription services, usually to reduce the cost of the service.

As EHR systems become more pervasive, the requirements for medical secretaries have changed. Instead of working for just one person, it is more typical for a secretary to provide support to an entire office or division, and to perform a wider range of administrative tasks. There were 471,000 people employed as medical secretaries in 2008, with average earnings of $29,680 (Bureau of Labor Statistics, Secretaries 2010–11).

Issues

As you have seen in this chapter, there are many, many more professions that provide health care services beyond physicians and nurses. In some fields, there are career ladders, so a person can obtain some education and training, go to work in the field, and then get more training and education to advance to a higher position. This practice, although providing opportunities for the individual, creates some concerns about the tradeoff between cost-effectiveness and quality. It is more cost-effective to utilize lower level professionals because they are not paid as much. They did not spend as much time training or being educated, so this preparation was also less expensive. The assistant or aide always works under supervision, but some still worry that the quality of care may suffer. Professional associations are also worried that the use of more assistants and aides erodes the professionalism and the earning potential of their specialty.

Related to the concern for cost-effectiveness is the concern about reimbursement. Some services and providers are reimbursed directly; others are not. Changes in reimbursement, especially by Medicare, have a ripple effect to other insurers and then impact the availability of personnel in that specialty.

Summary

In addition to services provided by physicians and nurses, health care services are provided by a wide range of other professionals. In fact, new career fields develop at a fast rate because of patient needs and new technology. In the office setting, the patient encounters physician assistants and medical assistants. The patient encounters surgical technologists in hospital and office-based surgical settings. The physician may order a variety of diagnostic tests such as X-rays, MRIs, and sonograms, as well as testing the patients' body fluids, tissues, and cells. The physician may also order the patient to receive therapy, such as physical or respiratory, and may write a prescription. In emergency care situations, the patient interacts with EMTs and paramedics. As part of a total health plan, the patient may seek assistance for dental, eye, spine, foot, and nutritional care.

In addition to medical professionals, offices, clinics, and hospitals employ many business professionals as well. Health information managers ensure the completeness and accuracy of the health information record, which contains a patient's personal, social, financial, and medical data. Coding and billing specialists ensure that reimbursements process promptly. Health administrators perform business function such as strategic planning, marketing, and accounting.

Questions for Review

1. What is the difference between the physician assistant and the medical assistant?
2. List three types of technologists and technician who provide diagnostic testing.
3. What types of services are provided by physical, occupational, and respiratory therapists?
4. What professionals provide care in emergency situations?
5. What services are provided by dentists, optometrists, chiropractors, podiatrists, and dietitians/nutritionists?
6. What activities are performed by the health information manager?
7. List three activities performed by billing and coding specialists.
8. Define health administration.

Questions for Discussion

1. Differentiate among a general practitioner, a nurse practitioner, and a physician assistant. What accounts for the difference in their compensation?
2. Were you surprised at the training levels and compensation of any of these professionals? Why?
3. Do you believe that the use of assistants and aides impacts the quality of care?
4. What factors do you believe drive which professionals receive direct reimbursement?
5. The speech pathologist in the chapter profile noted that Medicare will not pay for all of the services a person might need to regain functions. What might be a rationale for such a decision? Can you suggest other ways a health care system could achieve the same goal?
6. Differentiate among the MBA, MPH, and MHA. What accounts for the differences in these degrees?
7. Should clinical and non-clinical professionals be cross-trained? Would this improve either the level of patient care or the efficiency of the business?

8. Is there a profession that was not discussed in this chapter that is of interest to you? If so, do your own search for information. What are the education and training requirements? What can you expect to make?

Chapter References

Bureau of Labor Statistics, U.S. Department of Labor. 2010–11. *Occupational Outlook Handbook*. Available at www.bls.gov/oco/. See sections on Physician Assistant; Medical Assistant; Surgical Technologist; Radiologic Technologists and Technicians; Nuclear Medicine Technologists; Cardiovascular Technologists and Technicians; Diagnostic Medical Sonographer; Clinical Laboratory Technologists and Technicians; Physical Therapists; Physical Therapy Assistants and Aides; Respiratory Therapists; Occupational Therapists; Occupational Therapy Assistants and Aides; Recreational Therapists; Speech-Language Pathologists and Audiologists; Pharmacists; Pharmacy Technicians and Aides; Emergency Medical Technicians and Paramedics; Dentist; Dental Hygienists; Dental Assistants; Dental Laboratory Technicians; Optometrists; Dispensing Opticians; Ophthalmic Laboratory Technicians; Chiropractors; Podiatrists; Dietitians; Medical and Health Services Managers; Medical Records and Health Information Technicians; and Medical Transcriptionists.

American Academy of Physician Assistants Information Center (www.aapa.org)

American Association of Medical Assistants (www.aama-ntl.org)

Association of Surgical Technologists (www.ast.org)

American Society of Radiologic Technologists (www.asrt.org)

Alliance of Cardiovascular Professionals (www.acp-online.org/)

Society for Vascular Ultrasound (www.svunet.org)

American Society of Echocardiography (www.asecho.org)

American Registry of Diagnostic Medical Sonographers (www.ardms.org)

Society of Diagnostic Medical Sonographers (www.sdms.org)

American Physical Therapy Association (www.apta.org)

American Association for Respiratory Care (www.aarc.org)

American Occupational Therapy Association (www.aota.org)

American Therapeutic Recreation Association (www.atra-tr.org)

American Speech-Language-Hearing Association (www.asha.org)

American Academy of Audiology (www.audiology.org)

American Association of Colleges of Pharmacy (www.aacp.org)

American Pharmacists Association (www.pharmacist.com)

American Association of Pharmacy Technicians (www.pharmacytechnician.com)

National Association of Chain Drug Stores (www.nacds.org)

National Association of Emergency Medical Technicians (www.naemt.org)

National Registry of Emergency Medical Technicians (www.nremt.org)

American Dental Association (www.ada.org)

American Dental Hygienists' Association (www.adha.org)

American Dental Assistants Association (www.dentalassistant.org)

National Association of Dental Laboratories (www.nadl.org)

American Optometric Association (www.aoanet.org)

Opticians Association of America (www.oaa.org)

American Chiropractic Association (www.amerchiro.org or www.acatoday.com)

International Chiropractors Association (www.chiropractic.org)

World Chiropractic Alliance (www.worldchiropracticalliance.org)

American Podiatric Medical Association (www.apma.org)

American Dietetic Association (www.eatright.org)

American Academy of Medical Administrators (www.aameda.org)

American Academy of Professional Coders (AAPC) (www.aapcnatl.org)

American College of Healthcare Executives (www.ache.org)

American Health Information Management Association (AHIMA) (www.ahima.org)

Association for Healthcare Documentation Integrity (AHDI) (www.ahdionline.org)

Green, M., and J. Rowell. 2010. *Understanding health insurance: A guide to billing and reimbursement*. 10th ed. New York: Delmar Cencage Learning.

Haddock, C., R. Chapman, and R. McLean. 2002. *Careers in healthcare: How to find your path and follow it*. Ann Arbor, MI: Health Administration Press.

Smaltz, D., and E. Berner. 2007. *The executive's guide to electronic health records*. Executive Essentials Book

Thielst, C. 2010. *Social media in healthcare: Connect, communicate, collaborate*. Executive Essentials Book.

For Additional Information

Reference any of the Web sites just listed for additional information about these professions.

Brown, G., Stone, T., and T. Patrick. 2005. *Strategic management of information systems in healthcare*. AUPHA/HAP Book.

Thomas, R., and M. Calhoun. 2007. *Marketing matters: A guide for healthcare executives*. ACHE Management Series.

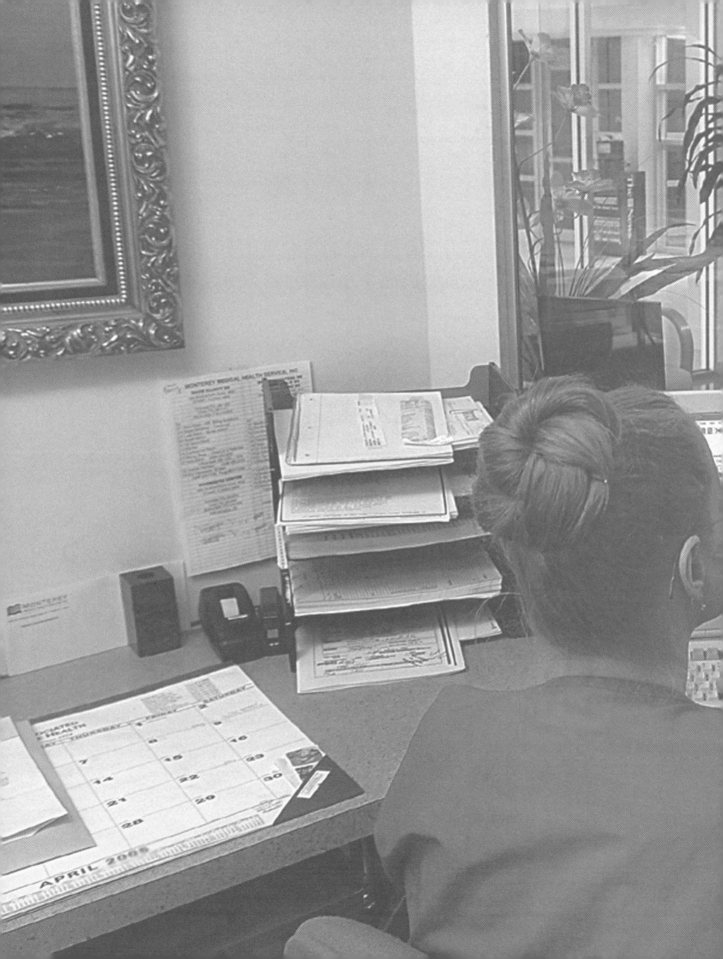

Offices, Clinics, and Hospitals

Learning Objectives

After reading this chapter, you should be able to:

1. Describe the ways a health care delivery system can be classified.
2. Describe the contents of a health information record.
3. Distinguish between the types of practice arrangements.
4. List the sources of physicians' revenues.
5. Describe the impact of legal issues and customer relations on practice management.
6. Classify the different types of hospitals.
7. List the role and function of the governing board, medical staff, and hospital administration.
8. Discuss the management, marketing, and finance functions that a hospital administrator must perform.
9. List the various utilization measures that hospital administrators use to evaluate performance.
10. List various measures of health care quality.

87

The Push Toward Electronic Health Records

The days of jokes about doctors' bad handwriting are coming to an end. Electronic health records (EHR) have replaced paper records in offices and hospitals around the country. Health care providers must implement electronic record systems in order to be in compliance with federal law. The majority of practices that have adopted EHR systems report a high level of satisfaction with the technology and the advantages it offers.

EHR offers some tremendous advantages. Most practitioners agree that EHR has improved the health of their patients. Errors caused by misreading handwriting or drug interactions can be dramatically reduced, both saving lives and money. The new system can also enhance communications with patients; a physician can link directly to clinical information while seeing the patient. Patients may be able to enter their own health information online and share this information with physicians. Using EHR creates staff efficiencies and patient-flow efficiencies. Since there's no need to pull charts, it may even be possible to add to practice revenues by seeing several more patients per day.

Although the advantages of integrated electronic records are widely recognized, implementing a new system requires effort and money. An effective EHR system combines hardware, software, and tech support and training to achieve the goal: all patient information is available at the point of care. As medical practices make the switch, they need to carefully evaluate the workflows in their practice to determine which system will do the best job for their needs. Critical workflows include: billing and accounts receivable, scheduling, in-house messaging, documentation of patient interactions, processing refill requests, reviewing and acting on lab results, and managing external correspondence about patients. One system may not do it all, so the system needs to be compatible with other programs. Sufficient time must be set aside for training. The budget must include funds for annual maintenance fees and future upgrades of software and hardware.

Once an EHR system is in place, offices must be aware of the need for enhanced security for those records. Like any electronically stored data, medical records are vulnerable to hackers. Records that a patient creates with a private vendor are also not covered under physician-patient privacy rules.

Practitioners and office professionals who have EHR systems generally find them beneficial. In a recent survey, 87 percent said they wouldn't go back to paper!

Sources: Edsall, R., and K. Adler. 2005. An EHR user-satisfaction survey: Advice from 408 family physicians. *Family Practice Management*, Oct; Medical Group Management Association. 2007. *Electronic health records: Perspectives from the adopters*, Oct.; Rowley, R. 2005. Practicing without paper charts: One clinic's experience. *Family Practice Management*, Feb.; Smaltz, D. and E. Berner. 2007. *The executive's guide to electronic health records*. Executive Essentials Book.

Introduction

In the previous chapters, you have learned about the health care professionals who deliver services to patients as well as other non-clinical employees. In the following chapters, you will learn more about the delivery systems. This chapter focuses on providers' offices, clinics, and hospitals.

There are a number of ways to classify delivery systems and the services that patients receive, and the categories often overlap. Systems can be classified by the physical location in which the services are delivered: office, clinic, hospital, and so on. That is the classification used in this chapter. As you will see, the distinction between which services are provided in an office and which services are provided in a hospital is less obvious than it was even 10 years ago.

The delivery system might also be classified by the patient's condition when the services are received. **Ambulatory care** means that patients are fully mobile—they

Ambulatory care
Medical care provided in an office setting to a mobile patient.

can bring themselves to the physician's office or to a clinic. **Acute care,** on the other hand, implies a level of urgency. This patient needs access to health care services immediately. Based on the seriousness of the illness, the patient may be admitted to a hospital; the services are then classified as **inpatient care.** Most primary care and even some routine surgery is performed on an **outpatient** basis, meaning there is no need for an overnight stay in a hospital. A third method of classification combines the location of care with a level of care; hence the terms primary, secondary, and tertiary. **Primary care** is defined as basic and routine care that can be delivered in an office or clinic by a primary care provider. **Secondary care** involves routine hospitalization and surgery, and **tertiary care** is complex and specialized care delivered in specific institutional settings. Primary care is the only term that is used with regularity.

Various data can be consulted to understand how many patients are served by each type of delivery system. According to the National Center for Health Statistics, there were more than 1.2 billion ambulatory care visits in 2007. Of these, the vast majority (994.3 million) were to physicians' offices. Almost 9 million visits were made to outpatient departments, and 117 million visits were made to emergency departments. Of the latter, 42.4 million were related to injuries and 13 percent resulted in hospital admission.

The data about ambulatory care visits indicate that primary care physicians provide almost 88 percent of all preventive care. Most of the visits made to physicians' offices (88%) were by established patients; 87 percent had made at least one previous visit in the past 12 months. More than half of visits involved a general medical exam, and 64 percent resulted in medication therapy (Hing, Cherry, and Woodwell 2006). These visits are critical for primary and preventive care—the uninsured have a much lower visit rate, putting them at risk for more serious health issues.

The U.S. Census Bureau gathers data on various industries every 5 years; the most recent data is from 2007. Comparative data about the business side of ambulatory care are presented in Table 7.1. Along with other segments of the health care industry, this segment is growing. Revenues, payroll, and employees have all increased over the 5-year time period in comparison with 2002 data.

acute care Short-term medical care provided to a patient with an immediate need for care.

inpatient care The patient needs care that requires being admitted to the hospital.

outpatient care Also referred to as ambulatory care. The patient does not require admittance to a hospital.

primary care Basic and routine care that can be delivered by a provider in an office or clinic.

secondary care Usually involves routine hospitalization and surgery on a short term basis.

tertiary care Complex and specialized care delivered in specific institutional settings such as burn treatment.

Providers' Offices and Clinics

When the patient visits the office or clinic, he or she interacts with many of the health care professionals whose roles and tasks were described in previous chapters. The patient is seen by the care provider, as well as by various nurses or physician's assistants. The patient may also receive services from an in-house laboratory or imaging center.

Table 7.1   *Ambulatory Health Care Services*

	All Ambulatory Providers	Physicians Offices	Outpatient Centers
Establishments (number in 1,000s)	547.7	219.7	30.0
Revenue (in millions)	$677.4	$339.3	$76.3
Employees (number in 1,000s)	5,733	2,112	671.7
Annual payroll (in millions)	$276.2	$147.2	$28.5

Source: U.S. Census Bureau. *2007 Economic Census. Sector 62:E076211: Health care and social assistance.* Release 3/26/2010.

The office or clinic is a business as well as a place to obtain health care services. Therefore, the patient will interact with non-clinical or administrative staff. An office manager is responsible for the business side of a professional practice. Depending on the size of the practice, the practice may employ receptionists, filing/record clerks, health information management specialists, coding and billing specialists, accounts receivable clerks, and payroll clerks.

Appointments must be scheduled, patients checked in, their records made ready, information from the current visit added, and the records stored appropriately, and further appointments scheduled. All of these processes must occur within the privacy guidelines as formulated in HIPAA.

In addition to the administrative tasks necessary to handle patients, the office or clinic must be managed like any other business. The business has facilities that must be paid for and maintained. Supplies and equipment, both for the office and for the needs of patients, are acquired and maintained. Appropriate information technology is used and upgraded as necessary. Employees must be hired and trained. Bills, payroll, and taxes need to be paid in a timely fashion. The office manager talks to all the sales reps that are marketing pharmaceuticals, new technology, or other product of interest. The business must be in compliance with the many state and federal laws that apply to all businesses, not just those in the health care industry.

The Health Information Record

As noted in this chapter's Profile, recording keeping is an important part of health care businesses. When you learned about the payment process earlier in this book, you learned how important billing and coding are to the reimbursement process. The health information record, however, serves a broader purpose than just payment.

health information record Contains the patient's personal, financial and social data as well as the medical data. The health information record replaces the term medical record.

Whether it is kept in paper or electronic form, the **health information record** contains two types of patient data. First, it contains the patient's personal, financial, and social data. Second, it also contains the patient's medical data, including descriptions of the patient's history, condition, diagnostic and therapeutic treatment, and the results of treatment (Smaltz and Berner 2007). Under the provision of HIPAA, it is mandated to protect the privacy of the entire record, but the second type of data is most sensitive and subject to regulation.

The office's health information manager is responsible for ensuring that the office's records are kept in compliance with state and federal regulations (Smaltz and Berner 2007). Many individuals in the office have a role in keeping the record accurate and up-to-date.

The health information record has both clinical and non-clinical uses. On the clinical side, the record provides information for patient care. It also provides data for research activities and public health monitoring, and can be used for quality improvement within the office. The record is also a legal document of the care a patient has received. Finally, as you learned early about the payment process in health care, the health information record provides the information necessary for billing and reimbursement (Green and Rowell 2010).

Practice Arrangements

solo practice A self-employed physician who practices alone.

In Chapter 2, you learned about the legal forms available to businesses in the United States. The operation of offices and clinics can be arranged in several ways: **solo practice,** group practice, or physician/provider employee. Although the solo practice arrangement has become less common for physicians, it is very typical for dentists and ophthalmologists and for some specialty physicians. Health care providers who are in solo practice are usually legally organized as sole proprietorships.

Group practice allows the individual provider to share facilities, equipment, and personnel. From a personal perspective, it also permits the provider to share the burden of providing care. The **partnership** is the traditional legal structure for a medical group practice. The partnership agreement can be written to handle all the details of how the physician/partners wish to manage the practice. However, each partner remains responsible, or legally liable, for the debts of the partnership. As with any business, these might be ordinary business debts. In a medical practice, they also may be incurred by a malpractice judgment against one of the physician/partners.

Many states now permit professional practices to organize a special type of partnership called a **limited liability partnership** (LLP). The advantage is that each partner's liability is limited to his or her capital contribution. However, the state requires the LLP to care liability insurance (at least $1 million's worth) to protect against malpractice and other wrongful acts of the partners or the employees of the LLP.

A medical practice can also be organized as a corporation, or a physician may be employed by a corporation. Many states permit the organization of professional corporations (PC) especially for professionals such as physicians; the PC often must carry individual malpractice insurance. In case where a physician is employed by a corporation, the physician provides health care services for which the corporation pays him a salary. This is how a Health Maintenance Organization (HMO) works. A group of physicians may also contract their services to a corporation for a fee, as is the case with some Managed Care Organizations (MCOs). In either of these cases, the physician remains personally responsible for his own malpractice, but the employer is not legally responsible.

Physicians and other providers entering this sort of arrangement work under an employment contract that specifies all the details of their employment, including compensation, work obligations, and terminations. It is typical for contracts to also include non-compete and non-solicitation clauses, both of which limit the physician's ability to leave that employer and take patients along or establish their own practice in the same geographic area.

group practice
A group of several physicians who practice as a group.

partnership A form of legal organization of a business involving at least two entities.

limited liability partnership
A specific type of partnership arrangement in which a partner's liability is limited to the amount of the capital contribution.

Issues in Practice Management

Physicians and other health care providers are trained to do just that, provide health care services. They are not trained to run businesses. Yet understanding the dynamics of running a successful business is an important part of the total package of primary health care delivery. Managing practice finances, legal compliance, and customer service are all important components.

Practice Finances

The financial health of a medical practice depends on several components. One component is revenue maximization. The other component is cost minimization. Taken together these two components achieve profitability.

The first step is to understand the revenue flows of a practice. As you can see in Table 7.2, physicians' offices receive the bulk of their revenue from patient care, with private insurance and Medicare providing the largest share of payments. At the same time, the office or clinic has expenses in the form of personnel, supplies and equipment, and services such as software, utilities, leases, and liability insurance.

If the provider knows the source of the revenues, then several strategies can be developed to maximize revenues. One strategy is to increase the number of patients

Table 7.2	*Revenues and Expenses for Physicians' Offices and Hospitals* 2008 Estimates in $ millions	
	Offices	**Hospitals**
Total Revenue		
Patient care		
Medicare	74.8	184.7
Medicaid	18.3	70.2
Other govt	5.3	36.9
Workers comp	7.4	7.2
Private insurance	185.7	307.6
Patient out-of-pocket	36.9	32.6
Other	19.4	23.8
Non-patient care	16.1	58.1
Total Expenses	320.6	667.7
Personnel	196.2	355.5
Supplies and equip.	35.5	120.4
Services	32.4	42.6
Other	56.5	149.0

Source: U.S. Census Bureau, *2008 Service annual survey: Health care and social assistance (NAICS 62),* Tables 8.9 and 8.11.

seen. This strategy can create ethical dilemmas for practitioners if they feel that an increased patient load is compromising care even as it improves the bottom line. Another strategy is to capture more revenue per patient. Practices can lose money through poor coding and billing practices. They can also lose money because their health plans have low reimbursement or because the practice doesn't keep it fee schedules up-to-date.

At the same time a medical practice works to increase its revenues, it must also understand, control, and reduce its costs. Practices should develop budgets and compare their expenses to national data such as that presented in Table 7.2.

Legal Compliance

antitrust law An area of federal law which prohibits monopolization and other activities which lessen competition in the marketplace.

Health Insurance Portability and Accountability Act of 1996 (HIPAA) A federal law that mandates insurance portability and sets up procedures for electronic data exchange.

All businesses operate in an environment that imposes legal restrictions. In addition to the general legal environment, businesses providing primary health care services also face regulation that is specific to the health care industry. One of the most significant legal areas that impacts all business is **antitrust law**. The federal antitrust laws are designed to prohibit activities that lessen competition in the marketplace. Health care providers are impacted by these laws whenever they purchase or merge practices. If two practices merge, no matter how much sense a merger makes from either a business or a patient care perspective, the fact remains that customer choice has been eliminated. The fewer medical practices there are in a geographic area, the more competition is reduced. The remaining practices are moving in the direction of a monopoly, which is prohibited by federal law. Health care providers can also be impacted by antitrust law in the way they set prices for their services. Businesses are not permitted to work together to set prices nor are they allowed to tie the sale of one service to another. Nevertheless, some of the negotiation in managed care contracts approaches this sort of prohibited collusion.

Another area of concern is compliance with regulations such as **HIPAA (Health Insurance Portability and Accountability Act)**. Under HIPAA, patients have the right to access and control their health records. In order to safeguard protected health information (PHI, or patients' individually identifiable information), health care providers must restrict access to the information and have patients' permission to disclose it. The provider has to give a patient a "Notice of Privacy Practice" on the patient's first office visit. The signed notice is kept in the patient's file. Patients also needed to sign an authorization/consent form in order for their PHI to be shared for reasons other than treatment, payment, and health care opportunities. Providers are also responsible for the security of electronic health information, whether that information was stored or transmitted. Realistically, this provision of HIPAA affects every office with a computer, Internet, and e-mail. The 2010 Patient Protection and Affordable Care Act contains additional provisions regarding the security of EHR.

A final area that has both financial and legal implications for providers is malpractice. **Malpractice** is the act of providing medical services that are below the standard of quality. Health care professionals carry malpractice insurance to protect themselves from financial loss in the event that they lose a malpractice lawsuit. Rising malpractice premiums are a concern for all health care professionals.

malpractice The act of providing professional services that are below the standard of quality for that profession.

Customer Service

In all businesses, improvements in customer service help to retain customers. Generally it is not the actual service, but the customer's perceptions of the service, that matters. Customers, patients in this case, can be surveyed so that the provider can understand what's important to the patient. A Harris Interactive poll found that the most highly rated characteristics were physicians' interpersonal skills. The following characteristics were rated "extremely important by more than 84 percent of respondents: "Treats you with dignity and respect," "listens carefully to your health care concerns and questions," and "is easy to talk to." Most respondents also felt their own physicians performed well in these areas. There was a gap between the training and expertise respondents expected and how they ranked their own care. More than 75 percent of respondents felt that being "up-to-date with the latest medical research and treatment" was extremely important; however, only 54 percent felt their physician met this standard (What patients want 2004).

A practice that values patient service can conduct similar surveys or use observation of its own practices to determine how it is doing on the features that patients value the most. Once this data is collected, service delivery strategies can be improved to meet patient expectations (Plesk 2002).

Hospitals

Like offices and clinics, hospitals are both a physical location for patients to receive care and also a business that must be appropriately managed to ensure that care is high quality and cost-effective.

Although hospitals were established in the United States as early as 1752, hospitals as we know them are a recent phenomenon dating from the 1920s (Grinney 1991). Prior to that time, the best medical care was obtained in the home. Even some surgical procedures were conducted in the home.

The first hospitals were charitable institutions created for the poor. At best, the hospital offered food, rest, and shelter. Patients were expected to help with nursing and cleaning and behave in morally appropriate ways. However, those who could afford home care stayed away from hospitals.

The discovery in 1846 that ether could be used as an anesthetic increased the use of surgical procedures, but hospitals were so unsanitary that one out of four patients died. It wasn't until 1865 that modern antiseptic surgery was developed, using carbolic acid to kill germs and heat to sterilize instruments (Grinney 1991). The advance of modern surgical techniques and the increasing use of technology in medicine changed the way doctors practiced. Now it made sense for the patient to come to the doctor rather than the other way around.

By the 1920s, surgery was the heart of the American hospitals. In addition to charity organizations, there were many for-profit, private institutions. They advertised and offered amenities such as semi-private rooms. Internally, hospitals were staffed by care givers, including nurses, and administrators who were increasingly professional (Grinney 1991).

The current trend is starting to go the opposite direction, again fueled by technological advances. Many procedures that used to require inpatient care are now performed on an outpatient basis, whether at the hospital, a clinic, or a physician's office. Some care that required specialized nursing can now be done with technology and home health. Still, certain types of care remain the province of the hospital. As discussed earlier, ambulatory patients may come directly to the hospital or they may be referred by their physician.

Types of Hospitals

According to the government's most recent analysis of the hospital industry, there are more than 6,500 hospitals currently operating in the United States (Census Bureau 2007). Basic operational data are presented in Table 7.3.

Although they share certain characteristics, hospitals are not all the same, either in the kind of business they are or in the kind of services they provide. The primary methods to classify hospitals are by the type of ownership or the type of services provided. However, hospitals may also be classified by size, location, length of stay, or any other measure that provides a meaningful way to compare one hospital to another.

Ownership Hospital ownership is one way to classify hospitals. Hospitals are owned either publicly or privately. **Public hospitals** are actually owned by the federal or state/local government. Federally owned hospitals are often operated for certain groups of patients. The Veteran's Administration hospitals are an example. State hospitals often specialized; for example, many states operate psychiatric hospitals. Cities and counties usually operate general hospitals that serve a broad spectrum of that local population. The Emergency Departments of public hospitals located in urban areas are often considered "safety nets" because they provide primary care for the indigent and uninsured (Bindman et al. 2009).

public hospitals
Hospitals owned by the federal, state, or local government.

Table 7.3	*Hospitals*			
	Establishments (number)	**Revenue ($million)**	**Annual Payroll ($million)**	**Employees (1000s)**
All hospitals	6529	$707.0	$264.8	5,544
General medical/Surgical	5159	663.6	245.0	5,116
Psychiatric/Sub. abuse	564	16.3	8.8	206
Other specialty	806	27.1	10.9	222

Source: U.S. Census Bureau. *2007 Economic Census. Sector 62:E076211: Health care and social assistance.* Release 3/26/2010.

Privately owned hospitals can operate on a not-for-profit or a for-profit basis. Formerly called the "voluntary" hospital, the private, not-for-profit hospital is owned by a community association or a nongovernmental entity. **Not-for-profit hospitals** benefit from provisions in state and federal tax regulations that allow them to avoid paying income and property taxes.

Private hospitals that operate on a for-profit basis are sometimes known as proprietary hospitals. As with any corporation, the shareholders own the business. Paying customers and cost-containment are critical to the financial success of a private hospital. Unlike the not-for-profit, they must pay income and property taxes. They also finance expansion with loans, rather than the tax-exempt bonds that are available to not-for-profits.

Services Provided Hospitals can also be classified by the types of services they provide for patients. Most hospitals are **general hospitals**—they provide a range of non-specialized services. Specialized services can include some of the federal hospitals noted above where services are provided only to certain categories of patients such as veterans. Specialized services also refer to hospitals that treat one type of disease or illness, such as psychiatric hospitals, drug or alcohol addiction treatment.

Other Categories Other ways to classify hospitals include size, length of stay, and location. Although there is no standard measure of size, the number of beds is one way to indicate hospital size. Small hospitals have fewer than 100 beds, while a large hospital might have more than 650 beds. Short-term hospitals refer to average patient stays of less than 30 days; **long-term care** is anything greater than 60 days. Hospitals classified by location usually focus on either rural or urban designations. Both locations face specific challenges in serving their populations. Some rural hospitals were able to covert to Critical Access Hospitals (CAH) under the Medicare Rural Hospital Flexibility Program of the 1997 Balanced Budget Act. Approximately 1,200 hospitals that meet the requirements are reimbursed on a cost basis for their Medicare patients. These additional funds have allowed rural hospitals to upgrade facilities, equipment, and staffing to better serve their communities (Roop 2008).

A final descriptor is the **community hospital**. If the facilities are available to the general public, this term includes all nonfederal short-term hospitals whether the services are general or special.

Hospital Organization

Regardless of the way a hospital is classified, hospitals are all structured in a similar fashion. As you can see from Figure 7.1, a typical hospital is organized in three main parts. These are the governing board, the medical staff, and the management team.

The Board of Directors The function of the **governing board** is to set institutional policy and goals. The board is responsible for the financial health of the hospital. Typical board decisions involve the purchase, transfer, or sale of hospital assets, changes in the hospital by-laws, and appointment of new board members. A key decision for the success of the hospital is to hire and evaluate the chief executive officer (CEO).

Who is chosen to be a board member depends on what type of hospital it is. In community hospitals, board members are active business people in their community. This helps them set policy that will serve the needs of the community. Often they serve voluntarily.

---

privately owned hospitals Hospitals owned by nongovernment entities.

not-for-profit hospitals The primary purpose of the hospital is something other than profit.

general hospitals Hospitals that provide a range of services.

long-term care The federal health care definition of long-term care is more than 60 days.

community hospital Non-federal hospital facilities available to the public.

governing board A group who sets the overall direction for a group or business.

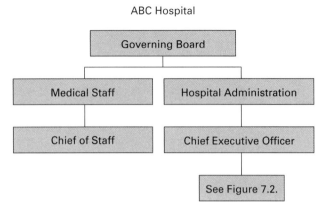

Figure 7.1   Hospital Organization

Boards meet monthly or quarterly. At their meetings, they review the financial performance of the hospital, hear reports from the committees, and vote on changes in policy. Boards do most of their work through specialized committees. The executive committee interacts with the medical staff. There might also be a finance committee, a buildings and grounds committee, or a public relations committee.

Medical Staff The governing board delegates the responsibility for patient care to the **medical staff**. It is their job to see that patients receive quality care. A physician applies to the hospital for staff membership and clinical privileges. The physician is not an employee of the hospital; he or she is usually in private practice outside the hospital. Membership and privileges simply allow the physician to admit patients to the hospital. In the last 12 years, there has been an increased trend toward the use of hospitalists. These physicians have an employment relationship with the hospital; they admit patients that would have been admitted by a primary care physician (Cors and Rohr 2010).

The chief of staff leads the medical staff. Usually the chief of staff is elected by the other medical staff according to the medical staff bylaws. The chief of staff interacts with the board and with the management team. The medical staff is organized by their area of medical specialty; each specialty has a chief. For example, the head of cardiology is referred to as the chief of cardiology.

The administrative work of the medical staff is carried out by committees. Key committees are the executive committee and the credentials committee. The executive committee governs the activities of the medical staff. The credentials committee focuses on the standards that will be used to grant staff membership and applies those standards to new applicants. Other committees focus on specific hospital departments, such as medical records, or on specific issues, such as quality improvement or utilization.

Management Team The board delegates authority to operate the hospital as a business to the hospital administrator. As in a private business, this person is often called the CEO. As you can see in Figure 7.2, many areas report to the CEO. The CEO delegates the necessary authority to each of the managers of these areas to complete their responsibilities. Unlike the medical staff, all of the personnel on the administrative side are employees of the hospital or independent contractors. Required job skills,

medical staff
Responsibility for quality patient care belongs to the physicians who make up the hospital's medical staff.

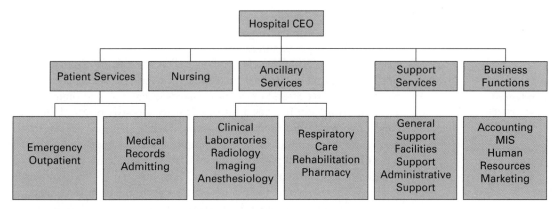

Figure 7.2   Organization Chart for ABC Hospital Administration

education, and training can range from low-skill to highly specialized positions. Pay rates vary accordingly.

Patient Services Patients enter the hospital for inpatient, outpatient, or emergency department care. In all cases, the patient's first contact is with the admitting department. Similar to the process in an office or clinic, a health information record is created. The admitting department enters the patient's personal data and insurance information into the hospital computer system. Once the patient has received medical care, a medical record is added to this information. HIPAA regulations regarding the privacy of health information records must be followed. The admitting personnel must have good customer relations skills as well as quick and accurate keyboarding skills.

Nursing Nurses play a vital role in patient care. The director or vice president of nursing is in charge of all the nursing areas; this person might be called the vice president for patient services. In addition to nursing education, the nursing department includes the various areas of patient care such as surgery, clinics, emergency room, and inpatient care. Each area is managed by a nursing supervisor. For more information about the professional training and job duties of the nursing staff, see Chapter 5.

Ancillary Services Key ancillary services include clinical laboratories, radiology, imaging, and anesthesiology. Additional services might include the pharmacy and respiratory or rehabilitative care. One of the difficulties in hospital administration is dual accountability. On the one hand, the ancillary services report to the hospital administrator. However, the physicians are also professionally accountable to the medical staff. Many of the health care professionals who perform these ancillary professional services for the patients and medical staff work as independent contractors. The imaging center, for example, might be located in or adjacent to the hospital facility. It hires and pays its own personnel. The facility contracts with the hospital to perform all of its imaging needs.

Support Service766s Keeping a hospital running requires the services of many people who are not health care professionals. There are three categories of support services: general patient Support Services, facilities support, and administrative support.

patient advocat
Hospital employee
whose role is to take
the side of the patient
in all discussions and
disputes.

- *General Patient Support:* While the nursing staff looks after the patient's medical needs, other groups assist in providing a pleasant stay. House-keeping cleans rooms and changes linens. The dietary department plans meals for the patients' special needs as well as running food service for the hospital employees and visitors. Social services, pastoral care, and the **patient advocate** attend to the other needs of patients and their families.
- *Facilities Support:* It takes a lot of effort to keep the physical facility in clean, safe working order. The laundry washes all those sheets, towels, and uniforms. Groundskeepers keep up the outside areas of the hospital. The maintenance department repairs all the mechanical systems like plumbing, electrical, and heat and air. If the hospital has its own parking facilities, these must be maintained and secured. Security is an increased concern for all businesses. A hospital must have security personnel to patrol the grounds and to man certain checkpoints to prevent unauthorized access. In addition, emergency plans are in place to evacuate the hospital in case of fire or other crisis.
- *Administrative Support:* This area is sometimes called materials management. If the hospital needs something, the purchasing department must contact the vendor and authorize the purchase. This is true whether the item is toilet paper or an MRI machine. The receiving department signs off that the item has arrived on site and passes the paperwork to the business office so that the vendor can get paid. All of the hospitals supplies must be warehoused until they are needed.

A trend in support services is to consider **outsourcing**. This means that the hospital no longer performs the function with its own personnel. Instead, it contracts with a private firm to handle those job duties. Laundry services and medical transcription are two areas that are often outsourced. The hospital can potentially realize large cost savings, particularly because it no longer pays benefits for these employees. However, the decision must be made carefully because the hospital loses some control over performance, and service can be interrupted.

outsourcing The
process of buying
goods or services from
another provider rather
than performing them
by the business.

Business Functions Business functions are those departments that take care of the business side of operating the hospital. These include accounting and finance, information services, human resources, and marketing.

Issues Affecting Hospital Administration

Hospital administration is concerned about patient care but also about profitability and other business issues. Furthermore, hospital administrators must be sure that the hospital maintains licensure and accreditation as well as legal compliance. Finally, all hospital employees must be concerned with the quality of care that is provided.

Performance Measurement Standards are used as a way to measure performance. Hospitals can set their own standards, and many use the standards established by TJC as benchmarks. Many organizations have undertaken initiatives such as TQM (Total Quality Management) or Six Sigma in order to improve their organization's performance (Dreachslin and Lee 2007).

Close attention to financial flows, such as those presented in Table 7.2, is another mechanism to improve enterprise performance. Many hospitals suffer financial losses because reimbursement schedules don't cover the actual costs of providing care.

Table 7.4	*Hospital Quality Web Sites*

www.hospitalcompare.hhs.gov
CompareYourCare.org

Leapfrog Group	leapfroggroup.org
California-Pacific Business Group on Health	healthscope.org
Dartmouth-Hitchcock Medical Center	dhmc.org
The Cleveland Clinic	clevelandclinic.org
Colorado Hospital Quality	Hospitalquality.org
New York State Hospital Report Card	myhealthfinder.com
Pennsylvania Health Care Cost Containment Council	phc4.org

According to the American Hospital Association, unreimbursed care cost hospitals $22.3 billion in 2002. Hospitals look for new ways to generate revenues such as an outpatient service like a fitness center. Hospitals have also grown increasingly concerned with managing costs.

In addition to monitoring overall expenses and margins, managers use a standard set of **utilization measures** to track and compare the performance of hospitals. Utilization measures include the average daily census, occupancy rates, capacity, average length of stay, inpatient days, and discharges. The average daily census is the average number of beds occupied per day. When that number is divided by the average number of bed, the occupancy rate is obtained. Capacity is the average number of beds available in the facility. Average length of stay is calculated by dividing inpatient days by discharges. Inpatient days is simply a night spent in the hospital, and a discharge is the release of an inpatient from the hospital.

utilization measures Measures that indicate whether an organization is being used to its full capacity.

Hospital quality can be measured in a number of ways. Quality has traditionally been determined by looking at patient outcomes. This was measured by mortality rates and long-term survival rates. Mortality rates are further broken down by type of procedure. Additional quality measures consider the volume of procedures, staffing levels, rates of infection, error rates, surgical complications, and infection rates. Surveys of patient satisfaction are also conducted. Data from the best performing hospitals can be used to benchmark performance. Consumers can access hospital quality at Web sites such as those listed in Table 7.4.

Licensure, Certification, and Accreditation Every hospital must be licensed to operate by the state in which it is located. Usually it is the department of health that sets the licensure standards. The licensure standards ensure that the physical facility complies with building codes, fire protection, and sanitation. Most states also set minimum requirements for personnel and equipment.

Hospitals can also be certified. This is necessary if the hospital wants to participate in Medicare and Medicaid. In order to become certified, the facility is inspected by the state health department. If the facility meets the "conditions of participation" developed by the Department of Health and Human Services, then it is certified.

In addition to licensure and certification, hospitals voluntarily participate in the accreditation standards of The Joint Commission (formerly referred to as JCAHO). The facility must pass a site survey visit in order to determine if it is in compliance with the TJC standards. In addition to being a respected measure of quality for the industry, TJC-accredited facilities are eligible for Medicare reimbursement (www.jointcommission.org).

Federal and State Law In addition to complying with the laws mentioned in this chapter, hospitals also must comply with laws that are unique to their operations.

Legislation aimed at improving rural access to hospitals mandated where new facilities could be built. The EMTLA (Emergency Medical Transfer and Active Labor Act) dictates policy in hospital emergency room.

Summary

Patient care can be characterized along many different dimensions. Primary care is the basic and routine care that can be delivered in an office or clinic by a primary care provider. Physicians can arrange their practices in several ways; solo, group, and physician employee are the most common. The primary source of physician revenue is patient care, and most is paid by private insurance, Medicare, and the patients themselves. Legal issues include antitrust, HIPAA, and malpractice. Office management requires attention to finances and customer service.

Hospitals are usually classified by the type of ownership or by the services provided. Hospitals may be publicly or privately owned, and may be operated on a not-for-profit or for-profit basis. Hospital organization includes the board of directors, the medical staff, and hospital administration. The board sets institutional policy and goals. The medical staff is responsible for patient care. Hospital administrators ensure that the business side of the hospital is operated effectively by reviewing numerous performance measures. Licensure is granted by the state authority. Certification is part of a Health and Human Services process that allows the hospital to receive Medicare and Medicaid payments. Accreditation is a voluntary process that assesses quality. Hospitals also use other methods to ensure quality.

Questions for Review

1. Describe some of the ways care delivered to patients is classified?
2. How are a solo practice and a group practice different?
3. What are the primary sources of physicians' revenues? How is this different for hospitals?
4. What are some of the legal issues facing offices, clinics, and hospitals?
5. Describe one way to classify hospitals.
6. Compare and contrast the role of the medical staff, the governing board, and the administrators in a hospital.

Questions for Discussion

1. What are your major complaints about visiting a physician's office? What suggestions would you make to improve the situation?
2. Is it ethical for a physician to see more patients in order to increase practice revenues?
3. Research the hospitals in your area. What form of ownership do they have? How many beds and how many employees do they have? How do their financials stack up against national data?
4. Research the use of EHR in your local offices and clinics? What do the users say are the pros and cons of their system? Are these the same as those mentioned in the chapter profile?
5. How do hospitals in your area compare on the quality measures listed in this chapter? Do you believe those measures really get at quality? Are there measures you would use instead?

Chapter References

Bindman, A. et al. 2009. Healthcare reform with a safety net: Lessons from San Francisco. *The American Journal of Managed Care*. October. Retrieved from MEDLINE.

Cors, W., and R. Rohr. 2010. The "ist" explosion: Driving forces, current trends, and future directions for hospitalists. *Physician Executive*, May-June. Retrieved from MEDLINE.

Dreachslin, J., And P. Lee. 2007. Applying six sigma and DMAIC to diversity initiatives. *Journal of Healthcare Management*, 52(6). Retrieved from MEDLINE.

Green, M., and J. Rowell. 2010. *Understanding health insurance: A guide to billing and reimbursement*. 10th ed. New York: Delmar Cengage Learning.

Grinney, E. (1991). *The hospital*. New York: Chelsea House.

Hing, E., D. Cherry, and D. Woodwell. 2006. National ambulatory medical care survey: 2004 summary. *Advance data from vital and health statistics*. Hyattsville, MD: National Center for Health Statistics.

The Joint Commission (www.jointcommission.org)

Plesk, P. 2002. Building a mind-set of service excellence. *Family Practice Management*, April.

Roop, E. (2008). A litmus test for critical access. *Hospitals & Health Networks/AHA*, January. Retrieved from MEDLINE.

Showalter, J. 2007. *The law of healthcare administration*. 5th ed. AUPHA/HAP Book.

Smaltz, D., and E. Berner. 2007. *The executive's guide to electronic health records*. Executive Essentials Book.

U.S. Census Bureau, *Statistical Abstract of the United States: 2010*.

U.S. Census Bureau. *2007 Economic Census. Sector 62:E076211: Health care and social assistance*. Release 3/26/2010.

U.S. Census Bureau, 2010, *2008 Service annual survey: Health care and social assistance (NAICS 62)*, available at www2.census.gov/series/sas/data/62/2008_NAICS62.pdf.

What patients want. 2004. *Family Practice Management*, November/December.

For Additional Information

American Academy of Medical Administrators (www.aameda.org)

American College of Healthcare Executives (www.ache.org)

Department of Justice, Health Care Antitrust Division (http://www.usdoj.gov/atr/public/health_care/health_care.htm).

Marcinko, D. (2000). *The business of medical practice: Profit maximizing skills for savvy doctors*. NY: Springer Pub.

Medical Group Management Association (www.mgma.com)

Pointer, D., and J. Orlikoff. 1999. *Board work: Governing health care organizations*. San Francisco, CA: Jossey-Bass.

Wenzel, F., and J. Wenzel. 2005. *Fundamentals of physician practice management*. AUPHA/HAP Book.

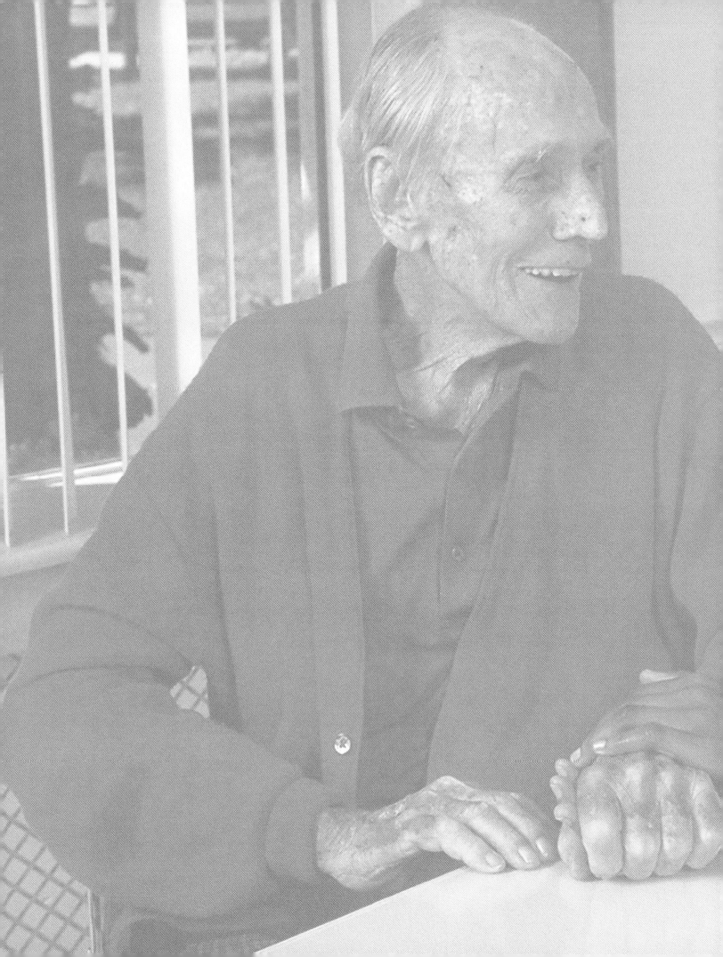

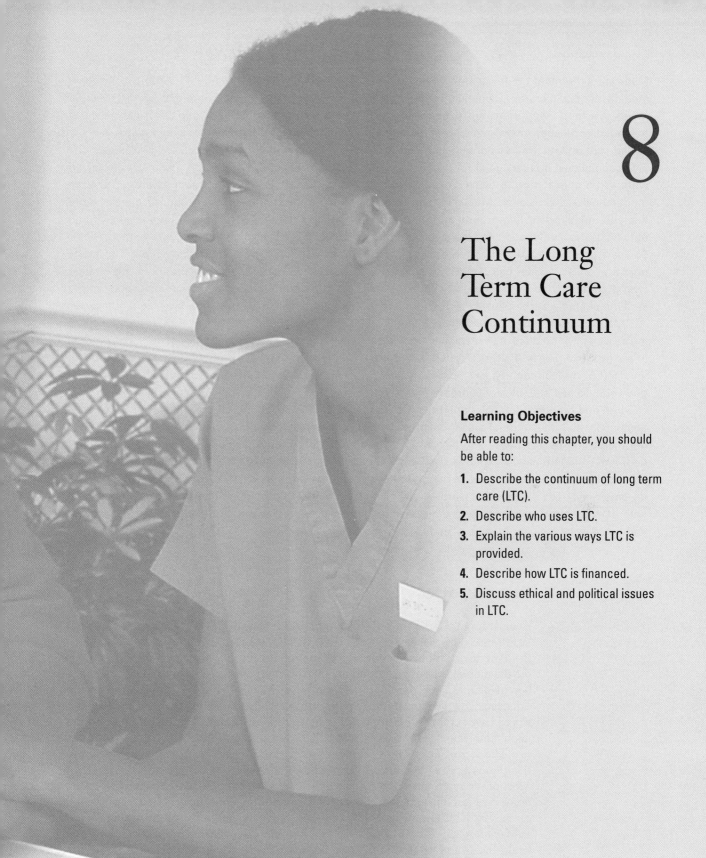

8

The Long Term Care Continuum

Learning Objectives

After reading this chapter, you should be able to:

1. Describe the continuum of long term care (LTC).
2. Describe who uses LTC.
3. Explain the various ways LTC is provided.
4. Describe how LTC is financed.
5. Discuss ethical and political issues in LTC.

The New Nursing Home Model

Madrona Retirement Center is a multilevel retirement center that features independent living apartments, assisted living units, an Alzheimer's unit, extended care unit, intermediate care unit, and skilled care unit, as well as home health and hospice capabilities. It is designed for residents who want to be able to age in place. Located near a moderate-size city, it sits on a 100-acre campus and has 100 independent living units and a 200-bed nursing center. In operation as a nursing center for 50 years, it is owned and operated by a religious organization. The center has 24-hour RN coverage, with a staffing ratio in the nursing center of 1.5 staff members for each resident.

Marge Segura moved into the independent living apartment at Madrona a year ago after the death of her husband. She is 78 years old, very active and involved in the community. Her apartment has a good-size kitchen and a spare bedroom for visiting children and grandchildren. Her apartment is also equipped with a multitude of aids to help her with her increasing heart disease and arthritis. All the door and cupboard handles are oversized and only require downward pressure, not twisting. She has an emergency call system in case she falls. The bathroom has a walk-in shower with a built-in chair, and the toilets are higher than usual and have a hip replacement seat. Night lights automatically come on when there is insufficient light, and all the light switches are motion sensors so that if she gets up at night there is no fumbling for a light switch.

As provided by her contract, Marge has one main meal in the dining room. The meals are served restaurant style with a full bar and wine list. She can have a guest for dinner or choose to take more meals in the facility restaurant on a pay-as-you-go basis. There is also a provision to have meals delivered if she cannot get to the dining room. The facility has a health club with an exercise room and a trainer specialized in geriatrics, a swimming pool, and a covered walking trail. There are frequent lectures and concerts at the facility. If at a later time she needs assistance with activities of daily living (ADLs) or instrumental activities of daily living (IADLs), it can be arranged in house. Should she need skilled nursing care, it is also available on site. Marge pays about $3,000 per month for all the services, and she can expect to age in place in this facility.

Contrast this with the nursing home of the past: what a huge difference! Many of these complexes are as large as small towns and have shopping, health care providers, banks, and beauty centers, as well as a full range of rehabilitation and preventative services.

Introduction

Long-term care (LTC) is and will continue to be one of the fastest growing sectors of health care. This is true for several reasons. The first is the aging of the baby boomers. By 2030, there will be an estimated 67 million people over the age of 65, almost double the number of this age group in 2000. Second, during this same period, the number of people over the age of 85 will also double because of the increased life expectancy of the current older population. Finally, the ability to treat diseases that would have resulted in death a few years ago for all ages will add significantly to the population who need the services of LTC (www.nih.gov/).

The term *LTC* means providing health care services to an individual for more than 90 days. A wide range of care facilities and professionals are involved in LTC. Most of the recipients (80%) of LTC assistance receive it in the community. Nursing homes are just one part of LTC, accounting for a small percentage (4.1%) of the total care given. LTC also includes hospitals, assisted living and community-based residential facilities, adult day care, respite care, hospice care, rehabilitation centers, mental health facilities (covered in Chapter 9), adult foster homes, children's chronic care facilities, and care provided by family and friends (http://www.aoa.gov/AoARoot/Aging_Statistics/Profile/2009/6.aspx).

Who Needs Long-Term Care?

The simple answer is anyone, child or adult, who has a **chronic condition** requiring assistance for more than 90 days. The U.S. Public Health Service definition is the standard used to determine if the service is in the LTC sector of health care. The period of time a person receives LTC assistance may range from a short time (90–100 days) after a surgery, accident, or chemotherapy to many years in an institutional setting.

The need for LTC is determined by assessing the ability of the person to perform what are called **activities of daily living (ADLs)** and **instrumental activities of daily living (IADLs).** The ability to perform these activities is assessed according to four categories: (1) totally independent, (2) requiring mechanical assistance only, such as a cane, hearing aid, or special eating utensils, (3) requiring assistance from another person, or (4) unable to do the activity at all. No matter what the disease or condition, if the person can manage most of the ADLs and IADLs alone or with mechanical assistance, they do not need LTC. For example, a person with multiple sclerosis may be able to dress themselves using assistive devices, be mobile using a motorized wheelchair, transfer from chair to bed and back using a hydraulic lift, and have adaptive bathing, toilet, and cooking facilities. This person is independent and may not need LTC services even though they live with a considerable degree of disability.

The activities of daily living (ADLs) are bathing, dressing, toileting, transferring (as in from bed to chair), continence control (bowel and bladder control), and eating. About 80 percent of those people receiving LTC assistance in the community demonstrate severe impairments in three to six of these activities. The activity impairments that most frequently cause people to move to a residential care form of LTC are continence control and transferring.

The instrumental activities of daily living (IADLs) are managing money, telephoning, grocery shopping, personal shopping, using transportation, housekeeping, doing chores, and managing medications. Family and friends often provide this care without charge to community residents. The frail elderly people who stay in their homes often have a very good support system in which friends or community volunteer agencies do chores, house and garden maintenance, shopping, and take the person to heath care appointments. Only when this network fails does the person have to either pay for the service in the community or move to a residential facility that provides these and other services.

In an ideal arrangement, the LTC services would be provided by a system that meets the needs of any person who needs assistance in the ADLs or IADLs. A system that would meet not only the physical needs of the person, but would provide social, mental health, and financial support is envisioned as a **continuum of care**. This ideal would emphasize the wellness or holistic approach rather than the illness or medical model currently used. An individual or family who needs assistance with the continuum of care now may have to interact with as many as 80 different agencies. This is hard enough to do when healthy and very difficult to do when someone is ill or frail.

Who Uses LTC?

People of all ages use LTC services for many reasons. LTC might be necessary because a person is aging, has a disability, or a chronic disease such as cancer, AIDS, multiple sclerosis, or diabetes. Those recovering from trauma or health events like a stroke or accident may need LTC services. Groups such as children with special needs or veterans may also utilize LTC services. The single largest age group using LTC is

chronic condition
An illness or injury lasting more than 90 days; a non-acute illness such as asthma.

activities of daily living Basic activities such as mobility, eating, toileting, dressing and bathing.

instrumental activities of daily living Activities like managing money, telephoning, grocery shopping, personal shopping, using transportation, housekeeping and managing medications.

continuum of care
The philosophy that the health care system should facilitate an individual's care from complete independence to dependence.

65 years and older. This segment represents about 80 percent of all LTC usage. However, children, young adults, and adults all use the LTC spectrum of care.

Older Adults

About one in every eight, or 12.8 percent (39 million), of the population is an older American. As discussed in Chapter 1, a demographic shift is occurring in the United States that will dramatically increase the number of older Americans; as a result, the LTC usage rate will inevitably increase. The data from the Administration on Aging are overwhelming: the older population (age 65 and older) numbered 39 million in 2008, an increase of 13 percent since 1998. The number of Americans ages 45 to 64 who will reach 65 over the next two decades increased by 31 percent during this decade. By 2030, the older population will more than double to 71.5 million. Members of minority groups are projected to represent 26.4 percent of the older population in 2030, up from 16.4 percent in 2000. The 85+ population is projected to increase from 4.7 million in 2003 to 9.6 million in 2030 (http://www.aoa.gov/prof/Statistics/profile/2008).

According to the Centers for Medicare and Medicaid Services, about 7 percent of the age group 65+ reports a need for outside assistance for either ADLs or IADLs. This percentage increases dramatically to 20 percent in the 85+ age group, although only about 5.5 percent of these are nursing home residents (http://www.aoa.gov/prof/Statistics/profile/2008).

The primary disease processes that affect this population and cause the need for assistance in the ADLs and IADLs are arthritis, complications of high blood pressure (e.g., stroke, heart disease), diabetes, pulmonary disease, cancers, fractures, and cognitive impairment from Alzheimer's or other dementias.

These demographic trends raise two questions. First, who will be available to care for an aging population? About 31 percent of non-institutionalized older people currently live alone; half of women age 75 and older live alone. This does not necessarily mean that they cannot access help from family and friends, but it is a more vulnerable population.

The second question is how we will fund that care? For a third of Americans older than 65 years, Social Security benefits constitute 87 percent of their income. The median income of older persons in 2008 was $25,503. About 3.7 million elderly persons (10%) were below the poverty level in 2008. Another 2.3 million, or 6.7 percent, of the elderly were classified as "near-poor" (income between the poverty level and 125 percent of this level). Major sources of income for older people in 2007 were: Social Security (87%), income from assets (52%), private pensions (28%), earnings (25%), and government employee pensions (13%). It is clear from these statistics that most older persons are on fixed or incomes with modest cost of living increases. As the numbers of elderly continue to rise, the number of people who cannot afford care will also increase (www.aoa.gov/agingstatsdotnet/Main_Site/Data/2008.../OA_2008.pdf).

Children

An estimated 17 percent of all children in the United States have a chronic condition that requires some LTC services. School-age children use these services more than the very young.

The nature of the condition varies by age group. Preschool children who require these services often have congenital abnormalities or birth trauma. The most common chronic conditions of the rest of the age groups requiring LTC services are, in order of occurrence, asthma, ADD/ADHD (attention deficit disorder with or without hyperactivity), severe mental disorders such as autism or depression, congenital abnormalities, developmental disabilities, and chronic diseases such as diabetes, cerebral palsy, and AIDS. Many children needing assistance have multiple problems. Families face incredible problems caring for these children ranging from care coordination between many parties, financial issues, and family dynamics.

People with Disabilities

Non-institutionalized people with disabilities represent about 19 percent of the American population. This is a very broad term that covers many types of conditions. These conditions include neurological disorders, blindness, paralysis, loss of limbs, chronic illness, mental illness, hearing and speech disorders, and developmental disabilities. The individual may have several conditions and need a wide spectrum of services to continue to live independently.

Veterans

The Department of Veteran Affairs (DVA) is the largest integrated health care system in the United States. It provides comprehensive health care to inactive members of the military and armed services based on the degree of their service-related disability. Fifty percent of men over the age of 65 are veterans. Since 1930, there has been an organization to oversee the provision of these services. The DVA has three main missions: medical care, training and education, and medical research. It also has the duty to act as backup for the Department of Defense during a war or national emergency for the care of injured military personnel. The military personnel (430,000) from the recent wars in the Middle East and United Nations peacekeeping actions have used this backup service.

In 2011, the DVA will treat 6.1 million people; this generates 800,000 hospital visits and 8.3 million outpatient visits. The DVA has Geriatric Research Education and Centers, which provide education and training in gerontology and the clinical care of geriatric patients. Each has a special focus, such as dementia, falls, diabetes, and delivery of health care.

The DVA also either operates or manages LTC facilities, which care for more than 100,000 veterans a year. The DVA also contracts for LTC with community-based home care, adult day care, inpatient and outpatient hospice care, homemaker/home health care, community residential care, and dementia/Alzheimer's special treatment programs. All parts of the LTC continuum are represented in the DVA system. It is also one of the leading educational and research organizations for chronic and aging care (www1.va.gov/health//).

Who Provides LTC Services?

There are many different providers of LTC. The largest group is unpaid caregivers. Most adults who live in the community rely on family and friends or voluntary organizations such as Meals on Wheels for assistance with ADLs and IADLs. Other community providers include home health care providers, adult day care, hospitals, LTC facilities, hospice, case managers, primary caregivers, and specialized organizations such as the American Lung Association, housing providers, prevention groups, and rehabilitation providers. Only 3.5 percent of the population needing LTC is served by nursing homes and other institutional providers (Older Americans 2008).

Unpaid Caregivers

Most adult people who need help with one or more ADLs or IADLs get that help from a network of family members, friends, church organizations, and voluntary organizations. This help is primarily supplied by women: daughters, daughters-in-laws, neighbors, and women's organizations.

Over 70 percent of all adults between the ages of 18 and 64 who require LTC receive it from unpaid caregivers. Another 11 percent are served by a combination of paid/unpaid care; only about 9 percent rely entirely on paid care.

The age group over 65 years relies more heavily on a combination of paid and unpaid caregiving. They receive about 41 percent of their care from a combination of unpaid and paid.

Unpaid caregivers account for about 57 percent of care received. The single largest group of unpaid caregivers is adult children, predominantly daughters. Spouses make up about 24 percent of the total and other relatives about 26 percent. Families then shoulder about 91 percent of the unpaid care, with friends accounting for the remaining 9 percent. These caregivers provide an average of 20 hours a week. Approximately three-fourths of these also work out of the household. One out of every three households (65.7million people) in America care for family members who need special assistance (Caregiving in the U.S. 2009). As the baby boomers move into old age, these proportions will change because there will be fewer adult children to give care. This will become a future policy discussion for financing LTC, which has relied on a huge voluntary base from family. Although there are volunteers and family help in nursing homes and other institutional settings, that help is not calculated in these figures. These figures reflect only community care giving.

Home Health Care

Home health care is the fastest growing segment of LTC. Although restrictions on reimbursement from Medicare and other factors have caused the actual number of agencies to decrease, the overall number of clients continues to increase at a rapid rate. This increase will continue into the 2020s because of demographic pressures. The home health industry is roughly divided into two categories: Medicare certified and private. The home health care spectrum also includes hospice care.

Home health care has been a part of the LTC continuum since the 1880s when a routine part of medical care was the visit by nurses in the home to those who could not afford a private nurse. It experienced a decline as the use of hospitals increased for extended stays. But with the decrease in long hospital stays that started in the 1980s, the use of home health visits began to increase dramatically. The increase in high-tech home therapy and the aging population, along with early release from hospital stays, fueled the increase. Since the 1980s, home health care has become a viable option to keep even the frail elderly in their homes as opposed to nursing home placement.

The funding of home health care is accomplished by a combination of federal, state, and personal dollars. Medicare reimbursement for home health visits requires the person to be enrolled in Medicare, be homebound as certified by a physician, and to require skilled nursing care or physical therapy. The person can need only intermittent care, not continuous care. These requirements limit the use of this type of home health care primarily to the 65+ age group.

The second type of home health care is provided by non-Medicare-certified agencies and is financed by out-of-pocket or insurance dollars paid by the patient or family. It is available to a much wider range of clients.

A snapshot of home health clients shows that the majority are 65+ for both categories, predominantly white, married, and women. Diseases of the circulatory system and heart top the list of diagnoses for home health care clients (35% of all visits), followed by cancer (17%) and injury (13%) (Evashwick 2001).

The ability to give high-tech treatments in the home that were once only possible in the hospital has made home health care a valuable part of the treatment of chronic disease. The most frequently given therapies include intravenous (IV) antibiotic therapy, chemotherapy, pain medication, total **parenteral nutrition** and **enteral nutrition**, renal dialysis, and respirator/ventilation therapy.

Staffing for home health agencies includes physicians, registered nurses, nutritionists, clinical pharmacists, social workers, home health aides, speech pathologists, and physical therapists, as well as managers, coders and billers, and other office staff support. Home health care agencies may also give hospice care and would then add grief counselors and family support to the staffing mix.

parenteral nutrition
Any method of delivering nutrition that is not by mouth, such as by an intravenous line or by a direct tube into the stomach or intestine.

enteral nutrition
Nutrition delivered by a tube to the intestines. Example–nasogastric feeding tube.

Adult Day Care and Respite Care

Adult day care allows clients to receive LTC services in a senior or other center for part of each day. Over half of the clients have significant cognitive impairments, and over 40 percent require assistance with three or more ADLs. These clients live at home and may come to the center for a few days each week or daily. The center may provide transportation services to and from the center as well as nursing, social services, rehabilitation services, meals, counseling, and a comfortable social setting. The average age of the clients is 76, and most clients are women, according to the Urban Institute report (Tilly, Goldenson, and Kasten 2001).

Respite care for caregivers is an important function of adult day care centers, allowing the caregiver to have scheduled times in which to do shopping, caring for their own health, and socializing with healthy friends and relatives. Nursing homes may also provide longer-term respite care for spouses and family. This might include caring for a person whose spouse becomes ill or a family that needs a vacation from the 24/7 care needs of a cognitively impaired family member.

Adult day care centers may be stand-alone centers or associated with senior centers, nursing homes, hospitals, or home health agencies. The funding for these centers is primarily from Medicaid funds and out-of-pocket dollars from the families. Other sources are Social Security, DVA, Title III funds, state funding, charitable organizations, and private giving funds.

This segment of LTC is growing because of the aging of America, the increased numbers of young adults with disabling chronic disease, the preference for noninstitutionalized care, and the cost savings afforded by this model of community-based care.

Hospitals

Hospitals are increasingly offering different types of LTC. A hospital may coordinate discharge services through a hospital home health agency. Many hospitals now operate a home health agency among the outpatient services provided by the hospital. Hospitals may designate beds as certified skilled nursing beds, so when a patient is discharged the patient can be admitted immediately to the skilled unit for rehabilitation services, ostomy management, or chemotherapy. Many hospitals provide the clinical pharmacy or respiratory care for patients under separate contracts with home health agencies. Hospital social services may do case management for some clients, particularly veterans or those covered under special funding sources. Hospitals are often the source for geriatric and psychiatric geriatric assessments and care services.

Increasingly hospitals have specific LTC services under their umbrella, such as adult day care services, hospice, intermediate and skilled nursing facilities, assisted living, and retirement housing. In a sense, the large multilevel hospitals offer cradle-to-grave services.

Nursing Homes

nursing home An old-fashioned word designating a chronic care facility.

A **nursing home** is defined by the National Center for Health Statistics as a facility with three or more beds that is licensed as a nursing home by its state, certified as a Medicare facility, or a designated nursing care unit of a retirement center to provide nursing or medical care. Nursing homes are a rapidly changing part of the LTC spectrum. In the past, the nursing home was a small, often family-owned provider of 24/7 care for the elderly and client with mental retardation. Now the reality is a corporate multilevel, multifacility modern system of care that may have more than 1,000 beds. In 2004, most nursing homes are proprietary (61.59%) and located in the Midwest and the South, but 30.8 percent were operated as voluntary nonprofit facilities and the remaining 7.7 percent were owned by government and other entities. Almost 1.5 million people live in the 16,100 nursing homes in the United States. Residents were 65 years and older (88.3%), female (71%), and white (85.5%). Residents were typically admitted from a hospital or other health care facility and had and advanced directive of some kind (Jones, Dwyer, Bercovitz, and Stranhan 2009).

proprietary Owned by an individual or group of individuals: a for-profit arrangement.

Nursing homes can be classified according to ownership characteristics. **Proprietary** nursing homes are for-profit organizations that may be owned by individuals, corporations, or be part of a chain. Not-for-profit nursing homes are institutions usually run by charitable organizations or religious groups. Governmental ownership includes county- and state-run facilities as well as the DVA facilities. Of the estimated 16,000 nursing homes in the United States, 88 percent are certified to accept Medicare or Medicaid reimbursements. Almost two-thirds of certified nursing homes are for-profit. The remaining third are not-for-profit or government sponsored (Jones et al. 2009).

The four categories of traditional nursing homes are the extended care facility (ECF), intermediate care facility (ICF), intermediate care for the mentally retarded (ICF-MR), and Skilled Nursing Facility (SNF). Each is defined by the type and level of nursing care given. This type of care delivery is essentially a medical model with nurses providing and supervising the ongoing care of the patient. The emphasis is on the physical care of the client. Cognitive impairment and the need for assistance with three or more ADLs account for over 64 percent of the residents (Older Americans 2008). The federal government defines the levels of care for reimbursement and certification by Medicare/Medicaid and other federal/state programs. Each level has criteria that have to be met to be certified. These criteria include the minimum type of care that is given in each level. In the SNF, the client receives types of care that range from ventilator care to medication assessment and intensive rehabilitation programs. The SNF must have a registered nurse on duty at least eight hours a day. Often there are registered nurses on duty 16 hours a day, with LPN coverage at night. The length of stay in the SNF has changed over the last decade as hospitals discharge patients earlier who still need skilled nursing care; the SNF has become an extension of the hospital. The ICF primarily maintains functional ability, assessing and monitoring medication administration and treating chronic conditions. The ECF is primarily for assisting in critical ADLs like eating and toileting. Many nursing facilities have special units for the cognitively impaired client or special rehabilitation units.

Unlike traditional nursing homes, **assisted living facilities (ALFs)** do not adopt the medical model. Rather they emphasis the social/cognitive care of residents. There are more than 36,000 assisted living facilities in the United States housing 910,000 people. The average age of all assisted living residents is 84. The average female-to-male ratio in assisted living residences is 3.5 women to 1 man (http://www.aarp.org/research/longtermcare/costs/).

Each unit is a full living unit; it must have a kitchen (often with microwave, small appliances, and refrigerator) and bath and sleeping quarters separate from a living space. Each apartment has special features to assist with ADLs and is specifically designed to increase the ability to maintain independence. These features include handrails, adaptive shelving and sinks to accommodate wheelchairs or other mobility assist devices, automatic lighting, intercom help system, and special fixtures. The residents eat at least one meal in a congregate dining area. They may get some assistance with medications and ADLs, but the purpose of the ALF is to allow the individual to remain functional and be able to make choices about independence without the restrictive safety regulations that the ICF must impose to keep licensed.

Estimates of the median cost for assisted living range from $1,800 to $2,200 a month. However, costs vary widely depending on the level of accommodations, geographic location, and range of services provided (http://www.aarp.org/research/longtermcare/costs/). In some states, these facilities may receive Medicaid funding with a federal waiver.

Independent living is just that, an apartment specially adapted so that the resident can live without assistance. However, these facilities include a very important restriction: age (usually 60). Independent living units are often part of a larger multilevel facility. They may actually have all the adaptive features of assisted living, but no nursing or other care is provided. Often these are cottages on large campuses or a separate wing of the facility.

A multilevel retirement facility that has independent living units, assisted living units, and all levels of traditional nursing home care demonstrates a concept called **aging in place**. This combination of services allows the client and spouse to begin in the independent living unit. Then, if either has a need for more assistance in either the ADLs or needs nursing, the services are delivered at the same facility, so there is no need to change facilities as the need for assistance with ADL increases or health status diminishes. The multilevel facilities also have home health and hospice services.

Financing of nursing home care is primarily by Medicaid and private individuals and families. Other sources are the DVA and private insurance. Medicare only pays for skilled nursing and accounts for 10 percent of the total spent on nursing homes. Nursing homes at the intermediate level, where the largest proportion of clients is in ICF, cost anywhere from $5,000 to $8,000 per month (Jones et al. 2009).

How Do We Pay for LTC Services

As you have learned in this chapter, LTC services are provided to many groups by many providers in many settings. As a consequence, it is very difficult to put a single dollar figure on the cost of LTC. As with other types of health care, payments are made by a combination of government programs such as Medicare and Medicaid and by private funding such as personal insurance and out-of-pocket payments. A great deal of LTC is unpaid assistance by family and friends.

assisted living facilities Homes or apartment-like living spaces that allow for independent activities such as cooking and bathing and also provide care such as medication or treatment delivery; a nonmedical model of chronic care living arrangements.

aging in place A philosophy that allows the aging person or couple to stay in their living situation while growing older with increasing levels of personal and medical assistance as needed. These are adult living communities where the range is from individual homes to a skilled nursing facility in one complex.

Government Programs

The primary insurance program for the elderly, Medicare, does not pay for LTC except under narrow circumstances. If a Medicare-eligible person who has been hospitalized moves to a nursing home, Medicare will pay for the first 20 days. Between 20 and 100 days, the patient must make a daily copayment. After 100 days, no further Medicare coverage is available. Medicare also will not pay for unskilled care or long-term home care. A guide to Nursing Homes and Skilled Facilities available at www. helpguide.org/elder/nursing_homes_skilled_nursing_facilities.

Medicaid will pay for nursing homes; however, the patient must meet Medicaid's income tests. The elderly often must spend down assets to become eligible, and they must do so within a time frame and in a manner that complies with Medicaid rules.

Private Funding

A great deal of information and advice is aimed at helping older Americans fund retirement, including their need for LTC services. Financial devices such as reverse mortgages and legal instruments such as living trusts are designed to protect assets in order to fund long-term living expenses (Matthews 2004). This is an area where an individual needs good professional assistance because the law changes frequently, and a bad decision can have devastating financial consequences.

Even those with overall good health insurance policies may not be adequately protected for a health problem that requires LTC. For this reason, LTC insurance policies have been developed. Before buying this type of policy, an individual should carefully examine it for the extent of coverage, the coverage conditions, and the exclusions. The cost of premiums should be weighed against the benefit amounts (Matthews 2004).

Some employers offer long-term disability insurance as part of their benefits package. This is insurance that will replace your income if you become disabled; it is not insurance that will pay for long-term health care.

Ethical and Political Issues in LTC

As you have seen in this chapter and previous chapters, a great number of agencies are involved in LTC. But most people are like Marge in the chapter-opening vignette and have only Medicare and Social Security benefits from the government. The person who needs more has to struggle with a very disjointed system of 60 government agencies and countless private organizations. One of the great political and health care delivery questions of the next 10 years is going to be how to make this system manageable and efficient and at the same time give people the assistance they need to maximize their physical/social potential and retain human dignity.

The great polity debate of the coming years will be the extent to which the government should finance, regulate, and deliver LTC services. The issues here revolve around resource allocation, including the competition for funding among age groups, guardianship and medical power of attorney issues, and end-of-life care.

Resource Allocation

The ethical dilemma of who will receive society's benefits will shape much of the LTC policy debate. LTC is very resource intensive, not just monetarily but also in terms of health care professionals' efforts. Staffing ratios in LTC facilities are relatively low, especially in comparison to a general hospital where the ratio can be over 100 people to each patient. Currently acute care is the major area funded by Medicare; as the need increases, will more resources be allocated to LTC?

If older citizens will need more resources, how do we take care of the children? Currently more children live in poverty than the 65+ age group, yet a much smaller proportion of federal spending goes to children. The elderly have powerful lobbying interests and are very politically active. After all, they can vote their interests. Children, however, have fewer spokespeople, and, as a rule, they do not have the lobbying or voting clout. This makes the question of intergenerational equity very one sided.

At the family level, caregivers often face the same dilemma as policymakers. Many families are caring for both children and grandparents. For adult children, this is called the **sandwich generation**, in between the two generations.

Health Care Power of Attorney/Guardianship

Many of the frail elderly cannot manage IADLs such as banking and health care decisions. In this case, a family member might apply to either have **medical power of attorney** for health care decisions or a full guardianship. In the health care power of attorney, the appointed family member or friend makes all the health care decisions for the elderly person. This includes treatment of acute and chronic conditions, going to a LTC facility, and end-of-life decisions.

It is easy to see that there could be some conflict between what health care providers and the decision maker would want to do. Economics could play a role in how much the family is willing to **spend down**, that is, how much money the elderly person has in assets such as a home that is available to spend for care. Should the family spend to care for the individual or should assets be conserved for the estate? This is an ethical dilemma for many families. The amount of money that families in the low- to middle-income ranges inherit has been decreasing over the last decades, in part related to spending down of assets to provide LTC.

End-of-Life Decisions

Utilization statistics consistently tell us that a person uses the most care in the last six months of life. This statistics refers not only to the financial costs but also to the use of specialized hospitals, skilled nursing, or medical technology. The use of physician directives and living wills, along with health care power of attorney, has become common. These tools allow the person to determine prior to an end-of-life decision what their wishes are concerning the use of medical technology such as ventilators, assistive cardiovascular devices such as a pacemaker, or feeding tubes.

The idea of death with dignity has a legal force at this time in several states; only Oregon has an actual assisted suicide law. These new options ideally allow the family to make very difficult decisions early in the disease process. They also give direction to caregivers. There are, of course, pros and cons concerning end-of-life decisions. There are opportunities for abuse and neglect that must be taken seriously by health care professionals. But according to many surveys, the American people want more personal control over the end of life process and how much technology is appropriate for the individual.

The ethical questions in LTC are complex and linked to our view of health care in general. How we treat the person who is chronically ill is a measure of our values as a country.

sandwich generation
The generation that is currently working and taking care of children and parents, thus sandwiched between two dependent age groups.

medical power of attorney A person appointed by another who can give consent for medical care or can withhold medical care. It is a legal document that empowers the surrogate decision maker in all health care decisions if the patient is unable to make decisions.

spend down
Redistributing assets so that the individual will be Medicaid eligible.

Summary

The continuum of long-term care (LTC) is the network of services available to the person needing it. It may include family and friends or paid caregivers. LTC is used by anyone young or old who needs medical care or assistance with ADLs or IADLs for more than 90 days. The older American uses the majority of LTC, which is provided in the home, community-based day care centers, hospitals, assisted living centers, veterans centers, specialized hospitals, and the many levels of nursing home care. Family and friends provide about 80 percent of all LTC. The role of the government is to fund some aspects of LTC, regulate LTC providers, and provide a policy framework to ensure that the needs of this population are met.

LTC is primarily financed by individuals, either as direct payment to providers or through LTC third-party insurance. More than 80 government agencies help fund LTC. The ethical and political issues in LTC revolve around the allocation of private and government resources.

Questions for Review

1. Who receives LTC in the United States?
2. To what extent are family, friends, and members of the community involved in LTC?
3. What is the relationship between IADLs and ADLs and the need for LTC?
4. Who besides the older American uses LTC and why?
5. What are the ethical issues involved in LTC?

Questions for Discussion

1. How would you advise your congressional representative to vote on a bill to provide some level of LTC to all who need it?
2. Would you be willing to raise your taxes to pay for the care of your parents, grandparents, or a chronically ill child?
3. What LTC options are available in your community?
4. In your community, is a facility like Madrona (as described in the chapter profile) available? What features are offered? What is the cost of such care? How does this cost compare to other options in your community, such as:
   a. Skilled Care Facility
   b. Intermediate Care – regular nursing home
   c. Assisted Living
   d. Foster Care
   e. Specialized care such as dementia.
   f. In home care
5. Review a policy for LTC insurance. What services are covered? What is the cost?
6. Review your state's provision for a medical power of attorney. What is included?
7. What features in a continuing care community would you want for yourself and/or your family members?

Chapter References

Department of Health and Human Services, Administration on Aging. 2008. *Profile of older Americans 2008*. Available at www.aoa.gov/prof/Statistics/profile/2008.

Evashwick, C., ed. 2001. *The long-term continuum of care*. 2nd ed. Albany, NY: Delmar.

Jones A.L., L. Dwyer, A. Bercovitz, and G. Stranhan. *The National nursing home survey: 2004 overview*. National Center for Health Statistics. Vital Health Statistics 13(167), 2009.

Matthews, J. 2004. *Long-term care: How to plan & pay for it*. 5th ed. Berkeley, CA: NoLo Press.

Tilly, J., S. Goldenson, and J. Kasten. 2001. *Long-term care: Consumers, providers, and financing—a chart book*. Urban Institute. Washington DC. (www.urban.org/health_policy/long-term_care)

A guide to nursing homes and skilled facilities. (www.helpguide.org/elder/nursing_homes_skilled_nursing_facilities)

Caregiving in the US 2009. (www.aarp.org/relationships/caregiving/info-12-2009/caregiving_09.html)

Department of Heath and Human Services, Administration on Aging (http://www.aoa.gov/AoARoot/Aging_Statistics/Profile/2009/6.aspx)

American Association of Retired People (www.aarp.org/research/longtermcare/costs/)

Older Americans 2008: Indicators of well being. (www.aoa.gov/agingstatsdotnet/Main_Site/Data/2008.../OA_2008.pdf)

United States Department of Veterans Affairs (http://www1.va.gov/health)

For Additional Information

Administration on Aging (http://www.aoa.gov/AoARoot/Aging_Statistics/future_growth/future_growth.aspx)

Agich, G. 2003. *Dependence and autonomy in old age: An ethical framework for long-term care*. 2nd ed. Cambridge, England: Cambridge University Press.

American Association of Retired Persons (AARP) (www.aarp.org)

American College of Health Care Administrators (www.achca.org)

American Geriatrics Society (AGS) (www.americangeriatrics.org)

American Geriatrics Society) (AGS) Foundation for Health in Aging (www.healthinaging.org)

American Society on Aging (www.asaging.org)

Centers for Disease Control and Prevention: Health Data Interactive (www.cdc.gov/nchs/hdi.htm)

Centers for Disease Control and Prevention: Health, United States, 2009 trend tables with data on older population age 65 years and over (www.cdc.gov/nchs/hus/older.htm)

Centers for Disease Control and Prevention: Summary Health Statistics for U.S. Adults: National Health Interview Survey, 2008 (www.cdc.gov/nchs/data/series/ser_10/sr10_242.pdf)

Centers for Disease Control and Prevention: National Ambulatory Medical Care Survey (www.cdc.gov/nchs/ahcd.htm)

Centers for Disease Control and Prevention: National Health and Nutrition Examination Survey (www.cdc.gov/nchs/nhanes.htm)

Centers for Disease Control and Prevention: National Nursing Home Survey (www.cdc.gov/nchs/nnhs.htm)

National Alliance for Caregiving in Collaboration with AARP (http://www.aarp.org/research/surveys/care/ltc/hc/articles/caregiving_09)

National Association of Area Agencies on Aging (www.n4a.org)

National Council on the Aging (www.ncoa.org)

National Hispanic Council on Aging (www.nhcoa.org)

National Institute on Aging (www.nia.nih.gov)

Older Women's League (www.owl-national.org)

Tepper, L., and T. Cassidy, eds. 2004. *Multidisciplinary perspectives on aging*. New York: Springer.

Young, H. 2003. Challenges and solutions for care of frail older adults. *Online Journal of Issues in Nursing* 8(2)(www.nurisngworld.org/ojin)

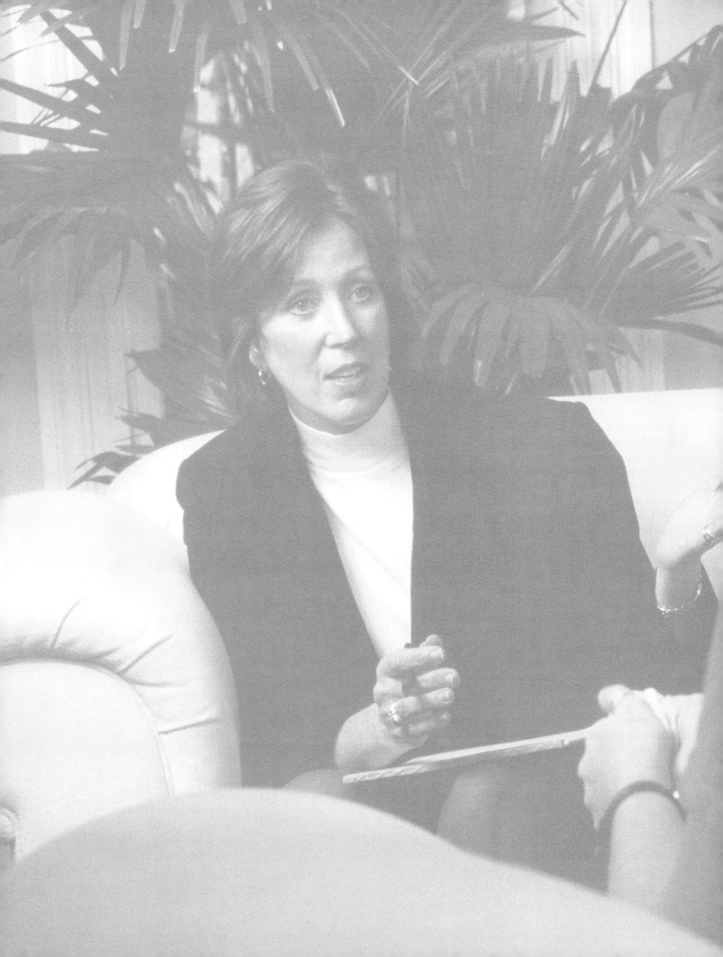

9

Mental Health Services

A Combination of Systems

Learning Objectives

After reading this chapter, you should be able to:

1. Define the scope of mental illness in the United States.
2. Compare the financing of the mental health system with the general health care system.
3. Identify the major human resource sectors of the mental health system.
4. Discuss the four eras of mental health in the United States.
5. Describe the major categories of mental illness and the populations affected.
6. Discuss the ethical issues in mental health service delivery.

A Young Adult with Mental Illness

Tad is returning to college after a 5-year break because of mental illness. When he was 18 years old, he began to experience audio hallucinations. Voices in his head started to drown out the people around him. He did not tell anyone what was happening to him for two reasons: first, he was pleased to be specially chosen to hear these instructions, and second, more important, no one asked him about them.

Although he had previously led an active social life and had played in a band as a teenager, Tad became increasingly withdrawn. His parents at first thought this change in behavior was just "those teenage years." But by the time he was 19 and had dropped out of college, they were worried. At his parents' insistence, Tad saw his primary care physician. His doctor took a detailed history that included Tad's self-reported use of recreational drugs and alcohol. The doctor attributed Tad's problems to his drug and alcohol history. In the next year, however, the symptoms became worse. Because he was no longer covered under his parents' insurance, he did not receive any medical intervention for his condition. Tad had frequent run-ins with the police; he was homeless, unemployed, and withdrawn. Finally, Tad was arrested and jailed for vagrancy and assault.

The court asked for a psychiatric exam because of his erratic behavior in jail. Tad was diagnosed with schizophrenia and released to an emergency treatment center where he was started on psychotropic drugs. After his discharge from the center, Tad was treated on an outpatient basis. His insurance plan covered his medication and provided follow-up care through the county mental health department.

Although Tad has returned to partial functioning, he faces a lifetime of chronic illness that will need treatment. Even so, he is lucky. Because the resources of most states are stretched thin, states are often unable to provide treatment for people like Tad. The less fortunate are thus often found in homeless shelters or living on the streets.

---

biochemical
Involving chemical substances present in living organisms, such as dopamine.

residential care
A living arrangement in which the person resides or lives full time at a facility.

somatic Affecting the body separate from the mind. For example, warm baths are a somatic treatment for calming the body.

talk therapy
Psychotherapy invented by Sigmund Freud that involves primarily talking rather than somatic or drug therapy.

burden of disease
The cost of a disease in terms of the individual, family, and community disability, including lost work, family relationships, and community participation.

Introduction

In the United States, the mental health system evolved as a system distinct from the general medical model of health care delivery. One of the reasons it became a separate system was the stigma attached to mental illness, which caused the care to be primarily in the home and in institutions and out of the public eye until the 19th century. Other reasons include the fact that mental illness was not regarded as a physical illness (such as appendicitis) until the late 20th century when scientists began to find a **biochemical** basis for some of the major categories of illness such as depression and schizophrenia. The treatment of mental illness at that point changed from **residential care** and physical, or **somatic**, treatments to treatments relying on drug and outpatient **talk therapy**.

This development had a profound impact on the delivery of mental health services; general practitioners and outpatient clinics could now manage mental illness. The care of people with mental illness now moved from the institutional model to a general delivery and business model like the rest of health care. In this chapter, the scope or **burden of disease**, history, diagnostic categories, delivery models, and the people who provide the services are described.

What Is Mental Illness and Mental Health?

According to the surgeon general of the United States, the term "mental illness" refers collectively to all diagnosable mental disorders. Mental disorders are health conditions characterized by alterations in thinking, **mood**, or behavior, or a combination of these associated with distress and/or impaired functioning. The precise cause, or etiology, of most mental disorders is not known. Researchers have found that the interactions among biological, psychological, and sociocultural factors are the major forces acting in both mental illness and mental health.

Mental health is not easily defined; like any definition of wellness, it has to be thought of in a framework that includes individual values and cultural differences. There are, however, indicators of mental health that can be assessed in an individual, such as the ability to cope with change, a positive outlook on life, the ability to interact with those close to us in a loving and supportive manner, and the general feeling of well-being. The mental health system addresses both mental health and illness with a wide variety of professionals, government and private programs, and **delivery models**.

Examples of mental illness include **mood disorders**, such as **major depression**; **cognitive**, or thinking, disorders, such as **Alzheimer's disease**; and behavior disorders, such as **eating disorders**. Mental illness is clinically diagnosed using a system that takes into consideration the observable signs and symptoms of the illness, the course and duration of the illness, the response to treatment, and the functional impairment caused by the illness. In the United States, mental illness is diagnosed by using the American Psychiatric Association's *Diagnostic and Statistical Manual of Mental Disorders*. It was first published in 1952; the current version is DSM-VI-TR-2000. This manual is updated every several years, with the next update scheduled for release in 2013, and establishes the criteria for a mental illness diagnosis. The manual is rapidly becoming the major diagnostic tool for mental illness around the globe.

These criteria are difficult to measure in absolutely objective terms, so the tracking of mental illness is not an exact science. The two best known comprehensive studies attempting to track the behavior and feelings of mentally ill people are the *National Comorbidity Survey* and the *Epidemiological Catchment Area* study. Both studies relied on extensive interviews to establish mental illness patterns.

Scope of Mental Illness

Mental illness is a global problem. It impacts the daily lives of the afflicted individuals, the family, friends, and employers, as well as the community as a whole. In the past, the toll of this disease process has been underrated significantly, according to the Murray and Lopez's *The Global Burden of Disease* (1996). In this study, the impact of mental illness over a lifetime was measured using the **Disability Adjusted Life Years (DALY)**. This study took into account loss of life, loss of work productivity, and loss of quality of life. It found that the worldwide burden of mental illness to society was second only to **ischemic cardiac disease** in its severity in selected world economies such as industrialized countries like the United States, Great Britain, Germany, and Japan (U.S. Department of Health and Human Services 1999, 411).

The availability and quality of mental health services affect every family and employer in the United States. Most mental illness is a chronic lifetime disease that interferes with an individual's ability to participate fully in family life, work, and school. Mental illness strikes one out of every five adults, or about 26 percent of the population. This figure includes both mental illness diagnosis and substance abuse. Approximately 19 percent of the adult population has a diagnosis of mental illness. Substance abuse of drugs and/or alcohol occurs in about 6 percent of the adult population. Dual diagnosis of both mental illness and substance abuse is responsible for the

mood The state of mind experienced at a particular time

etiology The study of the causes and origins of disease.

mental health The ability to cope with change, a positive outlook on life, ability to interact in close relationships in a loving and supportive manner, and the general feeling of well-being that can be assessed in the individual.

delivery models Systems to bring a type of care to individuals and groups.

mood disorders An altered state of mind, such as the continuous sadness known as depression.

major depression A depression that lasts for a significant period of time or recurs frequently; a medical diagnosis.

cognitive Relating to the process of thinking or acquiring knowledge. Cognitive diseases disrupt the ability to acquire or remember knowledge.

Alzheimer's disease A degenerative disorder that affects the brain and causes dementia.

eating disorders A group of diseases that describes a patient's focus on food, obsessive eating, or not eating, along with faulty perception of body image.

Disability Adjusted Life Years (DALY) The number of years a disease reduces the lifespan

ischemic cardiac disease A group of conditions characterized by a decreased blood flow to the heart.

final 3 percent. This translates to 57.7 million adults in any given year. Mental disorders are the leading cause of disability in both the U.S. and Canada for ages 15 to 44.

For children, the figures are not as well documented, but it is estimated that mild mental functional impairment occurs in 20 percent of children. Serious emotional disturbance is found in 9 percent of children between ages 9 and 17.

It is further estimated that only about half the people who have mental illness get adequate treatment. Part of this is because of economic and insurance status, cultural barriers, and the stigma of mental illness, and part is related to the inadequacy of the system itself (U.S. Department of Health and Human Services 1999, 405–7).

Financing the System

The total cost for the mental health system accounts for about 6.2 percent of all the dollars spent on health care. In 2001, this amounted to approximated $85 billion (Substance Abuse & Mental Health Services Administration <SAMHSA> 2003). The system is funded by a combination of public spending (63%), third-party insurance (22%), individual out-of-pocket spending (13%), and other (2%). Among the public payers, the bulk of the funds comes from Medicaid (44%), followed by other state and local agencies (37%), Medicare (12%), and other federal programs (7%). The other federal programs category includes those offered through the Department of Veterans Affairs (SAMHSA 2003).

The proportion each payer devotes to mental health as compared to total health spending indicates some interesting data. Of all private insurance payments, for example, only 4 percent is spent on mental health. Of all Medicare payments, only 3 percent is for mental health. A larger share of Medicaid dollars (10%) goes to mental health, and state and local payers spend close to 22 percent of their health care dollars on mental health.

Of that $85 billion, 21 percent is spent for prescription drugs. Medication plays an important role in mental health. More resources are spent for outpatient care (31%) than for inpatient (22%) or residential care (19%). Physicians accounted for 21 percent of expenditures for providers, with 72 percent of that for psychiatrists (SAMHSA 2003).

During the past two decades, there have been important shifts in which parties are responsible for mental health funding. Direct state funding of mental health care has been reduced, whereas Medicaid funding of mental health care has grown in relative importance. In part this is because of the substantial funding available to the states through the Medicaid program and public health block grants by the federal government. One consequence of this shift is that the Medicaid program design influences the delivery of each state's mental health care. Traditional state mental health agencies and departments of health and human services, however, continue to be an important force in making public mental health services policy.

Mental disorders and substance abuse are linked together for diagnostic and cost accounting purposes, but both third-party payers and providers handle them differently. A majority of private health insurance plans have a benefit that combines coverage of mental illness and substance abuse. However, many of the treatment services for mental illness and for substance abuse are separate and use different types of providers. The same is true for virtually all of the public funds for these services. This separation causes problems for treating the substantial proportion of individuals with both mental illness and substance abuse disorders who would otherwise benefit if both disorders were treated together.

Insurance coverage for mental health and substance abuse benefits differs among plans, employers, and states. State law may require insurers to provide a standard minimal offering of mental health and/or substance abuse benefits, and insurers can add additional coverage. In general, mental health benefits are not as extensive as medical/surgical benefits and require higher deductibles and copayments (www. mentalhealth.samhsa.gov).

Private insurance coverage has played a somewhat more limited role in mental health financing in the past decade. Various cost containment efforts have been pursued in the private sector through the introduction of managed care. This trend has increased the use of the general medical/primary care sector for mental health care. At the same time, private insurance coverage for prescription drugs has expanded dramatically. As a result of these efforts, insurance coverage for mental health drug therapy is moving toward parity with coverage for other illnesses.

The parity of payment to consumers is a major goal of mental health policymakers. **Parity** refers to the effort to treat mental health financing on the same basis or on par with financing for general health services. The fundamental motivation behind parity legislation is the desire to cover mental illness like any other physical disease. A parity mandate requires all insurers in a market to offer the same coverage, but as of 2006 only a handful of states require parity.

parity Equality; in this context it means equality of benefits between insurance coverage for mental health and medical coverage.

Organizing the Mental Health System

The U.S. mental health system is not a unified system at all. In this chapter, the *mental health system* means all services to those with a mental illness diagnosis, substance abuse, dementia, and children who have either cognitive impairment or a mental illness diagnosis. There are four ways to categorize this so-called system: (1) by who delivers services, (2) by treatment types, (3) by care setting, and (4) by human resource components.

Who Delivers Services

Mental health services can be provided by a wide variety of individuals from nonclinical self-help volunteers to psychiatrists. State and federal regulations vary widely on who can deliver services to people with mental health issues. Insurance companies reimburse some types of therapists and not others.

Treatment Types

The system also can be categorized by treatment types. These can include self-help, psychotherapy, talk therapy, behavioral therapy, drug therapy, and somatic device therapy such as electroshock therapy.

Care Settings

The mental health system is also defined by care settings. These include home care, community-based residential care, day care, sheltered work settings, outpatient facilities, and private psychiatric and recovery institutions. Care settings can even include public institutions for emergency and long-term care.

Human Resource Components

A common way to categorize the system is by its four major human resources components: the specialty mental health sector, the general medical/primary care sector, the human services sector, and the voluntary support network. This method of categorizing is popular because it recognizes that mental health problems are treated by a large variety of people who work in many different settings. The surgeon general's report on mental health estimates that these mental health sectors serve about 11 percent of the overall health care services provided in a year.

The specialty mental health sector includes mental health professionals such as psychiatrists, psychologists, counselors, psychiatric nurses, and psychiatric social workers. These professionals practice primarily in specialized mental health clinics, public and private psychiatric hospitals, and psychiatric beds in general hospitals. They also coordinate a wide variety of services to the seriously mentally ill through case management. It is estimated that 6 percent of adults and 8 percent of children access mental health care through this sector.

The general medical/primary care sector is composed of health care professionals such as primary care physicians, general internists, and nurse practitioners who practice in offices, general hospitals, and long-term care facilities. They are often the first health care provider contacted by an adult suffering from mental illness. Because the use of psychoactive drugs by primary care professionals has become widespread, adults with mild to moderate disease may use only this sector. Fewer children than adults use these professionals: only 3 percent as compared to 6 percent of adults.

The major sector that assesses, diagnoses, and treats childhood mental illness and cognitive disorders is the human services sector. Social services, school-based counseling, residential rehabilitation services, vocational rehabilitation, criminal justice/prison-based services, and religious counselors all belong to this sector. The school-based services are used by 16 percent of children, and child welfare and juvenile justice systems serve another 3 percent.

The last of the four sectors is the voluntary support network sector. Self-help groups, such as Alcoholics Anonymous (AA) and Al-Anon, and peer counseling are a rapidly growing part of the mental health services sector. There are 12-step type programs for many diagnoses, including those in the substance abuse category. In the 1980s, the *Epidemiological Catchment Area Study* estimated that 1 percent of the adult population used these services, but by early in the 1990s that had risen to 3 percent, as estimated by the *National Comorbidity Survey* (U.S. Department of Health and Human Services 1999, 415–17).

History of Mental Health Care in the United States

The history of mental health care demonstrates a shift in perception. Historically mental illness was seen as a problem of possession by evil spirits or as an imbalance in vital elements. Melancholy, now known as depression, was considered an imbalance in the vital humor until modern times. Epilepsy was a sign that visions and spirits visited the person. Freud began the modern era of psychiatry with what we now call psychotherapy or talk therapy. More important, he began to characterize the symptoms of mental illness. We still use a variant of the system Freud began over 100 years ago.

As the perception shifted from illness to wellness, so did the delivery systems for care. Prior to the 1950s, the emphasis was on housing people who were the most seriously mentally ill. The institutions for them were at best the sanitarium model where patients were housed comfortably but not allowed to leave. Some of these were very luxurious. At the other end of the spectrum were the huge charity and state-run institutions where people with mental illness were literally thrown into huge cells and food was pushed through doors. No attempt was made to cure or to see the individual as anything but subhuman.

The history of mental health care in the United States can be divided into four eras, each focused on reforming the problems not previously addressed. The four are the moral treatment era, the mental hygiene era, the community mental health era, and the current community support era (see Table 9.1).

The Moral Era

An era of "moral treatment" was introduced from Europe at the turn of the 19th century, representing the first of four reform movements in mental health services in the United States.

The first reformers, including Dorothea Dix and Horace Mann, imported the idea from Europe that mental illness could be treated by removing the individual to an asylum to receive a mix of somatic (physical treatment like baths, exercise, and special diet) and psychosocial treatments in a controlled environment characterized by "moral" sensibilities. The term *moral* had a different connotation than that of today. Then it meant the return of the individual to reason by the application of psychologically oriented therapy.

The building of private and public asylums characterized the moral treatment period. Almost every state had an asylum dedicated to the early treatment of mental illness to restore mental health and to keep patients from becoming chronically ill. Moral treatment accomplished the former objective, but it could not prevent chronic illness.

Mental Hygiene Era

Shortly after the Civil War, the failure of the early treatment moral era was recognized. Asylums were built for the untreatable chronic patients. The quality of care deteriorated in public institutions, where overcrowding and underfunding were the norm. A new reform movement, devoted to mental hygiene, as it was called, began in the late 19th century. It combined the newly emerging concepts of public health (which at the time was referred to as "hygiene"), scientific medicine, and social progressivism. Although the states built the public asylums, local governments were expected to pay for each episode of care. To avoid the expense, many communities continued to use local almshouses and jails for the mentally ill person. Asylums could

Table 9.1	*Historical Reform Movements in Mental Health Treatment in the United States*

Reform Movement	Era	Setting	Focus of Reform
Moral treatment	1800–1850	Asylum	Humane restorative treatment
Mental hygiene	1890–1920	Mental hospital or clinic	Prevention, scientific orientation
Community mental health	1955–1970	Community mental health center	Deinstitutionalization, social integration
Community support	1975–present	Community support	Mental illness as a social welfare problem (e.g., housing, employment)

Source: U.S. Department of Health and Human Services. 1999. *Mental health: A report of the surgeon general.* Rockville, MD: U.S. Department of Health and Human Services, Substance Abuse and Mental Health Services Administration, Center for Mental Health Services, National Institutes of Health, National Institute of Mental Health, Table 2.9.

not maintain their budgets, care deteriorated, and newspaper exposés revealed inhuman conditions both in asylums and in local welfare institutions.

The care of individuals with mental illness became the responsibility of state governments with the passage of the State Care Acts, passed between 1894 and World War 1. Local government took the opportunity to send everyone with a mental illness, including dependent older citizens, to state asylums. Dementia was redefined as a mental illness, although only some of the older residents were demented. For the past century, the states carried this responsibility at very low cost, in spite of the magnitude of the task. This was accomplished by centralizing the care into one or two state mental hospitals that cared for thousands of residents at a time. The movie *One Flew over the Cuckoo Nest* depicts life in such a hospital.

The reformers of the mental hygiene period formed the National Committee on Mental Hygiene (now the National Mental Health Association, NMHA) and called for an expansion of the new science, particularly neuropathology, in asylums, which were renamed mental hospitals. They also called for "psychopathic hospitals and clinics" to bring the new science to patients in smaller institutions associated with medical schools. They opened several psychiatric units in general hospitals to move mental health care into the mainstream of health care. The mental hygienists believed in the principles of early treatment and expected to prevent chronic mental illness. To support this effort, they advocated for outpatient treatment to identify early cases of mental disorder and to follow discharged patients.

Early treatment was no more successful in preventing patients from becoming chronically ill in the early 20th century than it was in the early years of the previous century. At best, the hospitals provided humane custodial care; at worst, they neglected or abused the patients. Length of stay did begin to decline for newly admitted patients, but older long-stay patients filled public asylums. Financial problems and overcrowding deepened during the Depression and during World War II.

Community Mental Health Movement

Enthusiasms for early interventions, developed by military mental health services during World War II, brought a new sense of optimism about treatment by the middle of the 20th century. Again, early treatment of mental disorders was championed; a new concept, community mental health, was born. The NMHA figured prominently in this reform, along with the Group for the Advancement of Psychiatry. Borrowing some ideas from the mental hygienists and capitalizing on the advent of new drugs for treating psychosis and depression, community mental health reformers argued that they could bring mental health services to the public in their communities. They suggested that long-term institutional care in mental hospitals had been neglectful, ineffective, and even harmful. The joint policies of community care and deinstitutionalization led to dramatic declines in the length of hospital stay and the discharge of many patients from custodial care in hospitals (U.S. Department of Health and Human Services 1999).

The Current Mental Health System: The Community Support Movement

The past 25 years have been marked by discrete defining trends in the mental health field, according to the Surgeon General's *Report on Mental Health*. There has been an extraordinary increase in the pace and productivity of scientific research on the brain and behavior. The introduction of a range of effective treatments for most mental disorders has changed clinical and client response dramatically.

In the modern era, the care of mentally ill people is decentralized. No longer do we have huge institutions that served as permanent homes for those diagnosed with mental illness and neurological disorders. The mental institutions of the 1950s and 1960s housed thousands of patients; those same institutions today house only a few hundred patients with the most serious mental illnesses. The number of people with mental illness in the community has not changed to any great degree, but the treatment is now outpatient and in small-group homes.

With the deinstitutionalization of people committed to psychiatric hospitals and changes in psychiatric treatment brought about by psychoactive drugs and managed care efforts, consumers developed self-help programs designed to improve outcomes for people with mental illness through peer support. Services offered include drop-in centers, vocational and housing programs, peer counseling, case-management services, crisis alternatives to hospitalizations, advocacy training, business ventures, and peer support groups. Although these programs have existed for over two decades, little formal evaluation has focused on the effectiveness of this mental health delivery model. A better understanding of existing consumer-operated service programs is needed to provide the empirical basis for creating effective partnerships between these programs and traditional mental health services.

The Consumer-Operated Services Program (COSP) Multisite Research Initiative is a federally funded national effort to discover to what extent consumer-operated programs as an adjunct to traditional mental health services are effective in improving the outcomes of people with serious mental illness. More than 2,200 racially and ethnically diverse consumers will participate in the 4-year study. It is designed to study the following:

1. Examine the effect of consumer-operated services on empowerment, housing, employment, social inclusion, and satisfaction with services
2. Determine how participation in COSP affects costs for in-patient hospitalization, crisis intervention, and emergency department utilization, as well as how it offsets costs in housing, criminal justice, vocational rehabilitation, physical health care, and income support (www.surgeon-general.gov/library/mentalhealth/home).

Secondary goals of the project include creating partnerships among consumers, service providers, and researchers and disseminating knowledge gained about the effectiveness of COSP and the specific components that contribute to its success. This large-scale research project will have major implications for future planning and policy decisions for the entire system.

Major Categories of Mental Illness

The scope and distribution of the most frequently occurring mental illness diagnoses are described here to provide a concrete idea of the wide variety of illnesses the mental health system addresses. According to the National Institute of Mental Health, the major categories of mental illness are mood disorders, schizophrenia, obsessive-compulsive disorders, anxiety disorders, posttraumatic stress disorder (PTSD), suicide, and cognitive impairments. Major depression is the leading cause of disability worldwide for people older than 5 years. For women, the major causes of disability are depression, schizophrenia, and bipolar disease. Many people suffer from dual disorder (more than one mental illness diagnosis). Table 9.2, "Major Mental Illness Categories at a Glance," will give you information about the types of mental illness, who is affected, and treatments.

Table 9.2	*Major Mental Illness Categories at a Glance*				
Disorder	**Description/ Symptoms**	**Demographics**	**Age of Onset**	**Treatment**	**Notes**
Mood Disorders, major depressive disorder, Dysthymic disorder, Bipolar Disorder	Prolonged sadness, changes in sleep and appetite, irritability, feelings of guilt and anxiety	Affects 9.5% of adult Americans 20.9 million, affects twice as many women as men, often co-occur with anxiety disorders and substance abuse	Between 15–30, median age 25–32, diagnosis in very young children and older people more common in last decade	Cognitive behavioral therapy, psychotherapy, social supportive care, pharmaco-therapy: antidepressants, tranquilizers, mood stabilizers, sleep aids or sedative mediation	Same genes suspected in both depression and bipolar disease
Suicide	90% have a diagnosable depressive disorder or substance abuse	In 2006, 33,300 people died, highest rates in white men over age 85, four times as many men as women	From early adolescence to old age	***PREVENTION Any person who talks about killing themselves needs help. If you or anyone you know is considering suicide get help!* Life Line – *1800273 8255 is available 24/7 to any one free***	Women attempt suicide three times more often than men. It is estimated that there are as many as 25 suicide attempts for every death
Schizophrenia	Loss of contact with reality, severe disturbance in social functioning, bizarre thoughts, withdrawal from social interactions, hallucinations, delusions	2.4 million adults age 18 and older, affects men and women with equal frequency, if one twin exhibits symptoms the other has a 45% chance of at some time becoming symptomatic	Men-appears in late teens or early twenties. Women- in twenties or early thirties Over 10,000 new cases are diagnosed every year	Pharmacotherapy: antipsychotic primarily, antidepressants, psychosocial treatments	Genes are being identified, but no specific set has been found. It seems that both a genetic predisposition and an environmental stressor are needed to trigger symptoms
Anxiety	Heightened feelings of dread, fear, apprehension, worry and/or uneasiness	13% of adults between 18–54 suffer an anxiety disorder		Psychotherapy and cognitive behavioral therapy; pharmacotherapy, tranquilizers, and sleep aids	Common to have more than one anxiety disorder coupled with substance abuse
Anxiety - Panic	Sudden onset of intense anxiety coupled with physical symptoms like hyperventilating and tachycardia	2.4 million Americans 18–54	Late adolescence or early adulthood	As above plus treatment for physical symptoms	About one in three people with panic attacks develop agoraphobia—afraid of open spaces

Table 9.2	*continued*				
Disorder	**Description/ Symptoms**	**Demographics**	**Age of Onset**	**Treatment**	**Notes**
Anxiety-Obsessive-Compulsive	Anxiety disorder characterized by recurrent, unwanted thoughts obsessions) and or repetitive behavior—compulsions	2.2 million Americans age 18 and older	Symptoms may begin in early childhood or adolescence median age of onset is 19	Pharmaco-therapy, Exposure psychotherapy, social support groups and deep brain stimulation	
Anxiety-Post-traumatic stress	Develops after a terrifying ordeal that involved physical harm or the threat of harm. Flash backs of the incident occur frequently causing intense stress	Affects about 7.7 million Americans. Affect women more than men. Some evidence of family susceptibility	Any age after a traumatic event.	Pharmaco-therapy, psychotherapy and social support groups all are effective	It often manifests within 3 months of the event, but may not surface for years. Often accompanied by depression, substance abuse, and other anxiety disorders
Eating-Anorexia nervosa, Bulimia, Binge eating	Anorexia-Fear of obesity and ritualistic food practices, loss of 15% of body weight, excessive dieting and self-induced vomiting. Bulimia-massive binge eating, use of laxatives and vomiting	Females 15–24 0.5%–3.7% of females experience anorexia and 1%–4.2% bulimia, while 205% of all Americans experience binge-eating disorder	35% of cases are male Mortality among people with anorexia is 12 times higher than the annual death rate of 15–24-year old from all other causes combined	Emergency medical maintenance for complications, Cognitive behavioral therapy, psychotherapy, social supportive care, pharmaco-therapy: antidepressants,	Bulimia had the highest morbidity—the purging may permanently damage the GI system and teeth. A colostomy may be needed and death may be caused by cardiac arrhythmias
Attention Deficit Hyperactivity ADHD	Inattention and/or hyperactivity and impulsivity	Most common mental disorder in children, also affects 4.1% of adults 18–44. Affects males more often than females	Becomes evident in preschool or early elementary years, median age of onset is 7 years old	Pharmaco-therapy: stimulants, Cognitive behavioral therapy, counseling, collaboration between providers and school/family/ friends/ employee	Etiology unknown, but twin studies suggest genetic susceptibility

(*continued*)

Table 9.2	*Major Mental Illness Categories at a Glance (continued)*				
Disorder	**Description/ Symptoms**	**Demographics**	**Age of Onset**	**Treatment**	**Notes**
Autism	Deficits in reciprocal language and social interactions, characterized by repetitive stereotyped behaviors— minimal eye contact, delayed language, disinterest in social interactions	Prevalence estimates difficult due to difference in the ways that cases are identified and defined, differences in study methods and changes in diagnostic criteria. But ¾ cases per 1,000 children is an acceptable estimate	Generally diagnosed by age 3- Four times more common in boys, but when girls affected symptoms are more severe and with greater cognitive impairment	No specific medications are approved for ASDs, but medications for behavior and mood may by used. Applied behavior analysis— individual intense one-to- one therapy has been shown to improve behavior and communication skills	Part of a group known as autism spectrum disorders (ASDs), autism being the most debilitating form, Asperger syndrome produces milder symptoms
Alzheimer's Disease	Progressive form of dementia that seriously disrupts activities of daily living, behavior and mood	Affects 4.5 million Americans, this number has doubled since 1980. Most common cause of dementia 65 and older. Increasing age is greatest risk factor	Symptoms first appear after 65, 1 in 10 individuals over 65 and nearly half of those over 85 are affected	Medications can slow progression and treat associated symptoms of depression, anxiety, and aggression. Social supports and occupational and physical therapy are important	From time of diagnosis, people with AD survive about half as long as those of similar age without dementia. Life span after diagnosis 8–10 years. Rare inherited forms can strike as early as 30s–40s.

Source: National Institute of Mental Health. *The numbers count: Mental disorders in America.* Bethesda, MD: National Institute of Mental Health, available at www.nimh.nih.gov/health/publications/the-numbers-count-mental-disorders-in-america/index.shtml.

Risk Factors and Prevention

Risk factors are those characteristics or hazards that, if present for a given individual, make it more likely that this individual, rather than someone selected at random, will develop a disorder. Some risks such as gender and family history are fixed; that is, the individual cannot change them. Other risk factors, such as a lack of social support, inability to read, and exposure to bullying, can be altered by strategic and potent interventions. Current research is focusing on the interplay between biological risk factors and psychological risk factors and how they can be modified. As explained earlier, even with a highly heritable condition such as schizophrenia, studies have shown that in over half of identical twins, the second twin does not have schizophrenia. This suggests the possibility of modifying the environment to eventually prevent the biological risk factor (i.e., the unidentified gene that contributes to schizophrenia) from being expressed.

Suicide Prevention

Any person who talks about killing themselves needs help!!!!

   If you or anyone you know is considering suicide, get help!

Life Line – 1 800 273 8255 is available 24/7 to any one free

Because mental health is so closely related to all other aspects of health, it is important to look at all the different types of interaction among the biological, psychological, and socio-cultural factors. For example, chronic illness, unemployment, substance abuse, racism, and violence can be risk factors or mediating variables for the onset of mental health problems. Yet some of the same factors can also be related to the consequences of mental health problems (e.g., depression may lead to substance abuse, which in turn may lead to lung or liver cancer).

Treatment

Mental disorders are treatable; new brain-based research increases the ability to diagnose and treat mental illness every day. A number of treatments are available that diminish symptoms and increase functionality. In fact, for most mental disorders, there is generally not just one but a range of treatments of proven value to patients. Most treatments fall under two general categories: psychosocial and pharmacological. Moreover, the combination of the two—known as multimodal therapy—can sometimes be even more effective than each individually.

The evidence for treatment being more effective than placebo is overwhelming. The degree of effectiveness tends to vary depending on the disorder and the target population. What is optimal for one disorder and/or age group may not be optimal for another. Furthermore, treatments generally need to be tailored to the client and to client preferences (www.mentalhealth.samhsa.gov).

If treatment is so effective, then why are so few people receiving it? Studies reveal that less than a third of adults with a diagnosable mental disorder, and even a smaller proportion of children, receive any mental health services in a given year. Systemic barriers, economics, stigma of disease, and cultural responses all contribute to the underutilization for persons with mental illness. The single largest barrier is socioeconomic class. The working poor and the underinsured have a very difficult time accessing adequate assessment and treatment. It is only in recent decades that the government has become the primary resource for mental health services.

Ethical Issues in Mental Health

The issues surrounding confidentiality, barriers to mental health services, parity in financing mental health and general health, and the uninsured are all ethical questions as well as policy questions. The ability of an individual or family to access mental health services is critical to the quality of life for the person with a mental illness as well as their family and social network, which makes access a key ethical issue when talking about the delivery of mental health services. The barriers that are culturally and ethnically centered require us to take action to decrease these barriers. This would include decreasing racism, looking at poverty as both an economic and an ethical issue, and reducing the stigma of mental illness. Only when these underlying causes have been addressed can we begin to have a system that is ethically responsive.

Another major issue in mental health services is confidentiality. Although it is also an important issue in general health care, there are special considerations in the mental health area. An individual with a mental illness might decide not to seek treatment for many reasons. Some might forgo treatment for financial reasons. Others might decide that the risk of stigma and discrimination still encountered by people with mental illness is too high a risk. Many people pay directly to the mental health provider rather than use the insurance provided by their employer because of fear that if it was known they had a mental illness, they would be fired or not considered for promotion.

Summary

Mental illness is a significant health concern in the United States; one in five Americans has a mental disorder in any given year, and 15 percent of the adult population use some form of mental health services during the year. In addition to adults, 21 percent of children ages 9 to 17 receive mental health services in a given year. The major categories of mental illness include mood disorders, schizophrenia, obsessive-compulsive disorders, anxiety disorders, PTSD, suicide, and cognitive impairments. The history of mental health treatment has moved from warehousing to individual treatment with a sophisticated mix of drugs and psychotherapy. The current mental health service system is complex and connects many sectors. As a result, care may become organizationally fragmented, creating barriers to access. The system is also financed from many funding streams, adding to the complexity. Although the United States spends $99 billion on the direct treatment of mental disorders, substance abuse, and Alzheimer's disease, there is concern that mental illness does not receive the equivalent amount of spending that physical illnesses receive. Parity legislation attempts to resolve this issue. In addition to access and resource allocation, there are ethical issues regarding confidentiality and discrimination.

Questions for Review

1. Define mental health.
2. Describe the most common mental health conditions in children, adolescents, adults and the elderly.
3. Compare the role of the individual patient, insurance companies, and the state and federal government in paying for mental health services.
4. Describe the current system used to deliver mental health services in the United States.
5. Compare and contrast the treatment for mental illness from the 1880s to the present.
6. Refer to the profile at the beginning of this chapter. How common is Tad's diagnosis, and who does it most commonly affect?

Questions for Discussion

1. Why is it so difficult to define mental health?
2. Do you believe that there is still a stigma attached to mental illness? What other factors might prevent a person from seeking treatment?
3. What mental health care facilities are available at your college?

4. Should mental health and substance abuse be treated together?
5. Should insurance treat mental health treatment the same way it treats any other illness?
6. Refer to the profile at the beginning of this chapter. Discuss Tad's case from two perspectives: as if he were your friend and if he was a stranger you heard talking to himself on the streets. How would you react differently? What is the general feeling about people who have hallucinations or talk to themselves? Do you think this perception exists in all cultures?
7. What is society's obligation to people with mental health problems, and how has that changed over the last 200 years?

Chapter References

Murray, C. L., and A. D. Lopez, eds. 1996. *The global burden of disease. A comprehensive assessment of mortality and disability frsom diseases, injuries, and risk factors in 1990 and projected to 2020.* Cambridge, MA: Harvard University Press.

National Institute of Mental Health. 2009. *The numbers count: Mental disorders in America.* Bethesda, MD: National Institute of Mental Health, (www.nimh.nih.gov/health/publications/the-numbers-count-mental-disorders-in-america/index.shtml).

Substance Abuse & Mental Health Services Administration. 2003. *National expenditures for mental health services and substance abuse treatment, 1991–2001.*

Substance Abuse & Mental Health Services Administration (www.mentalhealth.samhsa.gov).

U.S. Department of Health and Human Services. 1999. *Mental health: A report of the surgeon general.* Rockville, MD: U.S. Department of Health and Human Services, Substance Abuse and Mental Health Services Administration, Center for Mental Health Services, National Institutes of Health, National Institute of Mental Health.

For Additional Information

Alliance for Health Care Reform—Mental Health and Substance Abuse Chapter 11 available at http://www.allhealth.org/sourcebookcontent.

Conwell, Y. 1996. *Diagnosis and treatment of depression in late life.* Washington, DC: American Psychiatric Press.

Cowen, E. L. 1994. The enhancement of psychological wellness: Challenges and opportunities. *American Journal of Community Psychology* 22(2): 149–79.

Frasure-Smith, N., F. Lesperance, and M. Talajic. 1995. Depression and 19-month prognosis after myocardial infraction. *Circulation* 91: 999–1005.

Mental health: A report of the Surgeon General. (www.surgeongeneral.gov/library/mentalhealth/home).

Mental Health Disorders—statistics (www.cdc.gov/nchs/fastats/mental.htm)

National Institute of Mental Health (www.nimh.nih.gov)

National Institute of Mental Health. 2000. *Depression.* Bethesda, MD: National Institute of Mental Health, (www.nimh.nih.gov/publicat/depression.cfm).

National Institute of Mental Health. 2001. *Bipolar disorder.* Bethesda, MD: National Institute of Mental Health, (www.nimh.nih.gov/publicat/bipolar.cfm).

National Institute of Mental Health. n.d. *Schizophrenia.* Bethesda, MD: National Institute of Mental Health, (www.nimh.nih.gov/publicat/schizoph.cfm).

Secker, J. 1998. Current conceptualizations of mental health and mental health priorities. *Health Education Research* 13(1): 57–66.

Zisook, S., and S. R. Schucter. 1991. Depression through the first year after the death of a spouse. *American Journal of Psychiatry* 148: 1346–52.

Zisook, S., and S. R. Schucter. 1993. Major depression associated with widowhood. *American Journal of Geriatric Psychiatry* 1: 316–26.

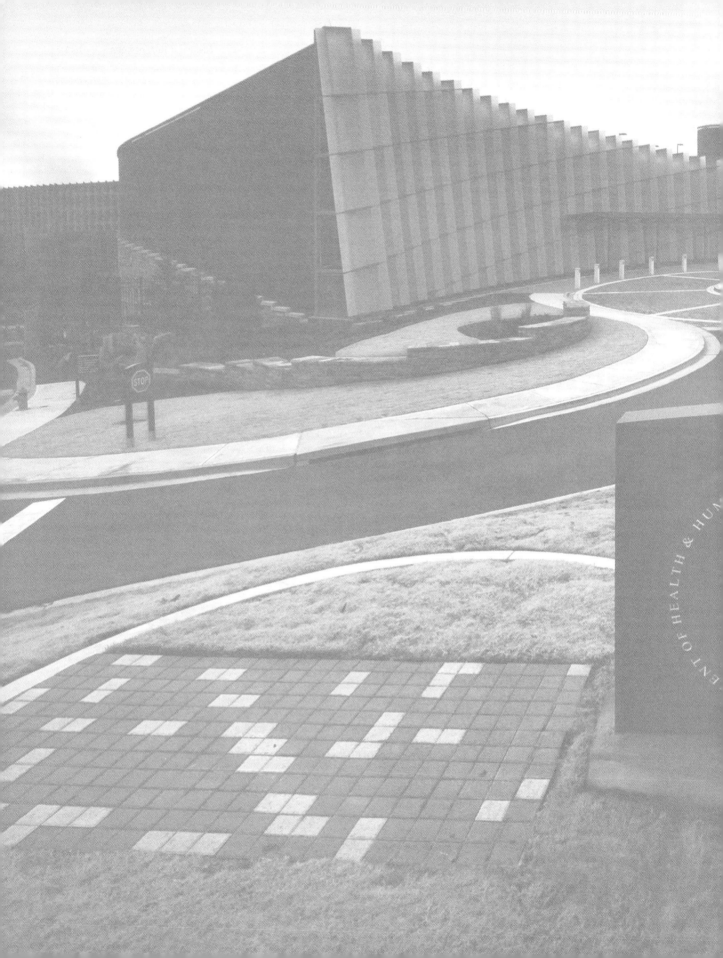

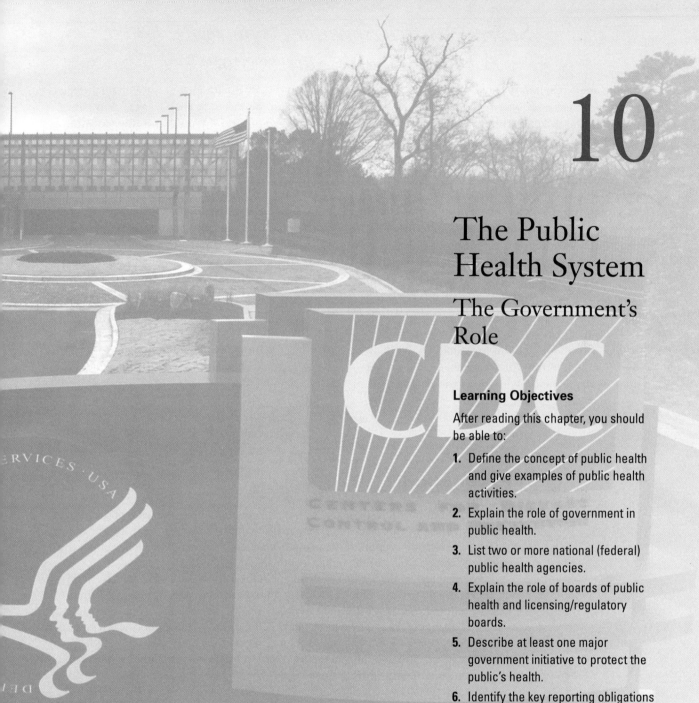

10

The Public Health System

The Government's Role

Learning Objectives

After reading this chapter, you should be able to:

1. Define the concept of public health and give examples of public health activities.
2. Explain the role of government in public health.
3. List two or more national (federal) public health agencies.
4. Explain the role of boards of public health and licensing/regulatory boards.
5. Describe at least one major government initiative to protect the public's health.
6. Identify the key reporting obligations that health professionals are mandated to uphold.

Severe Acute Respiratory Syndrome: A Public Health Success Story

Severe acute respiratory syndrome (SARS) is a respiratory illness that was recognized as a global threat in March 2003. The SARS virus can cause fever, headache, body aches, diarrhea, and respiratory problems that are related to low levels of oxygen in the blood. Many people with SARS develop pneumonia. It can also cause death. SARS appears to spread when infected persons cough or sneeze and spread small droplets of saliva and mucus that can land on the mucous membranes of a nearby person or on a surface/object touched by someone who later touches one of their mucous membranes. According to the World Health Organization (WHO), from November 2002 through July 2003, a total of 8,098 people worldwide became ill with SARS (many of them in China). Of this number, 774 died. In the United States, only eight persons were diagnosed with SARS and no one died.

How did the United States avoid a SARS epidemic? The Centers for Disease Control and Prevention (CDC) used strong surveillance techniques and monitoring to keep track of how many people were getting infected and their location. During the 2003 epidemic, the CDC worked with the Council of State and Territorial Epidemiologists to develop surveillance criteria and identify persons with SARS in the United States. Strong communication with state and local health departments helped supply local medical providers with information regarding the symptoms of SARS so that they could identify patients with the disease and report the information to the CDC. Then the agency could take appropriate action to protect the public's health. Epidemiologists investigated how the disease was spread so that prevention recommendations could be created. The science of public health helped prevent a SARS epidemic in the United States.

Source: cdc.gov/ncidod/sars

Introduction

As individuals, our health is important to us. Yet even though we take care of ourselves, we don't live alone or in isolation. Society is made up of millions of individuals. What affects one member of a community can often affect another member. The health of the nation is the responsibility of the public health system in the United States.

In this chapter, you'll learn about the public health system in the United States: what it is and who's responsible. The history and basic activities of public health are discussed, and the role of government in public health described. Finally, you'll learn about the challenges facing public health in the 21st century. The public health system is not a single system. It is made up of many different agencies coming together to improve the health and lives of Americans. This is a brief overview, highlighting some of the major components of the system.

What Is Public Health?

To define *public health*, we must first define *health*. The World Health Organization (WHO) defines health as "a state of complete physical, mental and social well-being and not merely the absence of disease or infirmity" (http://www.who.int/en/). According to this definition, being healthy is more than just not being sick. It is a state of well-being in our bodies, our minds, and our lives. Keeping this definition in mind, what happens when we place the word *public* in front of the word *health*? Public in this sense implies the government has primary responsibility for the social good of health, just as it does in public education. Public health, therefore, involves the well-being of all of us as we live together in neighborhoods, communities, states, and countries. It is anything and everything that relates to helping us collectively experience "a state of complete physical, mental and social well-being." It touches nearly every aspect of our lives. The large-scale goals of public health are to protect, promote, and restore health and to reduce the premature death and discomfort caused by disease. In short, the goal of public health is to protect the community from the hazards of group life.

Unlike **curative medical care**, which focuses on making us feel better when we are already ill, public health focuses on **prevention efforts** to keep us from getting sick in the first place. Because it focuses on prevention, public health has the power to impact the policies and laws that help us have a healthier society. It helps promote well-being on a societal level and often global level, and it makes the world a better place for all of us.

Public health can be seen in our everyday lives in things as simple as the crosswalk lines on a street that allow us to cross a roadway without getting hit by a car or the laws requiring construction workers to wear hard hats so that they are not injured by falling construction debris. It is also recognizable in state and nationwide campaigns to reduce smoking, heart disease, and cancer. Public health is actualized by activities such as nurses providing free immunizations to low-income children and police officers enforcing laws around seat belt and helmet use.

Most important, public health is the way a society reaches out to protect the health of its most vulnerable members. Using a system of **block grants** and specific public health initiatives, public health programs nationwide provide medical care for the elderly, substance abuse recovery programs, nutritional help for low-income women and infants, free dental care for children, medical care for the homeless, and so much more.

Public health is a wonderful idea, but does it really matter? Shouldn't it be enough for each of us just to take care of ourselves? Although our individual efforts to stay healthy do, in one sense, help us create a healthy community, some things require collective, organized efforts. For example, laws are needed to govern sanitation, waste disposal, food safety, and water purity. The quality of these services can affect an entire community. In the absence of public health efforts, it is easier for disease to spread and make more people ill.

Widespread illness affects not only people but also communities and economies. Think for a moment about the devastating effect of HIV infection in sub-Saharan Africa today. Of the 33 million AIDS **cases** (each case represents one person) worldwide, 22 million of them are in this one region (www.unaids.org). Young adults in the prime of life are dying. Not only are families devastated and children orphaned, but large sections of the population are not working because of premature death and illness. When people can't work, food is not grown, resulting in starvation, which leads to further problems, and the situation only worsens. Although some health programs are operating in Africa, they are clearly overwhelmed by the demands on their limited resources. The lack of a strong public health system can be the downfall of a society. Public health does more than keep us healthy; it makes civilization possible.

The History of Public Health

Public health is not a completely new concept in human society. Humans have tried to promote community health in a variety of ways at different points in history. One of the earliest ways was through sanitation efforts. The ancient city of Mojenjo Daro in northern India, built over 4,000 years ago, had paved streets covering sewers that drained waste from bathrooms in residential homes. The classical era of the Greek

curative medical care Medical care that helps cure an already ill or infected person.

prevention efforts Health programs and behaviors that prevent illness from occurring.

block grants Money granted by the national government to a state government with few restrictions on its spending. This can be contrasted with a categorical grant which has strict and specific provisions on the way it is to be spent.

case A term used in health statistics to refer to each person who has a disease.

quarantine Forced isolation of a person to prevent a disease from spreading.

and Roman civilizations also saw the creation of bathhouses to promote cleanliness and the building of drainage canals (Fairbanks and Wiese 1998). Early versions of **quarantine** were instituted in the Middle Ages (and earlier) when persons infected with leprosy were placed in leper colonies outside of town limits in an effort to keep the disease from spreading.

In the United States, public health efforts gained strength as the nation grew toward independence in the 1700s. Several key events helped shape public health. Some of the first efforts of organized action to protect community health were the creation of boards of health. These early boards of health were often created in response to an **epidemic** (Turnock 1997). For example, in 1793, a terrible epidemic of yellow fever broke out in Philadelphia, then the nation's capital. The epidemic was so devastating that it prompted not only the transfer of the national capital to Washington but also the establishment of Philadelphia's first board of health that same year.

epidemic A term used to describe a disease that is widespread in a population.

The NIH traces its roots to 1887 when a one-room laboratory was created within the Marine Hospital Service (MHS), predecessor agency to the U.S. Public Health Service (PHS). The MHS had been established in 1798 to provide for the medical care of merchant seamen. One clerk in the Treasury Department collected 20 cents per month from the wages of each seaman to cover costs at a series of contract hospitals. In the 1880s, Congress had charged the MHS with examining passengers on arriving ships for clinical signs of infectious diseases, especially for the dreaded diseases such as cholera and yellow fever, in order to prevent epidemics. During the 1870s and 1880s, moreover, scientists in Europe presented compelling evidence that microscopic organisms were the causes of several infectious diseases. In 1884, for example, Koch described a comma-shaped bacterium as the cause of cholera. Officials of the MHS followed these developments with great interest. In 1887, they authorized Joseph J. Kinyoun, a young MHS physician trained in the new bacteriological methods, to set up a one-room laboratory in the Marine Hospital at Stapleton, Staten Island, New York. Kinyoun called this facility a "laboratory of hygiene" in imitation of German facilities and to indicate that the laboratory's purpose was to serve the public's health. Within a few months, Kinyoun had identified the cholera bacillus in suspicious cases and used his Zeiss microscope to demonstrate it to his colleagues as confirmation of their clinical diagnoses. "As the symptoms . . . were by no means well defined," he wrote, "the examinations were confirmatory evidence of the value of bacteria cultivation as a means of positive diagnosis" (history.nih.gov/exhibits/history).

One of the key events to shape public health in America was the signing of the Act for the Relief of Sick and Disabled Seamen by President John Adams in 1798 (see Table 10.1). The act provided for a tax of 20 cents a month on the salary of sailors. The funds were used to build and staff hospitals to care for sailors. Over time, this system of hospitals and the person appointed to oversee it became the government body on which we rely today to protect our nation's health: the U.S. Public Health Service, headed by the surgeon general (Fairbanks and Wiese 1998).

In 1850, Lemuel Shattuck published the *Report of the Sanitary Commission of Massachusetts*. It outlined the existing and future public health needs for that state and became America's blueprint for the development of public health systems. Shattuck's report called for the establishment of state and local health departments to engage in sanitary inspections, **communicable disease** control, food sanitation, vital statistics, and services for infants and children. Although it took several decades for his ideas to catch on, Massachusetts established the first state health department in 1869. By 1900, there were 40 such state health departments (CDC 1999a). The public health

communicable disease A disease that spreads from person to person; another term for infectious disease.

Table 10.1	*Abbreviated Historical Development-National Institutes of Health*
1798	President John Adams signed "an Act for the relief of sick and disabled Seamen," which led to the establishment of the Marine Hospital Service.
1803	The first permanent Marine Hospital authorized to be built in Boston, Massachusetts.
1836	Library of the Office of Surgeon General of the Army established.
1870	President Grant signed a law establishing a "Bureau of the U.S. Marine Hospital Service," Treasury Department, which created central control over the hospitals, and a Supervising Surgeon (later Surgeon General).
1887	Laboratory of Hygiene established at Marine Hospital, Staten Island, New York, for research in cholera and other infectious diseases.
1891	Rocky Mountain Spotted Fever Laboratory established in Hamilton, Montana, as field station of Public Health Service.
1922	Congress authorized National Cancer Institute (NCI) and the awarding of research grants. Rocky Mountain Laboratory became part of NIH.
1938	National Institute of Health moved to land donated by Mr. and Mrs. Luke I. Wilson at Bethesda, Maryland. Cornerstone for Shannon Building laid.
1949	Mental Hygiene Program of Public Health Service transferred to NIH and expanded to become National Institute of Mental Health.
1950	"Omnibus Medical Research Act" authorized the establishment of the National Institute of Neurological Diseases and Blindness and the National Institute of Arthritis and Metabolic Diseases, and the latter absorbed the Experimental Biology and Medicine Institute.
1957	The Center for Aging Research established.
1961	The Center for Research in Child Health established in Division of General Medical Sciences.
1964	Division of Computer Research and Technology established.
1966	Division of Environmental Health Sciences created.
1970	National Institute on Aging created.
1990	National Center for Research Resources was created by consolidating the Division of Research Services and the Division of Research Resources.
1991	National Center for Medical Rehabilitation Research established within the National Institute of Child Health and Human Development.
1992	National Institute on Alcohol Abuse and Alcoholism, National Institute on Drug Abuse, and National Institute of Mental Health were transferred to NIH from the Alcohol, Drug Abuse, and Mental Health Administration.
1993	National Center for Nursing Research was re-titled as the National Institute of Nursing Research.
1994	The Dietary Supplement Health and Education Act of 1993 mandated establishment of an Office of Dietary Supplements within NIH to conduct and coordinate NIH research relating to dietary supplements and the extent to which their use reduces the risk of certain diseases.
2000 to present	The international Human Genome Project public consortium—funded by NIH, DOE, and others—assembled a working draft of the sequence of the human genome.
2003	The International Human Genome Sequencing Consortium, led in the United States by NHGRI and the Department of Energy, completed the Human Genome Project
	The complete genetic blueprint of Bacillus anthracis—the microbe that gained notoriety during the 2001 anthrax mail attacks—has been completed by NIAID-funded researchers.
	President George W. Bush visits NIH on Feb. 3 to unveil Project BioShield, a $6 billion, 10-year effort to protect the public from various weapons of bioterrorism.
2004	NIH opens the Mark O. Hatfield Clinical Research Center, a 240-bed successor to the NIH Clinical Center, which opened in 1953
2008	Through legislation enacted by Congress, NICHD was renamed the Eunice Kennedy Shriver National Institute of Child Health and Human Development at the institute's 45th anniversary celebration. In the early 1960s, Shriver persuaded her brother, President John F. Kennedy, to include the proposal for an NIH institute focusing on child health and human development in his first health message to Congress. NICHD was then established in 1963.

Source: http://www.nih.gov/about/almanac/historical/chronology_of_events.htm

system was expanded considerably in the period just after the great influenza epidemic in 1918 (Berry 2004). Today, every state has a health department and a public health laboratory.

Key Public Health Functions

In 1988, the Institute of Medicine released a report called *The Future of Public Health* that outlined these three key functions of public health: assessment of the health of the community, policy development, and assurance of the public health. **Assessment** means determining the health needs of the community by surveying disease incidence and prevalence, identifying needs, analyzing why health outcomes are not met, collecting and interpreting data, monitoring health trends research, and evaluating outcomes.

Policy development is the collective decision about what actions are most appropriate for the health of the state or nation. **Assurance** is making sure that the necessary actions are actually taken. To carry out these three functions, information is needed. Public health officials engage in three key activities to satisfy this need: epidemiology, surveillance, and monitoring. These activities provide them with the information they need to assess and assure a community's health and to make policy decisions.

Epidemiology is the study of the history of a disease and its distribution throughout a society. It permits understanding and rational decision-making regarding actions that need to be taken. Epidemiologists investigate where a disease outbreak occurred, who it affected, and how and when. Popularized recently as "disease detectives," epidemiologists help determine not only where a disease came from but also how to protect people from it. For example, in 1993 in the state of Washington, 477 people became ill from *Escherichia coli*, a deadly bacterium that causes severe intestinal problems and sometimes death. Epidemiologists kept track of who had the disease. They investigated what activities the infected persons had engaged in up to the time when they got sick. Their research led them to a local fast-food restaurant that had been undercooking ground beef. Thanks to epidemiologists, the cause of the problem was discovered and further illness prevented. To learn more about the career of epidemiology, see the Career Box.

The term *surveillance* is used to describe the actions of police as they watch a suspect and take note of what takes place. Similarly, in public health, **surveillance** refers to the continuous search for and documentation of disease. If public health departments were not always on the lookout for new diseases or outbreaks of disease, diseases could run rampant. Surveillance keeps track of all kinds of things, from sexually transmitted infections, to episodes of violence, to the number of cases of the flu.

Monitoring refers to the use of surveillance data to determine changes in the number of infected persons so that the appropriate action can be taken when the infection rate gets too high. Monitoring helps answer questions about whether or not there is more or less of a particular disease present now than in the past.

Several basic measurements can help us understand the information uncovered through surveillance and monitoring activities. Often you hear these terms used in the news or in reports about a current health concern. These measurements are used to create a picture of how a disease is affecting society. Table 10.2 lists some key public health terms.

Where do the data for surveillance and monitoring come from? State health departments are required by law to report on cases of specific diseases or conditions.

assessment The process of determining the health needs of a community.

policy development The process of making a collective decision about what needs to be done to protect the community's health.

assurance The process of making sure that correct actions are taken to protect community health.

epidemiology The study of the nature, cause, control, and determinants of the frequency of disease, disability, and death in human populations. Also the study of the history of a disease and its distribution throughout a society (public health).

surveillance The continuous search for and documentation of disease in public health.

monitoring The regular review of disease data to determine changes in disease levels.

Career Profile: Epidemiologist

Epidemiologists are sometimes called "disease detectives." Like any good detective, their primary duty is to carry out investigations, in this case of a disease. They study where a disease outbreak occurred, who it affected, and how and when. They examine the relationships among various factors such as lifestyle, environment, person-to-person contact, and geography. They collect information from people using surveys and interviews. They also look at existing health information such as local disease statistics or insurance claims information.

Epidemiologists can work in health departments, laboratories, hospitals, and government agencies, such as the CDC. Because disease outbreaks can occur anywhere at anytime, some epidemiologists travel the nation, or even the world, for their investigations.

Other epidemiologists investigate disease outbreaks closer to home. When not investigating a disease, epidemiologists work at their computers cataloging all the information they have collected.

The conclusions reached by epidemiologists and the data they collect are important in several ways. First, in determining how a disease is spread, epidemiologists can make recommendations about how to avoid further infections. Second, their conclusions can help boards of health and health departments develop policies to protect the community's health. Without the work of epidemiologists, our understanding of diseases and how they pass from person to person would be severely limited. Thanks to epidemiologists, our path to health gets clearer, and a little bit easier, all the time.

Some of this data, such as the number of persons infected with a particular disease, are collected for statistical purposes and to alert health authorities to a possible epidemic. Other conditions, such as child abuse, are reported because it allows someone to intervene in the situation and ideally prevent any further abuse from occurring. Whenever health or social service providers come across one of these conditions or diseases, they are required to report the information to the state. This information can be reported confidentially. For example, although the number of people infected with HIV is reported to the state, their names are not. As of 2009, 72 diseases had to be reported at the national level, including HIV, cholera, rabies, sexually transmitted infections, tuberculosis, hepatitis, and anthrax exposure (see Table 10.3).

Table 10.2	*Key Terms in Public Health Measurement*
Incidence	Number of new cases of a disease or event such as a motor vehicle accident in a specific population
Morbidity	Number of cases of a specific disease in a specific period of time per unit of population, usually expressed as a number per 1,000
Mortality rates	Number of people who have died from a given disease or event
	These rates are collected and analyzed from death certificates.
	Morbidity and Mortality Weekly Report is published by the CDC and reports illness and death rates for a variety of diseases.
Prevalence	Total number of infected/affected people (cases) over a given period of time
Relative risk	How an individual's risk may change relevant to a specific factor (e.g., a smoker has a higher relative risk of getting lung cancer than a person who does not smoke)
Risk	Likelihood that someone will become infected/affected

Table 10.3   *Infectious Diseases Designated as Notifiable at the National Level During 2007*

Acquired immunodeficiency syndrome (AIDS)	Meningococcal disease
Anthrax	Mumps
Domestic arboviral diseases	Novel influenza A virus infections
California serogroup virus disease	Pertussis
Eastern equine encephalitis virus disease	Plague
Powassan virus disease	Poliomyelitis, paralytic
St. Louis encephalitis virus disease	Poliovirus infection, nonparalytic
West Nile virus disease	Psittacosis
Western equine encephalitis virus disease	Q fever
Botulism (foodborne, infant, other)	Rabies (animal, human)
Brucellosis	Rocky Mountain spotted fever
Chancroid	Rubella (congenital syndrome)
Chlamydia trachomatis, genital infection	Salmonellosis
Cholera	Severe acute respiratory syndrome-associated
Coccidioidomycosis	coronavirus
Cryptosporidiosis	Shiga toxin-producing Escherichia coli (STEC)
Cyclosporiasis	Shigellosis
Diphtheria	Smallpox
Ehrlichiosis (human granulocytic, human monocytic,	Streptococcal disease, invasive, group A
human with other or unspecified agent)	Streptococcal toxic-shock syndrome
Giardiasis	Streptococcus pneumoniae, invasive disease (drug
Gonorrhea	resistant—all ages, nondrug resistant—age <5years)
Haemophilus influenzae, invasive disease	Syphilis (congenital)
Hansen disease (leprosy)	Tetanus
Hantavirus pulmonary syndrome	Toxic-shock syndrome (other than streptococcal)
Hemolytic uremic syndrome, postdiarrheal	Trichinellosis
Hepatitis A, acute	Tuberculosis
Hepatitis B (acute, chronic, virus—perinatal infection)	Tularemia
Hepatitis C (acute, virus infection—past or present)	Typhoid fever
Human immunodeficiency virus (HIV) infection (adults	Vancomycin-intermediate Staphylococcus aureus
age > 13 years, pediatric age < 13 years)	infaction (VISA)
Influenza-associated pediatric mortality	Vancomycin-resistant Staphylococcus aureus infection
Legionellosis	(VRSA)
Listeriosis	Varicella infection (morbidity)
Lyme disease	Varicella (mortality)
Malaria	Vibriosis (non-cholera Vibrio infections)
Measles	Yellow fever

Source: www.cdc.gov/mmwr/preview/mmwrhtml/mm5653a1.htm (latest available data).

Role of Government in Public Health

The government plays a key role in assuring the public's health. Government in action can be seen at the local (county, neighborhood), state, and federal levels. Prior to the Great Depression (1929–41), U.S. citizens did not think the federal government should intervene in people's health. Health is not a power granted to the federal government in the Constitution. Therefore, individuals, with some help from the state government, took care of their health themselves. But the situation was so desperate during the Great Depression that the federal government was expected to take action (Turnock 1997).

Since then, the federal government's role in health has expanded. Two sections of the Constitution have been interpreted as allowing the federal government to intervene in the nation's health. The first is the ability to tax people to provide for the "general welfare." This allows for the collection of money to be used in support of health programs. In fact, today the government's main role in public health is financial support of public health programs.

Second, the federal government has the ability to regulate commerce. Only the government can enforce policies that limit the personal and property rights of individuals or businesses. This power allows for the regulation of restaurants, sewage and water companies, product and drug safety, and other businesses that sell products to consumers.

Federal Government

Public health at the federal level is represented by numerous agencies, each dedicated to a specific aspect of the public's health. The Department of Health and Human Services (DHHS) is the U.S. government's principal department protecting the health of the nation. As of 2004, DHHS included over 300 programs and several key agencies (Berry 2004). Here is a list of some of these key agencies:

- The Food and Drug Administration (FDA) assures the safety of foods, cosmetics, and medications.
- The CDC works with state health departments and other community organizations to monitor disease, help prevent outbreaks, maintain national health statistics, and operate disease prevention and health promotion programs.
- The Health Resources and Services Administration (HRSA) provides access to health care services for low-income and uninsured people or for people who live in areas where health care is not easily available. HRSA-funded health care centers provide medical care for more than 13 million people in over 3,600 health centers across the nation.
- The Centers for Medicare and Medicaid Services (CMS) provides health care insurance through third-party carriers for about one in every four Americans. Medicare provides insurance for more than 41 million elderly and persons with disabilities. Medicaid additionally covers 44 million low-income persons, including 19 million children. State children's health insurance programs administered by CMS cover an additional 4.2 million children (see Chapter 4 for a more detailed discussion).
- The Substance Abuse and Mental Health Services Administration (SAMHSA) works to improve the availability and quality of substance abuse prevention, addiction treatment, and mental health services. Funding from SAMSHA helps more than 650,000 Americans with serious substance abuse problems or mental health problems.

As mentioned earlier in the chapter, public health is the way a society cares for its most vulnerable citizens. The government's financial involvement is clearly crucial to this effort. Without this support, literally millions of individuals would be without adequate medical care. Our ability to control disease would be severely hampered. A government's investment in public health is a symbol of how much it supports and cares for its citizens.

State Government

At the state level, there are two kinds of public health bodies: boards of health and state health departments. Boards of health are the policymaking bodies for a state's

Department of Health. Twenty-four states have boards of health that oversee financing and policy development (Fairbanks and Wiese 1998). States that do not have boards of health have other mechanisms to make policy. They have the power to adopt and amend rules and regulations and to make recommendations. State health departments are charged with promoting the public's health and implementing public health laws. States regulate things like newborn screening. Forty-eight states and the District of Columbia have regulations requiring PKU and other genetic disorders screening. Many have provisions for treating these defects with special formulas and other necessary interventions through the Health Departments (http://www. hrsa.gov).

Additional responsibilities of state departments of health include:

- Carrying out national and state mandates designed to protect health
- Managing environmental education and personal health services
- Collecting, analyzing, and disseminating information on threats to the community's health
- Responding to statewide health crises such as hepatitis and flu outbreaks
- Setting policies and standards for health care and medical professionals
- Conducting inspections of restaurants and factories
- Conducting the planning and evaluation of health programs

There are two models of a state health department. In most states, the health department is a freestanding agency that reports directly to the state governor. In other states, the health department is part of a larger institution, such as the state's Department of Health and Human Services. The Affordable Health Care Act of 2010 will impact the scope and responsibility of state health departments (http://www. healthcare.gov/).

In addition, licensing and regulatory boards help protect the public's health by assuring that health care professionals and others, such as food handlers, are held to basic standards of care, cleanliness, and safety. For example, state health inspectors evaluate whether or not laboratories are using proper techniques, if restaurants have adequate food safety efforts, or if a factory has strong enough pollution control measures. As you read in the chapters about health professionals, licensing boards assure consumers that their health or service professionals have been tested and trained on specific knowledge. Not only are health professionals licensed, but in many states so are service personnel such as food handlers and cosmeticians.

Local Health Departments

Local health departments can serve an individual county, city, or region. They are responsible for the delivery of services mandated by the state or by local statute. They can be independent or part of a state department of health.

In 1999, the National Association of County and City Health Officials surveyed 1,100 local public health agencies nationwide in an effort to better understand their activities. They determined that the most common programs and services included adult and child immunizations, communicable disease control, community assessment, community education, environmental health services, epidemiology and surveillance, food safety, restaurant inspections, and tuberculosis testing. These local agencies rarely provided direct medical care. Because state government has so many administrative, legal, and inspection responsibilities, it is important to have local health systems that can provide more direct service to community members.

Other Public Health Partners

Public health is not solely in the hands of the government. Organizations like the Red Cross, March of Dimes, and the American Cancer Society play an important role. In addition, smaller local social service organizations are able to work directly with the community members whose health they want to protect. These may be not-for-profit organizations or community-based organizations. They provide services in their local communities for specific populations and for one or two targeted health problems. For example, an organization could choose to help inner-city homeless youth or young women with substance abuse problems. **Foundations** are a particular kind of not-for-profit organization. They raise funds to support a cause of their choice and then distribute the funding to other community-based organizations in support of their work.

> **foundation** A type of non-profit organization that raises money and then distributes it to other organizations in support of their programs.

The importance of these nongovernmental partners cannot be underestimated. In particular, community-based organizations often go directly to the person needing services. Sometimes this means visiting people in their homes or finding them in parks or on the street. Thus many people who might not make it to the health department receive the help they need. By specializing in a specific health issue, these organizations can also provide expert advice to their patrons. Nongovernmental efforts help complete and strengthen the public health system.

Past Successes and Future Challenges

According to the CDC, the life expectancy of persons living in the United States has increased by 30 years since 1900; 25 years of this gain are attributable to successful public health interventions. Although the successes of public health are many, the CDC selected key program areas as having the most impact on lowering death rates and decreasing illness and disability in the United States (CDC 1999b). These 10 great achievements are related to the following areas:

1. Vaccination: The development of vaccines and vaccination campaigns has led to decreased incidences of many illnesses such as diphtheria. Also, vaccinations have eradicated diseases such as smallpox and, in the Western Hemisphere, polio.
2. Safer workplaces: New safety standards in industries such as mining, construction, manufacturing, and transportation have led to a 40 percent reduction in the rate of job-related injuries.
3. Healthier mothers and babies: Improvements in hygiene, nutrition, and availability of antibiotics, greater access to health care, and technological advances have helped reduce infant and maternal mortality.
4. Control of **infectious diseases**: Improved sanitation and clean water have helped control many diseases such as cholera and typhoid. Also, new medications have helped control the spread of diseases like tuberculosis and sexually transmitted infections.

> **infectious disease** A disease that can spread from person to person (versus a genetic disease or a disease that is not contagious).

5. Coronary heart disease and stroke prevention programs: Education regarding smoking cessation, blood pressure control, and the importance of early detection has led to a 51 percent decrease in death rates since 1972.
6. Safer and healthier foods: The identification of essential nutrients and food fortification programs (e.g., adding iodine to salt or vitamin D to milk) has nearly eliminated diseases such as rickets and goiter.

Medical Reserve Corps

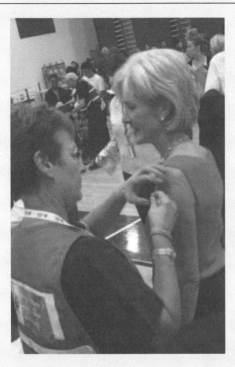

The Medical Reserve Corps (MRC) was founded after President Bush's 2002 State of the Union Address, in which he asked all Americans to volunteer in support of their country. It is a partner program with Citizen Corps, a national network of volunteers dedicated to ensuring hometown security. The U.S. Surgeon General assigns MRC units specific areas to target that strengthen the public health infrastructure of their communities each year. These reflect the priorities for the health of individuals, and the nation as a whole. The goal, in addition to providing well-trained volunteers in an emergency, is to improve health literacy, and in support of this, she wants us to work toward increasing disease prevention, eliminating health disparities, and improving public health preparedness. Units are community-based and function as a way to locally organize and utilize volunteers who want to donate their time and expertise to prepare for and respond to emergencies and promote healthy living throughout the year. MRC volunteers supplement existing emergency and public health resources.

MRC volunteers include medical and public health professionals such as physicians, nurses, pharmacists, dentists, veterinarians, and epidemiologists. Many community members—interpreters, chaplains, office workers, legal advisors, and others—fill key support positions.

MRC volunteers can also choose to support communities in need nationwide. When the southeast was battered by hurricanes in 2004, MRC volunteers in the affected areas and beyond helped communities by filling in at local hospitals, assisting their neighbors at local shelters, and providing first aid to those injured by the storms. During this 2-month period, more than 30 MRC units worked as part of the relief efforts, including those whose volunteers were called in from across the country to assist the American Red Cross (ARC) and the Federal Emergency Management Agency (FEMA).

During the 2005 hurricane season, MRC members provided support for ARC health services, mental health, and shelter operations. MRC members also supported the HHS response and recovery efforts by staffing special needs shelters, community health centers, and health clinics and by assisting health assessment teams in the Gulf Coast region. More than 1,500 MRC members were willing to deploy outside their local jurisdiction on optional missions to the disaster-affected areas with their state agencies, the ARC, and HHS. Of these, almost 200 volunteers from 25 MRC units were activated by HHS, and more than 400 volunteers from more than 80 local units were activated to support ARC disaster operations in Gulf Coast areas. During the 2009 flu pandemic, volunteers set up vaccination stations in schools, public meeting places, and fire stations.

MRC volunteers attend training sessions and must be certified in Incident Command Strategy to facilitate the integration of the volunteers with Emergency Response teams to avoid some of the confusion found in early large-scale disasters.

Sources: http://www.medicalreservecorps.gov/; Photo: http://www.medicalreservecorps.gov/image/PhotoGallery/Training/ExerSep09-006.jpg

7. Family planning: Access to family planning has provided health benefits such as smaller family sizes and longer intervals between the births of children. In addition, the use of barrier contraceptives (condoms) has helped prevent unwanted pregnancies and the transmission of HIV and other sexually transmitted diseases.

8. Motor vehicle safety: Improvements in both car and highway design and successful education programs to change personal behavior (e.g., wearing seat belts, helmets, not drinking and driving) have led to large reductions in vehicle-related deaths.

9. Fluoridation of drinking water: Since 1945, fluoride has been added to drinking water and has helped to reduce tooth decay in children (40% to 70%) and tooth loss in adults (40% to 60%).

10. Recognition of tobacco as a health hazard: Antismoking campaigns have helped prevent initiation of tobacco use, promoted quitting, and reduced environmental tobacco smoke. The prevalence of smoking among adults has decreased, and millions of smoking-related deaths have been prevented.

Even with all these successes, there remains much work to be done. What are the new challenges for public health in the next 100 years? Public health must meet several new challenges in the future, such as changing patterns of disease, increasing numbers of chronic conditions, new and emerging infections, injuries, violence, and curable genetic diseases (Turnock 1997). Diseases once thought under control, like tuberculosis, are making a comeback because of global travel in and out of countries where these diseases are common and in specific populations such as those with compromised immune systems. Antibiotics, one of our most powerful weapons in the fight against disease, are becoming increasingly ineffective as many bacteria become **drug resistant** (i.e., the bacteria are no longer killed by the antibiotic). Global travel allows for the quick spread of disease across borders. The United States faces a range of wholly preventable diseases and conditions that have reached epidemic proportions, such as HIV/AIDS, obesity, and stress-related conditions. In the next 100 years, public health must continue to adapt and expand its capacity to address these new health concerns.

drug resistant The term used to describe when a disease or bacteria is not affected or stopped by the use of common antibiotics and other drugs.

Summary

In this chapter, you read about the history of public health both globally and in the United States. Public health refers to any and all organized and collaborative efforts that are undertaken with the goal of protecting community health. The basic public health activities are assessment of the health of the community, policy development, and assurance of the public health. Health professionals who study disease and monitor key data perform these activities. The government is involved at the federal, state, and local level to carry out these activities. Foundations and other private partners also play a role in assuring the nation's health.

Questions for Review

1. Define public health.
2. List the three key functions of public health.
3. Name a public health agency and define its role.

4. Define incidence, morbidity, and mortality rate.
5. List one public health achievement.
6. See the profile at the beginning of the chapter. What public health measures were taken to protect the United States from SARS? Were they effective?
7. Compare and contrast the public health response to SARS and H1N1 flu epidemics.
8. Explain what an epidemiologist does to help control disease.

Questions for Discussion

1. What do you think the role of the federal government should be in public health? Are public health efforts worth all the tax dollars you pay for them?
2. If public health is really so successful, why are people still getting sick and engaging in behaviors that are bad for their health?
3. What do you think are the most important problems for public health to address today?
4. Why do we need so many types of health departments at the federal, state, and local levels? Does public health help create too much of a government bureaucracy? Why or why not? Does it matter?
5. Is it more important for the government to invest in curative medical care or in prevention efforts? What are the benefits and drawbacks of each?
6. Would you volunteer for the Medical Reserve Corps in your community? Why? Why not?

Chapter References

Berry, J. 2004. *The great influenza: The epic story of the deadliest plague in history*. London: Penguin Books.

Centers for Disease Control and Prevention. 1999a. Achievements in public health, 1900–1999: Changes in the public health system. *Mortality and Morbidity Weekly Report* 48(50): 1141–47.

Centers for Disease Control and Prevention. 1999b. Ten great public health achievements: United States 1900–1999. *Mortality and Morbidity Weekly Report*. 48(12): 21–243.

Centers for Disease Control and Prevention (http://www.cdc.gov).

Fairbanks, J., and W. Wiese. 1998. *The public health primer*. Thousand Oaks, CA: Sage.

Health Resources and Services Administration (http://www.hrsa.gov/heritabledisorderscommittee/correspondence/NBStreatmentStatutesRegs.htm).

HealthCare.gov (http://www.healthcare.gov/).

Medical Reserve Corps, (http://www.medicalreservecorps.gov/).

National Institutes of Health (http://www.nih.gov/about/almanac/historical/chronology_of_events.htm).

National Institutes of Health. *A short history of the National Institutes of Health*. (http://www.history.nih.gov/exhibits/history).

Turnock, B. 1997. *Public health: What it is and how it works*. Gaithersburg, MD: Aspen.

UNAIDS: The Joint United Nations Programme on HIV/AIDS (www.unaids.org).

World Health Organization (http://www.who.int/en/).

For Additional Information

Mullan, F. 1989. *Plagues and politics: The story of the United States public health service*. New York: Basic Book.

National Association of County and City Health Officials. 2001. *Local public health agency infrastructure: A chartbook*. Washington, DC: National Association of County and City Health Officials.

Centers for Disease Control and Prevention, Emergency Preparedness and Response (http://www.bt.cdc.gov/).

International Network for the History of Public Health (http://www.liu.se/tema/inhph/).

State and Local Government on the Net (http://www.statelocalgov.net/).

United States Department of Health and Human Services (http://www.hhs.gov).United States General Accounting Office. 2004. *HHS bioterrorism preparedness programs: States reported progress fell short of program goals for 2002*.

Medical Technology, Pharmaceuticals, and Pharmacological Research

Learning Objectives

After reading this chapter, you should be able to:

1. Define medical technology.
2. Discuss the impact of medical technology on modern health care.
3. Identify the ethical issues in new technologies.
4. Discuss the size and scope of the pharmaceutical industry.
5. Explain how a new prescription drug gets to market.
6. Identify how new prescription drugs are marketed.
7. Discuss the ethical issues in pharmaceuticals.

Stem Cells for the Future Treatment of Parkinson's Disease

Parkinson's disease (PD) is a neurodegenerative disorder that affects more than 2 percent of the population older than 65 years. PD is caused by a progressive degeneration and loss of dopamine (DA)-producing neurons, which leads to tremor, rigidity, and hypokinesia (abnormally decreased mobility). It is thought that PD may be the first disease to be amenable to treatment using stem cell transplantation. Factors that support this idea include the knowledge of the specific cell type (DA neurons) needed to relieve the symptoms of the disease. In addition, several laboratories have been successful in developing methods to induce embryonic stem cells to differentiate into cells with many of the functions of DA neurons.

In a recent study, scientists directed mouse embryonic stem cells to differentiate into DA neurons by introducing the gene Nurr1. When transplanted into the brains of a rat model of PD, these stem cell-derived DA neurons reinnervated the brains of the rat Parkinson model, released dopamine, and improved motor function.

Regarding human stem cell therapy, scientists are developing a number of strategies for producing dopamine neurons from human stem cells in the laboratory for transplantation into humans with PD. The successful generation of an unlimited supply of dopamine neurons could make neuro-transplantation widely available for Parkinson's patients at some point in the future.

Source: http://stemcells.nih.gov/info/basics/

Introduction

technology
The application of knowledge based on inventions, innovations and discoveries in science

medical technology
Therapeutic and diagnostic devices used to prevent, treat, diagnose, and assist patients medically. The X-ray machine is an example of medical technology.

pharmaceuticals
Bioactive agents in the human body for therapeutic purposes (e.g., antibiotics).

Medical technology and pharmaceuticals are an increasingly important and expensive part of modern health care. **Technology** is the application of knowledge based on inventions, innovations, and discoveries in science. Table 11.1 presents a picture of technological advances in health care from the 1800s to the present. Just as Pasteur's proof that microorganisms cause disease fundamentally changed the ways physicians treated patients in the 19th century, today's technological advances have changed who treats patients, how health care professionals are trained, how they interact with patients, and health care economics.

This chapter addresses advances in medical technology and in the pharmaceutical industry. **Medical technology** in this chapter means those therapeutic and diagnostic devices used by health professionals to prevent, treat, and diagnose illness and assist patients medically. This includes everything from ordinary items such as stethoscopes and blood pressure monitors to the latest in imaging machines and *in vitro* diagnostic tests. **Pharmaceuticals** are the research, production, marketing, and dispensing of agents (drugs, genes, molecules, etc.) that are bioactive in the human body for therapeutic purposes. Each of these has produced global industries and impacts the delivery of health care.

Medical Technology

medical devices The range of medical technologies that are used for therapeutic purposes such as cardiac pacemakers and thermometers

Medical technology is a growth area of health care, from both a business perspective and delivery perspective. According to the Annual Survey of Manufacturers, production of **medical devices** and diagnostics was valued at $135.9 billion in 2008, about 6 percent of the total revenues for the health care industry. The industry employs about 423,000 people, with a total payroll of $24.6 billion (Lewin Group 2010). Industry components are presented in Table 11.2. The surgical supplies and instruments categories

Table 11.1	*Technological Advances in Health Care*

1819	René Laennec invents the stethoscope
1846	American dentist Dr. William Morton uses ether as anesthetic
1847	Dr. James Simpson uses chloroform as anesthetic
1879	Louis Pasteur proves microorganisms cause disease
1865	Joseph Lister uses disinfectants and antiseptics during surgery to prevent infection
1892	Dimitri Ivanovski discovers viruses
1895	Wilhelm Roentgen discovers X-rays (roentgenograms)
1896	Almroth Wright develops vaccine for typhoid fever
1901	Carl Landsteiner classifies ABO blood groups
1923	Frederick Banting and Charles Best discover and use insulin to treat diabetes
1932	Sir Alexander Fleming discovers penicillin
1944	First kidney dialysis machine is developed
1952	Jonas Salk develops polio vaccine
1953	Francis Crick and James Watson describe the structure of DNA
	First heart-lung machine is used for open-heart surgery
1954	Joseph Murray performs first successful human kidney transplant
1960	Birth control pills are approved by the FDA
1963	Thomas Starzl performs first liver transplant
1964	James Hardy performs first lung transplant
1968	Christian Barnard performs first successful heart transplant
1975	CT (computerized axial tomography) scan is developed
1980s	Vaccines against hepatitis, herpes simplex, and chicken pox are developed with genetic engineering
1981	AIDS (acquired immune deficiency syndrome) is identified as a disease
1987	First laser surgery on human cornea
1990	First gene therapy is developed to treat disease
1990s	Rapid increase in identification of genes causing disease occurs
1995	Lasik eye surgery approved by FDA
2000	First robotic system for general laparoscopic surgery approved by FDA
2001	RNAi: RNA interference is a process to deactivate selected genes
2003	Drug-eluting stent for clogged arteries approved by FDA
2006	First vaccine to protect against cervical cancer
2008	Commercial hybrid PET/MRI scanner produced

Source: Bryan 1996 and *Chartbook* 2009, Figure 23.

account for more than 50 percent of the industry's sales, which means that every visit to an office, clinic, or hospital is impacted by the medical technology industry.

Medical technology is an innovative industry. The industry invests about 11 percent of sales in **research and development (R&D)**. By comparison, the auto industry invests 4 percent and the aerospace industry invests 3 percent. Because companies rigorously protect their investments, there is considerable patent litigation concerning medical technology.

research and development (R&D)
The process of examining and bringing a product to market.

Although there continue to be advances and major breakthroughs daily, the last 20 years have seen advances in four areas that have made enormous differences in health care outcomes. These four areas are medical devices, medical imaging, minimally invasive surgery, and genetic mapping and testing.

Table 11.2	*Medical Technology Industry*		
Sector Payroll	Revenue ($ billion)	Employees (# in 1,000s)	Annual ($billion)
Surgical appliance/supplies manufacturing	35.3	114.5	35.3
Surgical/medical instrument manufacturing	33.6	109.3	6.2
Electromedical/therapeutic apparatus manufacturing	27.6	65.3	4.8
In vitro diagnostic substance manufacturing	12.7	27.0	2.2
Irradiation apparatus manufacturing	11.6	16.8	1.5
Ophthalmic goods manufacturing	5.8	23.5	1.0
Dental laboratories	4.7	50.0	1.8
Dental Equipment/supplies manufacturing	4.7	16.3	0.8
Industry TOTAL	136.1	422.8	24.6

Source: Adapted from Lewin Group 2010, Exhibit 1, and 2008 Annual Survey of Manufacturers.

Medical Devices

Medical devices cover a wide range of technologies from medical implants (cardiac pacemakers) to fetal or heart monitors to a simple manual blood pressure cuff. The modern hospital utilizes hundreds, perhaps thousands, of medical devices. The stock of many medical device companies is publicly traded on the New York Stock Exchange, an indication of the profitability of this segment of the health care industry.

implants Medical devices that are placed inside the human body for therapeutic purposes, such as an insulin pump or artificial knee joint.

Implants are one part of this growing medical device sector. Cardiac pacemakers are just one of many implantable devices designed to enhance or replace injured or nonfunctioning tissue. Others include bionic limbs, eyes, cochlear ear implants, nerve stimulators, medication pumps (insulin and pain medication), and whole organs such as the heart.

medical imaging Viewing the inside of the human body using a variety of techniques such as X-rays and CT scans.

These devices have the potential to dramatically improve the quality of life. And once the new technology is developed, physicians and patients want to use it. This is creating a huge technology divide between the insured and uninsured population. Those who can afford these devices experience a much improved quality of life with far less morbidity (Jacobs 1999).

CAT scans (computer axial tomography) Machine that visualizes the inside of the human body using a combination of X-ray technology and computerized axial tomography; results are viewed on the computer.

Medical Imaging

Medical imaging includes a wide variety of techniques to provide visual images of the inside of the body. Nothing since the invention of the X-ray has changed medical diagnosis as much as the computer. New computer-enhanced tools allow us not only to visualize what is going on inside the body but to watch body processes in real time. This technology will continue to advance rapidly as computer capability increases and the tools to visualize at a molecular level are developed. These new tools will improve the diagnostic ability of the physician but will come at a high economic cost.

magnetic resonance imaging (MRI) Technology that uses electromagnetic radiation to visualize the body's soft tissues, such as the brain and spinal cord.

A number of different energy sources are currently used for medical imaging. These include traditional X-rays, **CAT scans (computer axial tomography)**, ultrasound, electron beams, positrons, and magnets and radio frequencies (**magnetic resonance imaging**, or **MRI**). As these sources are combined with improved contrast materials and improved computer displays, the ability to diagnose abnormalities and to study the body functions will be vastly enhanced. This will in turn lead to even more sophisticated imaging than currently possible.

For example, instead of using the traditional X-ray, **electron beam computer tomography** can be used. This technology creates images using electrons instead of X-rays. Patient care is improved by reducing the time and discomfort a patient experiences being immobile and confined for a conventional CT scan. Patients and health care payers will have to decide whether the benefit outweighs the increased cost.

Minimally Invasive Surgery

Minimally invasive surgery refers to the use of fiberoptics, guided images, microwave, laser, high-intensity focused ultrasound, cryotherapy, and the newest addition—radiofrequency—to do operations without the traditional open surgery. Through the use of miniature cameras, image-guided surgery now makes possible the intraorgan repair of tissue. In the past, the patient would have to undergo major open surgery with ribs, cartilage, muscle, and soft tissue being disturbed, cut, or removed. Now single or multiple scopes are inserted through small openings, and whole organs are then removed, explored, or repaired. It is even possible to perform surgery on the fetus using intrauterine technology to repair heart and spinal defects before birth.

The techniques for thermal destruction of tissue began with **electrocautery** for small-size tissue like blood vessels. The field has progressed to microwave therapy and destruction of tumors using laparoscopic techniques combined with thermal technology. Until recently, the technique could not be used for large tumors because a large mass of tissue could not be heated. The use of **radio frequency ablation (RFA)** overcame that limitation; RFA is being used safely for tumors of the liver, heart, kidney, and more (http://www.cc.nih.gov/drd/rfa/background.html/).

Other forms of less invasive surgery combine thermal, radio frequencies, and mechanical ablation with fiberoptic visualization. The recovery times have decreased from several months to days. Although the medical devices to achieve these results are very expensive, the cost in terms of patient outcome and loss of work productivity has been lowered. This leads to recommendation for some types of surgery as both therapeutic and preventative (e.g., in the case of cardiac angioplasty). Indications for surgery have changed in the light of the recent developments in less invasive techniques.

Genetic Mapping and Testing

The **Human Genome Project** has provided the driving force behind the explosion of genetic testing possibilities. Geneticists have been able to predict the possibility of genetic disease in a few special circumstances like Huntington's chorea for a long time. Now genetic mapping has given practitioners valuable early information about the possibility of delivering a baby with certain diseases like Down syndrome or Tay-Sachs disease. Genetic mapping can also trace familial history in diseases such as hemophilia. The ability to test for common diseases and disease predisposition and susceptibility for more and more diseases and chronic conditions is becoming available as researchers use the information provided by the Human Genome Project. This will ultimately lead to information about the causes of certain diseases. Even now we have valuable information about the relationship between certain genes and a greater predisposition or susceptibility to disease.

A good example is breast cancer. We now know that women with the genes BRCA1 and/or BRCA2 have a higher probability of getting breast cancer than those women who do not have these genes. Each year more than 192,000 women learn they have breast cancer; 5 percent to 10 percent of those have the hereditary form of breast cancer. According to estimates of lifetime risk, about 13.2 percent (132 out of 1,000 individuals)

---

electron beam computer tomography Uses electron beams instead of X-rays for computerized axial tomography and also viewed on computer. Compared with the traditional CT scan, it does not require the patient to be completely still, is less enclosed, and costs more.

minimally invasive surgery Use of fiber optics, guided images, microwave and other technologies to do surgery rather than cutting large sections of tissue.

electrocautery The process of destroying tissue by an electrically heated instrument.

radio frequency ablation (RFA) Uses microwaves to destroy tissue.

Human Genome Project An international cooperative scientific project to map the 60,000 human genes that make up the human genetic code.

of women in the general population will develop breast cancer, compared with estimates of 36 percent to 85 percent (360 to 850 out of 1,000) women with an altered BRCA1 or BRCA2 gene. In other words, women with an altered BRCA1 or BRCA2 gene are three to seven times more likely to develop breast cancer than women without alterations in those genes. Women with the genes BRCA1 and/or BRCA2 also have a higher probability of getting ovarian cancer. Lifetime risk estimates of ovarian cancer for women in the general population indicate that 1.7 percent (17 out of 1,000) will get ovarian cancer, compared with 16 percent to 60 percent (160 to 600 out of 1,000) of women with altered BRCA1 or BRCA2 genes (http://www.cancer.gov/cancertopics/types/breast).

Approximately 500 human genetic diseases can currently be identified by genetic testing. The ability to test for the predisposition to a disease raises important ethical concerns. Insurers would like very much to know who may get a specific disease—it would mean much less risk if the industry could deny insurance to someone on the basis of genetic testing (Jeffrey 1999; Langreth 1999). It may be important to people contemplating marriage or business partnerships to know if partners test positive for a specific genetic disease. For the individual, knowing what disease potential he or she has inherited may alter life decisions. In short, genetic testing may result in genetic discrimination. The Task Force on Genetic Testing was created by the National Institutes of Health (www.nih.gov) to study the medical, legal, and ethical issues raised by genetic testing.

Gene Therapy

gene therapy The treatment of disease using normal or altered genes to replace or enhance nonfunctional or missing genes.

Gene therapy is a technique for correcting defective genes responsible for disease development. Stem cell therapies, DNA manipulation, genetic alteration through introduction of vector virus, and the repair, replacement, and translocation of genetic material are all covered in this definition. Although to date (2010) there are no FDA-approved gene therapies, there is ongoing clinical research on both animals and humans.

Researchers may use one of several approaches for correcting faulty genes. The most common approach is to insert a normal gene to replace a nonfunctional gene. This is the line of research currently being focused on for type 1 diabetes and Parkinson's disease. Another approach is to swap an abnormal gene for a normal gene through

recombination The genetic process of new gene combinations that gives rise to offspring that have a combination of genes different from those of either parent.

recombination. Selective reverse mutation may allow the repair of an abnormal gene, returning it to normal function. The regulation (the degree to which a gene is turned on or off) of a particular gene could be altered. Gene therapy works by using a carrier molecule, called a vector, to deliver the normal gene to the cells. The most common vector is a virus. The virus is introduced to a target organ like the liver where it injects the new DNA material, theoretically repairing or replacing the defective gene.

As of February 1998, 200 therapeutic protocols for gene therapy had been formally reviewed by the Human Genome Program: 23 dealing with HIV infection or AIDS; 33 with single-gene diseases, especially cystic fibrosis; 138 with cancer; and 6 with other diseases (Human Genome Program 1998). Because of several reports of the introduction of leukemia-type diseases with the introduction of viral vectors, human research was halted in 2003. Genetic therapy research is continuing in several other areas, and discussions are under way to allow the viral vector studies to continue with appropriate safeguards. But the deaths of two patients in France and one in the United States underscore the fact that genetic therapy is not without substantial risks.

The safety issues in gene therapy are one aspect of the ethical debate. There are several other serious ethical issues in genetic therapy that are complex and involve the way human beings are defined as normal or abnormal. Serious questions have also been raised about the cost of gene therapy and how affordability will restrict access to the therapy.

None of the questions have been adequately answered. Much more study and research into the bioethics of gene therapy must be done. The U.S. Department of Energy (DOE) and the National Institutes of Health (NIH) have devoted 3 percent to 5 percent of their annual Human Genome Project (HGP) budgets toward studying the ethical, legal, and social issues (ELSI) surrounding the availability of genetic information. This represents the world's largest bioethics program, which has become a model for **ELSI programs** around the world (http://www.ornl.gov/sci/techresources/Human_Genome/elsi/elsi.shtml).

ELSI programs
Programs around the world that study the ethical, legal, and social aspects of the availability of genetic information.

Cost/Benefit Analysis

The ability to compare patient outcomes with both the specific costs of equipment and training and overall costs of treatment is a vital part of health care economics and policy. The shorthand way of talking about this comparison is a **cost/benefit analysis.** In many countries, a new technology undergoes a formal cost/benefit analysis before being adopted by health care professionals.

cost/benefit analysis
The process of comparing the specific costs of a treatment to the benefits obtained by that treatment.

In the United States, the development of new technology is market driven. A survey of medical technology companies indicates that their ability to develop new products is influenced by FDA requirements and by the availability of insurance coverage for the use of the new technology (AdvaMed 2004). However, the lure of that $135 billion market is strong.

On the surface, advanced technology seems like a very expensive way to provide health care. But is it really? In one possible scenario, the new technology can improve individual patient outcomes that make the overall price of the advance to society lower. The second possible scenario is that the use of advanced technology increases the price of care with no improvement of outcomes for patients.

Several examples illustrate these scenarios. The use of laparoscopy surgery has in most cases reduced the overall cost of the procedure by decreasing the hospitalization time from 3 to 7 days down to 1 to 2 days. The cost of the equipment and special training of the physicians and operating room staff is compensated for by the shorter stays. In particular, the overall cost of repair of torn knee cartilage—anterior cruciate ligament repair—using laparoscopic techniques is 75 percent less than the tradition method of repair. However, some of this savings have been possible because the patient now bears a greater burden for postoperative care and rehabilitation. What was once done in the hospital before the patient was discharged is now done at home (Henderson 2005).

In another example, the cost of treating childhood earaches has increased in the last two decades with no significant change in outcomes (Follard, Goodman, and Stano 2004). More consistent application of cost/benefit analysis would help determine if the new technology was really worth it.

Pharmaceuticals

Pharmaceuticals play a key role in modern medicine. The modern drug industry has researched millions of substances looking for new drugs to cure old diseases. Drugs have been used and distributed for thousands of years. Evidence of healing compounds has been found in the archeological remains of most civilizations. The current pharmaceutical industry began with the discovery of insulin in 1920, the beginning of antibiotics with sulfa and penicillin in the 1930s, and the polio vaccine in the 1950s. It would be hard to imagine life today without the many drugs that save and enhance lives. The other side of the life-saving coin, however, is people spending their life savings for those very drugs.

Picture of an Industry

prescription drug
A drug that must have a health care provider's written order (prescription) to be dispensed.

generic drug A drug sold or dispensed under a name that is not protected by a trademark, usually a chemical name or description (e.g., acetaminophen instead of Tylenol).

over-the-counter (OTC) Drugs and medical devices that may be sold without a written health care providers order. Aspirin and crutches are examples.

Three major types of drugs produced can broadly categorize the pharmaceutical industry: prescription, generic, and over-the-counter (OTC). **Prescription drugs** are those available when a physician prescribes them for a patient and a pharmacist fills the prescription. Because the manufacturer of the drug holds a patent on the drug that gives the manufacturer the sole right to produce that drug, the sale of prescription drugs is enormously profitable. In fact, manufacturers rely on their so-called blockbuster drugs for as much as 45 percent of their company profits.

Generic drugs are those drugs that no longer have patent protection; therefore, any company can manufacture essentially the same drug under its company name. Generics are generally much cheaper than a brand-name alternative. **Over-the-counter (OTC)** medications are those that consumers can buy for themselves without a prescription, and they include both brand name and generic equivalents. Examples are Tagamet (cimetidine), Benadryl, cortisone topical ointment, and Motrin. Many prescription drugs are also available in an OTC form.

To bring a prescription drug to market, three major functions occur in a pharmaceutical company: research and development (R&D), production, and sales and marketing. In the R&D function, scientists work to develop new drugs (the complete process is described later in the chapter). Most of these researchers are highly trained, holding PhDs or MDs, and companies invest in additional training so that their researchers stay current in their fields. In 2009, companies spent an estimated $65.3 billion on R&D, reinvesting 16 percent of sales revenue into this critical activity (Pharmaceutical Research and Manufacturers of America <PhRMA> 2010). As the R&D process identifies candidates for potential drugs, the production function begins to analyze whether the drug can be produced in sufficient quantity and quality to be profitable. Many of the personnel involved in this function have engineering backgrounds. The sales and marketing function designs a strategy to get the word out about the drug. Specific strategies are discussed later in the chapter. Companies recruit sales representatives with bachelor's degrees in the sciences and then extensively train them about the company's products.

According to data from the Centers for Medicare and Medicaid, the United States spent $227 billion on prescriptions in 2007; Medicare/Medicaid picked up $70 billion of that (U.S. Census Bureau 2010). This level of spending translates into an industry that is extremely profitable. Table 11.3 describes the largest pharmaceutical companies. According to the **Fortune Global 500**, the global pharmaceutical industry was the 27th most profitable. The top companies remain the same, although their exact rankings vary from year to year (Fortune 2009).

Fortune Global 500
The top earning 500 companies globally as listed by *Fortune* magazine.

All of these companies are publicly traded and must file quarterly reports, known as 10-ks, with the Securities and Exchange Commission. The reports are available online and provide significant disclosure of the company's financials.

Industry Regulation

The pharmaceutical industry is one of the most heavily regulated industries in the United States. The Food and Drug Act of 1906 was passed in response to public

Table 11.3	Largest Pharmaceutical Companies 2008			
Company (Country)	Sales	R&D Spending	Profits	Employees
Johnson & Johnson (USA)	63.7	6.9	12.3	118.7
Pfizer (USA)	48.3	8.6	8.6	81.8
GlaxoSmithKline (UK)	44.7	6.4	8.6	99.0
Roche Group (SVZ)	44.3	14.7	8.3	80.1
Sanofi-Aventis (FR)	42.2	5.5	7.4	98.2
Novartis (SVZ)	41.5	7.5	8.4	96.7
AstraZeneca (UK)	31.6	4.4	7.5	65.0
Abbott Labs (USA)	29.5	2.7	5.7	68.8
Merck (USA)	23.8	5.8	12.9	55.2
Wyeth (USA)	22.8	NA	4.4	47.4
Bristol-Myers Squibb (USA)	21.4	3.6	10.6	35.0
Eli Lilly (USA)	20.4	NA	(2.1)	40.5

Source: Global 500, Pharmaceuticals, *Fortune*, July 20, 2009, and company reports
Note: Sales, R&D, and Profits in $billions; Employees in 1,000s.

outcry against dangerous food additives and drugs. The act did not require testing or safety, only that drugs and food additions be labeled with their major ingredient. In 1938, the federal Food, Drug and Cosmetic Act began requiring testing for safety. The act left the responsibility for the testing to the drug companies, requiring only reporting of testing. It was not until 1959 and the Kefauver Senate hearings on the questionable practices of drug companies that further legislation was introduced.

The thalidomide tragedy occurred shortly after these hearings. Thalidomide was a tranquilizer used in early pregnancy to control nausea and vomiting. It was widely used in Europe prior to its introduction to the United States. Soon there were reports of severe birth defects. The drug was available for experimental use in the United States. The FDA withdrew approval for the drug but not before some children were born with these defects.

In response to the tragedy, in 1962 Congress passed amendments to the 1938 Act to give much more control to the FDA over the introduction of new products. The new powers required more extensive testing of new drugs and controlled the pre-market distribution of new drugs more tightly. The process for new drug distribution has become a multistage process that takes a number of years and is quite expensive. In addition, the FDA also has the authority to regulate drug advertising.

Getting a New Drug to Market

The road from a molecule discovered in a plant or animal to a marketable drug is a long one. Table 11.4 presents the complete process, described in detail next.

Through the new tool of **gene sequencing**, scientists can examine millions of compounds in a year to screen for good ideas or drug leads. Out of these come perhaps 10,000 that are tested; 1,000 of these show bioactivity; of these maybe 100 are worth investigating; from there, 10 go to clinical trails; maybe then one of those millions of compounds ends up as a drug on the shelf.

Once a drug company decides a new drug has potential, it must file an **investigational new drug (IND) application** with the FDA to begin clinical tests on

gene sequencing The process of determining the individual arrangement of nucleotides that compose a given gene. Used extensively in drug research.

investigation new drug (IND) application The notice to the FDA (Food and Drug Administration) that they intend to begin clinical tests on humans.

Table 11.4 *The Drug Development Process*

Stage of Development	No. Compounds	Years	R&D costs	No. Employees
Drug discovery	Millions	5	$12.8 billion	26,113
Preclinical	250	1.5	to IND	
IND (investigational new drug) application submitted to FDA				
Clinical trials				
Phase I	1–5	2–10	$3.9 billion	6,409
Phase II		total for	6.1 billion	9,526
Phase III		trials	15.4	21,356
NDA (New Drug Application) submitted to FDA				
FDA review	1 drug approved	2	$2.2 billion	5,025
Large-scale				
manufacturing Phase IV		2	$6.8 billion	11,739

Source: R&D expenditures and employees based on 2010 member survey of PhRMA (Pharmaceutical Research and Manufacturers of America).

human subjects. The three phases of clinical tests are designed to answer three primary questions:

1. Is the new drug safe?
2. Does it work?
3. Is it better than the standard treatment already in place?

Scientists who want to test drugs on people to answer these questions must follow strict rules to make sure that the drug is as safe as possible. The NIH Web site provides the information that volunteers must receive before they are selected for a **clinical trial** (www.nih.gov). The clinical trial is designed and then must be approved by an **Institutional Review Board (IRB)**. These boards review all human experimentation. The volunteers must give informed consent and sign a form that says they understand the risks and benefits of the study.

To this point, the process has taken several years. The three-phase testing process required by the FDA can now begin and will take several more years to complete. Currently hundreds of drugs are in process. Table 11.5 shows a number of drugs either in clinical trials or awaiting FDA approval.

Phase I tests the drug to figure out what happens to the drug in the body. How is the drug absorbed, metabolized, and excreted? Blood, urine, and timing tests are done on the volunteers; there may be as few as a dozen or as many as 100. This phase takes several months. If there are no serious adverse effects, then after review, the next phase begins.

Phase II studies whether the drug produces the desired effect. For example, does it stop the pain of a migraine or reduce the size of a tumor? This phase may take several years and involves several hundred patients. Patients are carefully monitored for both the desired effect and side effects such as nausea, headaches, or heart irregularities.

Tests in Phase II and III are often conducted in **blind random trials.** The volunteers do not know whether they are receiving the drug, a placebo, or the standard treatment. Neither does the physician who examines the volunteers. This type of trial prevents preconceptions from biasing the results.

clinical trial The process of testing a new drug, treatment, or medical device on humans in a controlled manner.

Institutional Review Board (IRB) The group of people appointed by the government or a university to oversee any research on animals or humans.

blind random trials A clinical trial method in which no one knows which drugs the participants are receiving until the trial is finished.

Table 11.5 *Drugs in the Pipeline for Human Use*	
Therapeutic Category & Examples	**No. of Products**
Autoimmune & Inflammatory Diseases (Allergy, Graft Versus Host Disease, Lupus, Rheumatoid Arthritis)	1,105
Blood and Lymphatic Diseases (Anemia, Hemophilia, Thrombocythaemia)	415
Cardiovascular & Circulatory Disorders (Congestive Heart Failure, Angina Pectoris, Atherosclerosis)	846
Cancer (Leukemia, Colorectal Cancer, Small Cell Lung Cancer, Melanoma)	5,390
Central Nervous System (Alzheimer's Disease, Parkinson's Disease, Depression, epilepsy)	2,080
Dental (Caries, Dental Implant Systems, Dental Pain)	35
Dermatology (Psoriasis, Acne, Diabetic Ulcers)	530
Digestive System (Duodenal Ulcer, Gastroesophageal Reflux Disease, Ulcerative Colitis)	477
Genetic Diseases (Gaucher's Disease, Mucopolysaccharidosis-I, Turner's Syndrome)	71
Infections (AIDS/HIV, Bacterial Infections,Hepatitis)	1,843
Kidneys & Genito-Urinary System (Urinary Incontinence, Nephritis, Erectile Dysfunction)	308
Metabolic/Endocrinology Disorders (Diabetes, Growth Hormone Deficiency, Acromegaly)	865
Musculoskeletal Disorders (Bone Diseases, Muscle Pain, Osteopetrosis)	335
Ophthalmology (Cataract, Choroidal Neovascularization (CNV), CMV Retinitis)	488
Respiratory Disorders (Asthma, Chronic Obstructive Pulmonary Disease, Respiratory Syncytial Virus (RSV) Infection . . .)	699
Substance Abuse (Alcoholism, Drug Abuse, Methanol Poisoning, Smoking Cessation . . .)	107
Women's Health (Ovarian Cancer, Breast Cancer, Endometriosis, Menopausal Symptoms . . .)	247

Source: www.medtrack.net/research/lstats.asp

Phase III typically lasts several years and involves thousands of patients in different parts of the country. The safety and effectiveness of the drug compared to both the standard treatment and placebos are carefully analyzed and studied. Occasionally a clinical trial is halted and the trial unblinded, if the results indicate either the drug could save lives or there are serious complications.

If all phases go well, the drug company submits a **New Drug Application (NDA)** to the FDA for approval to market the drug. During Phase IV, the FDA continues to monitor the drug. After the drug is on the market, if any problems arise, the manufacturer is required to file adverse incident reports with the FDA. The responsibility of physicians and health care facilities to report is voluntary. The FDA receives between 300,000 and 400,000 reports of possible adverse reactions each year; about 10 percent are actual adverse reactions (Mathews and Abboud 2005).

New Drug Application (NDA) The formal request from the FDA to be allowed to market a new drug.

The FDA can recall a drug when a clear threat to patient safety exists. For example, the anticholesterol drug Baycol was recalled after several patients died from complications caused by the drug. Additional recent recalls are presented in Table 11.6.

The FDA's efforts to protect the public once a drug has been approved have come under increased criticism, particularly after the drugs Vioxx and Celebrex proved problematic. The FDA acknowledges that the current system has limitations. Although the FDA can request manufacturers to conduct follow-up studies, it has no power to enforce that request. Likewise, when the risks and benefits are balanced, the best the FDA can do is to press the manufacturer to change the label and thus advise consumers of the risks (Mathews and Abboud 2005).

Sales and Marketing Efforts

After a drug is approved for market, the drug company must get it into the patient's hands. Typically there are three major ways to market a new drug in the United States. Two strategies target the physicians who prescribe the drug, and one targets patients directly.

The first way to market a new drug is by medical journal and conference reporting on the new drug. This approach is targeted to the physicians who specialize in the disease for which the drug is under investigation. *The New England Journal of Medicine* and *Lancet* (in Great Britain) are examples of juried publications that report on drug research. Reports of the benefits of the drugs in medical journals may begin while the drug is in phase III testing.

The second major tool is personal selling by drug representatives of pharmaceutical companies. Drug representatives call on physicians to solicit their use of the drug. This may be accompanied by free samples of the drugs for patients and literature and promotional material advertising the drug. Many offices never purchase pens or note pads because so many are given away by the drug representatives. Members of the Pharmaceutical Research and Manufacturers of America, an industry trade group, have adopted a voluntary code that governs interactions with

Table 11.6   *Recent Safety-Based Drug Withdrawals*

Drug	Use	Year Approved	Year Withdrawn	Reason
Vioxx	Pain	1999	2004	Cardiovascular risk
Baycol	Cholesterol	1997	2001	Muscle damage; sometimes fatal
Propulsid	Heartburn	1993	2000	Heart rhythm abnormalities; sometimes fatal
Rezulin	Diabetes	1997	2000	Liver toxicity
Duract	Pain	1997	1998	Liver damage
Posicor	Blood pressure	1997	1998	Drug interactions
Redux	Weight loss	1996	1997	Heart valve damage
Seldane	Allergies	1985	1997	Drug interactions; fatal heart rhythm abnormalities

Source: FDA, as reported in Fuhrmans 2005 and Mathews 2004.

health care professionals. Giveaway items that bear a company or product name are allowed if the items "entail a benefit to patients" and "are primarily associated with the health care professional's practice." Although the code allows members to provide informational presentations to health care professionals, the code prohibits entertainment/recreational events, takeout meals, and the inclusion of spouses or guests. Because these codes are voluntary, there is no enforcement mechanism if a member violates the code.

The third way is to reach patients directly by paid advertising. The United States is the only country that allows advertising of prescription drugs. Advertising was confined to the professional journals but is now common in popular magazines like *Newsweek* and *People*. A comprehensive advertising campaign includes television and the Web as well as print ads.

Despite the fact that various universities and government agencies have studied the question, it is unclear whether drug advertising drives up the cost of pharmaceuticals. Only a handful of the most popular drugs are advertised in the popular media, but those have advertising budgets in the millions. Claritin, Lipitor, and Viagra are examples of drugs advertised in popular print and television media. Generic drugs are not advertised. According to surveys of physicians, patients often now ask for drugs by brand name. These drugs are usually more expensive than the lesser-known drugs of the same family.

The FDA regulates direct-to-consumer advertisements of prescription drugs; in addition, the Federal Trade Commission (FTC) regulates truth in advertising generally. The FDA requires that direct-to-consumer advertising be accurate and not misleading, make claims only if supported by substantial evidence, reflect a balance of risks and benefits, and be consistent with FDA-approved labeling (PhRMA 2005).

The Cost of Prescription Drugs

The economic success of pharmaceutical companies and the skyrocketing cost of prescription drugs have caused considerable media attention to be focused on the industry. The data are alarming. The United States pays 50 percent to 75 percent higher drug prices than any place in the world. A prescription drug that would cost $150 in Canada or Australia costs $481 in America even through a managed care plan. One company alone, GlaxoSmithKline, earned $2.3 billion on the sale of the HIV/AIDS drug AZT in 2003. In response to rising prices, many U.S. citizens began obtaining their prescription drugs in Canada beginning in 2002 despite Congress's opposition and claim that the drugs were unsafe (made by the same drug companies that made the American drugs). Although the United States began a prescription discount card benefit for Medicare recipients in 2003, the drug price inflation index rose so fast that the gain that would have occurred was negated by the higher prices.

Cost containment strategies are being used in all countries to try to slow down the upward spiraling of drug costs. The strategies include switching to generic drugs, more cost/benefit analysis, and awareness by practitioners of costs.

The switch to generic drugs instead of brand names is one major way to control costs. The savings to individual state Medicaid budgets by this tactic alone can be up to 5 percent of the total budget. Generic's share of the market has grown from 49 percent in 2000 to 74 percent in 2009 (IMS 2009). The 2010 Patient Protection and Affordable Care Act includes changes to Medicare and Medicaid to cover prescriptions, as well as a number of initiatives to encourage the use of generics.

Another strategy is for independent research facilities to do serious cost/benefit analysis by comparing drugs in the same family to determine if the more you pay, the more you get. Most of these studies have shown that price is not the quality determinant. In one Australian study, the least expensive drug showed no significant difference in patient outcomes among three drugs in the same family for gastric reflux and esophageal reflux. Changing to the least expensive drug that gives a good outcome can save millions of dollars a year.

Finally, health practitioners need to be aware of pricing when prescribing. One National Institutes of Health study demonstrates that physicians rarely ask the patients if they can afford the drug they are prescribing; consequently, patients often do not fill the prescription because they cannot pay for it. For instance, the top-selling drug for gastric reflux, pantoprazole, may cost $541 for a month's supply, whereas a generic pump inhibitor may only cost $100 per month. For a person on a fixed budget, this is the difference between eating or paying the rent and buying the drug. If the physician or nurse practitioner is not sensitive to drug pricing, the patient may not get needed medication. As noted in Chapter 4, changes to Medicare Part D have increased the access of older Americans to prescription medications. Of the 26 million who have enrolled for this benefit, it is estimated that 14 million were previously uninsured or lack coverage for prescriptions (CMS 2009).

Social and Ethical Questions

The high cost of drug therapy not only spurs efforts to contain costs, but raises the issue of whether industry profits are excessive. The industry has argued that patent protection and profitability are the return they receive for the investment they made in the research and production process. Some research indicates that only 20 percent of marketed drugs earn revenues that exceed their R&D costs (Vernon, Golec, and DiMasi 2009). As you have read earlier in this chapter, the process to bring a new prescription drug to market is both long and costly. The industry argues that without patent protection (essentially a short-term monopoly), they would be unable to afford the cost and risks associated with the process. The industry also argues that the price they charge is a way to recover those costs, as well as the legal and financial risks once a drug is available to the market. As many primary patents expire, the drug companies are just now experiencing the pressures of competition. Consumers, the media, and politicians question pricing policies and may not accept the industry's arguments.

There is an urgent need for the increased research and development of new drugs. The emergence of worldwide epidemics such as HIV/AIDS, SARS, avian or bird flu, and West Nile disease requires new vaccines or new antibiotics. The rise in numbers of patients with antibiotic-resistant tuberculosis (TB) and staphylococcus infections are also pharmaceutical emergencies. These conditions have a high mortality rate and are not responding to traditional drug therapy. How should drug companies be reimbursed for the research and development of vaccines and drugs to combat these and new emerging epidemics?

The controversy over HIV/AIDS drugs is only the first in a long line of social and ethical questions about drug therapy. Should millions die because the drugs to treat AIDS are too expensive for most countries, let alone individuals, to afford? The cost for a year of AIDS drugs in the United States is over $40,000, many times over the average annual income worldwide. More than 1 million people in the United States and 40 million worldwide have AIDS. Most of the new cases are in developing nations and minority populations in the developed countries (http://www.niaid.nih.gov/about/organization/daids/).

Many advocate that patents on certain drugs, such as those for AIDS, malaria, and TB, should be cancelled. The research should be available to everyone, following the model of the Human Genome Project. The pricing of drugs that only have a very limited market for distribution for people with rare diseases is another area of concern. The price of the generation of drugs that brings together genetic research and targeted cell response will probably remain high. These and many more questions are issues for those making social policy around the world.

Summary

Medical technology is those therapeutic and diagnostic devices used by health professionals to prevent, treat, and diagnose illness and assist patients medically. Pharmaceuticals are the research, production, marketing, and dispensing of agents (drugs, genes, molecules, etc.) that are bioactive in the human body for therapeutic purposes. Medical technology and pharmaceuticals have had a huge impact on modern health care, both in improving individual patient outcomes and in the increase in spending on health care.

New medical technologies include medical devices such as pacemakers, insulin pumps, new imaging techniques, computer-assisted imaging, new drugs, and genetic mapping and testing. New types of pharmaceuticals will use DNA manipulation and stem cell research. Pharmaceuticals can now target individual receptors and cells.

The pharmaceutical industry is a global industry with a huge financial impact. Companies research millions of possibilities to arrive at one marketable drug. A new drug gets to market through a three-phase testing and research process that may take 10 to 12 years. Ethical issues include the cost of prescription drugs and new medical technologies as well as the decision to research and develop drugs for certain diseases and not for others.

Questions for Review

1. Define the terms and give examples of medical technology and pharmaceuticals.
2. Describe four new medical technologies.
3. What is the difference between prescription, generic, and over-the-counter (OTC) drugs?
4. Describe two ways pharmaceuticals are marketed.
5. Using a flow chart, explain how a new drug gets to market.

Questions for Discussion

1. What is the impact of medical technology and pharmaceuticals on modern health care? Use comparisons in your answer.
2. How is the pharmaceutical industry regulated? Do you believe that this process safeguards the public's health?

3. Do some cost research of your own. Pick a drug, and compare the cost of at least two suppliers. What accounts for the differences?
4. Should patents be available on drugs that can save peoples' lives?
5. Who should decide which medical technologies and which pharmaceuticals are developed?
6. Should stem cell research for diseases like Parkinson's be available scientists all over the world like the Human Genome Project—why/why not?

Chapter References

AdvaMed. 2004. *The medical technology industry at a glance—2004.* Advanced Medical Technology Association. Available at www.advamed.org.

Bryan, J. 1996. *The history of health and medicine: Advances that have changed the world.* Austin, TX: Raintree Steck-Vaughn.

Centers for Disease Control and Prevention (www.cdc.gov).

CDC, Health Statistics. 2009. *Chartbook. Health, United States. Special Feature: Medical Technology.*

Centers for Medicare and Medicaid Services. 2009. *Enrollment Report.*

Follard, S., A. Goodman, and M. Stano. 2004. *The economics of health and health care.* New York: Macmillan.

Fortune. 2009. Global 500, Pharmaceuticals. July 20.

Fuhrmans, V. 2005. Early-warning tool for unsafe drugs. *Wall Street Journal*, April 28, p. D4.

Henderson, J. 2005. *Health economics & policy.* 3rd ed. Mason, OH: Thomson/Southwestern.

Human Genome Program, U.S. Department of Energy. 1998. *Human Genome News* 10 (1–2).

Human Genome Project Information (http://www.ornl.gov/sci/techresources/Human_Genome/elsi/elsi.shtml).

IMS. 2009. *Nation prescription audit.* December.

Jacobs, K. 1999. Left behind: Technology has the potential to narrow the gap between the haves and have-nots—or to widen it. *Wall Street Journal*, October 18, p. R14.

Jeffrey, N. A. 1999. A change in policy: Genetic testing threatens to fundamentally alter the whole notion of insurance. *Wall Street Journal*, October 18, p. R15.

Langreth, R. 1999. Early warnings: Genetic tests will allow people to take steps to delay—or prevent—the occurrence of disease. *Wall Street Journal*, October 18, p. R7.

Lewin Group. 2010. *State economic impact of the medical technology industry.* Available at www.advamed.org.

Mathews, A. 2004. As drug-safety worries grow, looking overseas for solutions. *Wall Street Journal*, December 31, pp. A1, A9.

Mathews, A., and L. Abboud. 2005. New FDA board set up to review approved drugs. *Wall Street Journal*, February 16, p. A1.

National Institute of Allergy and Infectious Disease, National Institutes of Health, Division of Acquired Immunodeficiency Syndrome (www.niaid.nih.gov/daids/).

National Cancer Institute (http://www.cancer.gov/cancertopics/types/breast).

National Institute of Health, Stem Cell Information (http://stemcells.nih.gov/info/basics/).

National Institutes of Health (www.nih.gov).

National Institutes of Health, Clinical Center, Diagnostic Radiology Department (www.cc.nih.gov/drd/).

Oak Ridge National Laboratory (www.ornl.gov/sci/techresources/Human_Genome/elsi/).

Pharmaceutical Research and Manufacturers of America. 2010. *Pharmaceutical industry profile 2010.* Available at www.phrma.org/.

Pharmaceutical Research and Manufacturers of America. 2005. *PhRMA guiding principles: Direct to consumer advertisements about prescription medicines.* August. Available at www.phrma.org/.

U.S. Census Bureau. 2010. *Statistical Abstract*, Tables 131 and 133.

Vernon, J., J. Golec, and J. DiMasi. 2009. Drug development costs when financial risk is measured using the Fama-French three-factor model. *Health Economics Letters.*

For Additional Information

Cassels, C., R. Purtillo, and E. McParland. 2004. Contemporary ethical and social issues in medicine. *2005 Health Affairs* 23(6): 149–56.

Danis, M., C. Clancy, and L. Churchill. 2003. *Ethical dimensions of health policy*. New York: Oxford University Press.

Genetics Home Reference (http://ghr.nlm.nih.gov/).

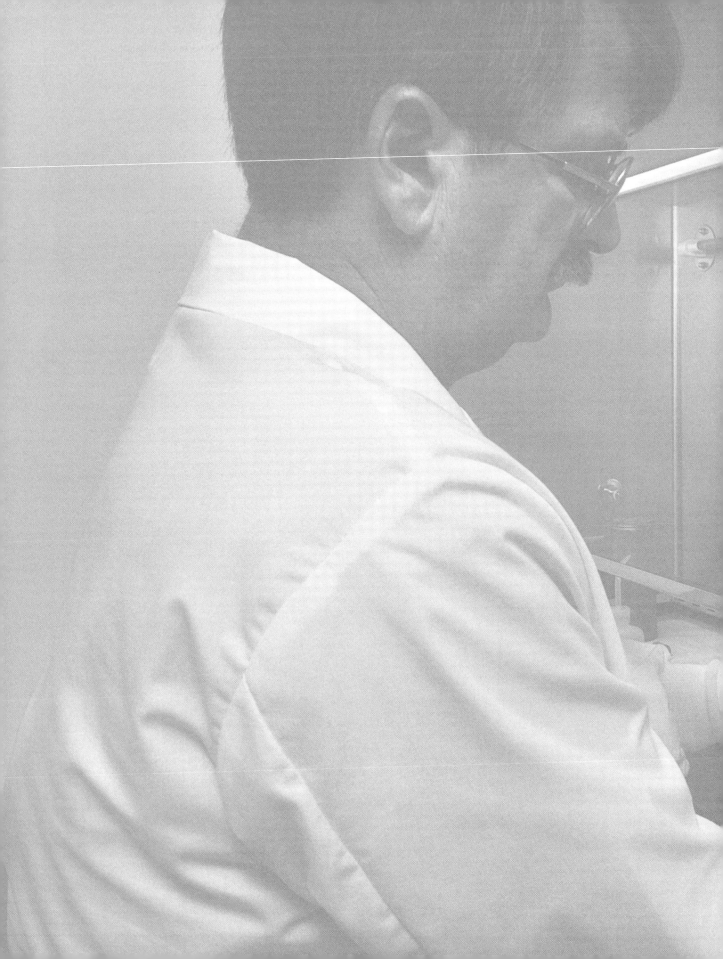

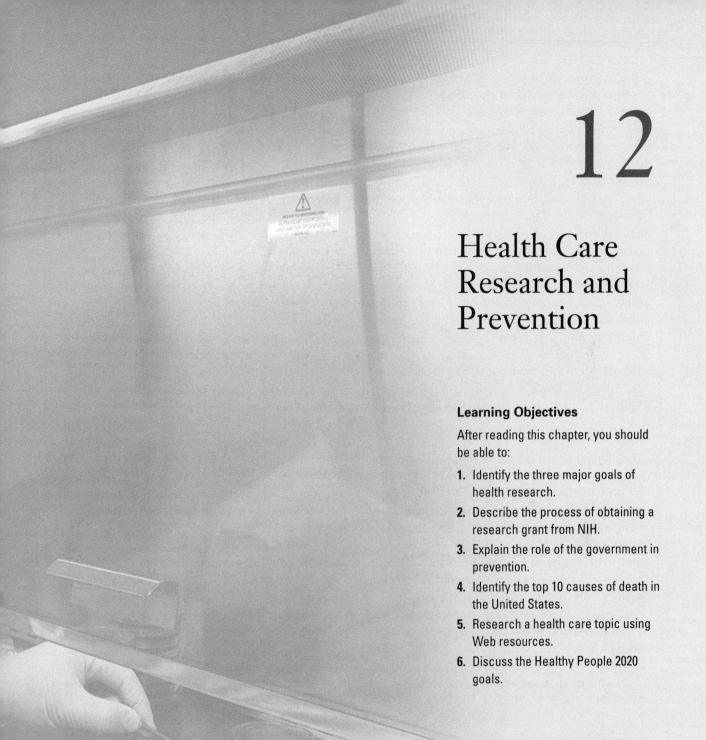

12

Health Care Research and Prevention

Learning Objectives

After reading this chapter, you should be able to:

1. Identify the three major goals of health research.
2. Describe the process of obtaining a research grant from NIH.
3. Explain the role of the government in prevention.
4. Identify the top 10 causes of death in the United States.
5. Research a health care topic using Web resources.
6. Discuss the Healthy People 2020 goals.

Fighting the Flu

One of the types of prevention most of us have practiced is the annual flu shot. This is one of the most common preventive pharmaceuticals in the world. Each year, millions of people line up to be vaccinated for the flu. In 2009, 126 million people were vaccinated against the new H1N1 influenza (www.flu.gov).

The flu or influenza is viral infection caused by a specific virus. The Centers for Disease Control and Prevention (CDC) estimates that 10 percent to 20 percent of Americans come down with the flu during each flu season, which typically lasts from the beginning of November through March. Children are two to three times more likely to than adults to contract the disease and are often the means by which the disease is spread to both other children and adults. The CDC further estimates that 100,000 people are hospitalized and 36,000 people die annually from the flu and its complications. Table 12.1 lists the major pandemics.

The Influenza virus

The influenza virus is wound with eight segments of single-strand RNA inside, which is responsible for copying the virus. When viewed under an electron microscope, the most striking feature of the virus is a layer of spikes projecting from its surface. There are two different types of spikes: one is the protein hemaglutinin HA(H), which allows the virus to stick to a cell and begin infection; the other is a protein called neuraminidase NA(N), which enables newly formed viruses to leave the host cell and infect new cells. These spikes allow the virus to shed or drop from the body of the infected person or animal and easily infect other people or animals.

Depending on their protein composition, influenza viruses are classified as type A, B, or C. Found in many kinds of animals, including chickens, ducks, pigs, whales, and humans, type A is not only the most common flu virus, but the most deadly of the three types. Type A was responsible for the global human pandemics of 1918, 1957, 1968, and 2009/2010, which killed millions of people. The avian, or bird, flu is a type A virus; it kills millions of wild migratory and domestic chickens and ducks, and when it mutates, it causes worldwide human flu epidemics.

Type A viruses are divided into subtypes depending on the host (chicken, duck, etc), the place first found, a laboratory identification number, the year of discovery, the place of origin, and, in parentheses, the surface spikes; the Hong Kong flu of 1997 is thus known as A/Chicken/Hong Kong/G9/97 (H9N2). This scientific notation allows the scientific community to communicate rapidly about which flu is being researched and to identify new strains quickly. This ability to track new viruses is important because the type A virus periodically undergoes sudden and dramatic changes that create new subtypes. Because the change is so sudden, people have no immunity to the new subtypes. Severe epidemics are the result, as in 1918, 1957, 1968, and 2009/2010.

The H1N1 pandemic of 2009 was a type A virus. In April 2009, human infection with a new strain of H1N1 influenza was confirmed in Mexico. Within weeks, human infections spread to the United States, and cases begin occurring in other regions around the world. In the United States, the CDC estimated there were 57 million cases of H1N1 flu between April 2009 and January 2010, with 275,000 people hospitalized and 11,600 deaths in that period. The number of children affected, hospitalized, and died was the highest since the CDC began keeping statistics.

The type B virus causes epidemics, but the disease it produces is milder than those caused by type A. A new vaccine must be developed each year because B viruses have gradual and continuous changes, called **antigenic drift**. Although these changes are not dramatic, they make the new virus unrecognizable to the human immune system. Type C virus has been found in humans, pigs, and dogs (dog flu). This virus causes a mild respiratory infection but does not spark epidemics.

The flu virus has been in the wild aquatic bird population for millions of years and normally does not harm the birds. However, when the virus mutates, it can quickly jump from wild birds to the domestic duck and chicken population. From there, the next step is for the virus to jump species and infect a new host, usually the pig. This is because pigs, ducks, and chickens are frequently found together on domestic farms around the world. Humans, chickens, ducks, and pigs may all carry any one of the three flu viruses. If the pig gets the human and the avian virus together, a genetic exchange takes place and a new virus is formed. This resulting form of the virus may then spread from the pigs to humans and then from humans to humans. In 1997, scientists found the first instance of the avian flu skipping the pig stage and going straight to humans. The severity of the flu is determined by the ability of the virus to be spread from human to human.

The symptoms of the flu don't actually begin until about 4 days after a person has been exposed and infected. During this period and for the first 3 to 4 days after the first symptoms, the person is contagious. Because the person doesn't realize he or she is sick, it is easy to see why the flu spreads so quickly in schools and workplaces. The symptoms usually start quickly with a fever, body aches, chills, dry cough, headache, sore throat, and stuffy nose. The fever is the highest for the first 3 days. The respiratory symptoms may last several weeks, depending on the type of virus. The stomach flu is not influenza. The diagnosis is usually made on the basis of the symptoms and the known extent of the epidemic. Laboratory tests are not often used for routine diagnosis, but they can be used early in the epidemic to determine which type of virus is responsible for the epidemic.

The best way to prevent the flu is to get a flu shot 6 to 8 weeks before the season starts. The yearly flu vaccine is made up of the killed A and B type viruses the scientists feel will most likely be in circulation that year. This determination is made about 9 months before the North American flu season begins in November. The better the tracking of the flu virus, the better the vaccines are against it.

How are the viruses selected to make flu vaccine? The viruses used in making seasonal flu vaccines are chosen each year based on information collected over the previous year about which influenza viruses are spreading and what vaccine viruses would offer the best protection against circulating viruses. Viruses gathered by 130 national influenza centers in 101 countries as well as information on disease trends are further analyzed by the four World Health Organization (WHO) Collaborating Centers for Reference and Research on Influenza located in Atlanta, United States (CDC); London, United Kingdom (National Institute for Medical Research); Melbourne, Australia (Victoria Infectious Diseases Reference Laboratory); and Tokyo, Japan (National Institute for Infectious Diseases). The seasonal flu vaccine is usually a trivalent vaccine (a three-component vaccine) with each component selected to protect against one of the three groups of influenza viruses circulating most commonly in humans. However, the 2009 H1N1 vaccine made to protect against the pandemic virus first detected in April was a monovalent (one-component) vaccine that only protected against the 2009 H1N1 viruses.

In a trivalent vaccine, the three vaccine viruses are chosen to maximize the likelihood that the main circulating viruses during the upcoming flu season will be well covered by the vaccine. WHO recommends specific vaccine viruses for vaccine production, but then each individual country makes its own decision for licensing of vaccines in its country. In the United States, the US Food and Drug Administration (FDA) determines what viruses will be used in U.S.-licensed vaccines.

What flu viruses are included in the seasonal vaccine for 2010-2011? WHO recommended that the Northern Hemisphere's 2010–2011 seasonal influenza vaccine contain the following three vaccine viruses:

an A/California/7/2009 (H1N1)–like virus,

an A/Perth/16/2009 (H3N2)–like virus, and a

B/Brisbane/60/2008–like virus

(http://www.cdc.gov/flu/about/qa/1011_vac_selection.htm).

Even though you have been vaccinated, you may still get the flu; the symptoms are milder in those who have had the shot.

Since 2004, there have been periodic shortages of the vaccine, particularly in 2009 for the H1N1 flu vaccine. Other methods for prevention have been recommended. In 2003, the FDA approved a live virus nasal spray vaccine called FluMist, which can be used for healthy people between the ages of 5 and 49. There are also antiviral medicines available by prescription, such as Tamiflu (oseltamivir), Flumadine (rimantadine), and Symmetrel (amantadine), that will help prevent flu infection if you take them for at least 2 weeks during the outbreak. Rimantadine and amantadine can be used in persons 1 year or older, but oseltamivir is for adults and teenagers 13 years and older. There have been reports of drug resistance to the H1N1 virus.

New research suggests that increased dietary use of whole grains and exercise helps in preventing the flu. Nevertheless, the treatment for the flu has not changed much in the last 50 years. Doctors recommend bed rest, fluids, and acetaminophen for fever and body aches. But prevention is actually the best medicine.

Source: http:www.flu.gov

antigenic drift
Describes the gradual and continuous changes in the genetic make-up of some viruses such as the Type B flu virus.

Table 12.1 *Influenza Timeline*
Appearance of a New Influenza Strain in the Human Population

1918   Pandemic
"Spanish flu" H1N1

The most devastating flu pandemic in recent history, killing more than 500,000 people in the United States, and 20 million to 50 million people worldwide.

1957–58 Pandemic
"Asian flu" H2N2

First identified in China, this virus caused roughly 70,000 deaths in the United States during the 1957–58 season. Because this strain has not circulated in humans since 1968, no one younger than 30 years old has immunity to this strain.

1968–69 Pandemic
"Hong Kong flu" H3N2

First detected in Hong Kong, this virus caused roughly 34,000 deaths in the United States during the 1968–69 season. H3N2 viruses still circulate today.

1977   Appearance of a new influenza strain in humans
"Russian flu" H1N1

Isolated in northern China, this virus was similar to the virus that spread before 1957. For this reason, individuals born before 1957 were generally protected; children and young adults born after that year, however, were not because they had no prior immunity.

1997   Appearance of a new influenza strain in humans
H5N1

The first time an influenza virus was found to be transmitted directly from birds to people, with infections linked to exposure to poultry markets. Eighteen people in Hong Kong were hospitalized, six of whom died.

1999   Appearance of a new influenza strain in humans
H9N2

Caused illness in two children in Hong Kong, with poultry the probable source.

2002   Appearance of a new influenza strain in humans
H7N2

Evidence of infection is found in one person in Virginia following a poultry outbreak.

2003   Appearance of a new influenza strain in humans
H5N1

Caused two Hong Kong family members to be hospitalized after a visit to China, killing one of them, a 33-year-old man. (A third family member died while in China of an undiagnosed respiratory illness.)

H7N7

Eighty-nine people in the Netherlands, most of whom were poultry workers, became ill with eye infections or flu-like symptoms. A veterinarian who visited one of the affected poultry farms died.

H7N2

Caused a person to be hospitalized in New York.

H9N2

Caused illness in one child in Hong Kong.

2004
H5N1

New influenza strain icon Appearance of a new influenza strain in humans

Caused illness in 47 people in Thailand and Vietnam, 34 of whom died. Researchers are especially concerned because this flu strain, which is quite deadly, is becoming endemic in Asia.

H7N3

Is reported for the first time in humans. The strain caused illness in two poultry workers in Canada.

H10N7

Is reported for the first time in humans. It caused illness in two infants in Egypt. One child's father is a poultry merchant.

2005
H5N1

The first case of human infection with H5N1 arises in Cambodia in February. By May, WHO reports four Cambodian cases, all fatal. Indonesia reports its first case, which is fatal, in July. Over the next 3 months, seven cases of laboratory-confirmed H5N1 infection in Indonesia, and four deaths, occur.

On December 30, WHO reports a cumulative total of 142 laboratory-confirmed cases of H5N1 infection worldwide, all in Asia, with 74 deaths. Asian countries in which human infection with H5N1 has been detected: Thailand, Vietnam, Cambodia, Indonesia, and China.

2006
H5N1

In early January, two human cases of H5N1 infection, both fatal, are reported in rural areas of Eastern Turkey, while cases in China continue to spread. As of January 25, China reports a total of 10 cases, with 7 deaths. On January 30, Iraq reports its first case of human H5N1 infection, which was fatal, to WHO.

In March, WHO confirmed seven cases of human H5N1 infection, and five deaths, in Azerbaijan. In April, WHO confirmed four cases of human H5N1 infection, and two fatalities, in Egypt.

In May, WHO confirmed a case of human H5N1 infection in the African nation of Djibouti. This was the first confirmed case in sub-Saharan Africa. Throughout 2006, 115 human cases of H5N1 infection occur, with 79 deaths.

2007
H5N1

In early January, two human cases of H5N1 are confirmed in Indonesia. By the end of 2007, 88 confirmed cases occur in Indonesia, Cambodia, China, Lao People's Democratic Republic, Myanmar, Nigeria, Pakistan, and Vietnam, with 59 deaths.

H7N7

In May, four cases of H7N7 avian influenza were confirmed in the United Kingdom among individuals exposed to infected poultry.

2008
H5N1

On May 28, Bangladesh reports its first case of human H5N1 infection to WHO. By the end of the year, 40 cases are confirmed in Bangladesh, Cambodia, China, Egypt, Indonesia, and Vietnam.

2009
H5N1

On January 7, Indonesia confirmed a new case of human infection with H5N1 influenza. Since that time, new cases have been identified in Egypt, China, Indonesia, and Vietnam.

H1N1

In April, human infection with a new strain of H1N1 influenza is confirmed in Mexico. Within weeks, human infections spread to the United States, and cases begin occurring in other regions around the world.

Source: http://www3.niaid.nih.gov/topics/Flu/Research/Pandemic/TimelineHumanPandemics.htm.

Introduction

Throughout this text, you have learned that the function of the health care industry is to diagnose and treat illness. As indicated in the chapter profile, research and tracking of disease play an important role in being able to control and cure illness. In this chapter, the research side of health care is presented. And because it is better if people don't get sick to begin with, the chapter looks at prevention as an increasingly central health care strategy.

Health Care Research: A Pound of Cure

predisposition
In medicine, a susceptibility to a disease or condition because of hereditary or other factors.

To know what to do to prevent a condition or disease, a person must first know what are the causes, or **predispositions**. That is the job of health care research. Researchers not only find the cures for bacterial diseases like strep throat or bacterial meningitis, but they also learn how to control symptoms and prevent the condition in the first place.

Medical research is conducted in several settings in the United States. Faculty at the major research universities, such as the University of Washington, Harvard University, and the University of Maryland, are one group who conduct research. The research can be government sponsored or supported by funds from private industry or from not-for-profit organizations. Research is also conducted by scientists at the National Institute of Health laboratories, the CDC laboratories, and other research-based public institutions. As you saw in Chapter 11, private industry also conducts research.

Types of Research

curative research
Research whose major aim is to find a cure for a specific disease.

Research can be classified by its goal. Generally, the three goals are cure, control, and prevention. **Curative research** is designed to eliminate a disease altogether. This type of research may be either done through physical treatments or pharmaceuticals. Physical treatments include various surgical procedures, such as those that either eliminate tumors or correct abnormalities. Correction of congenital heart abnormalities is an ongoing type of curative surgical research. The use of laser robotic surgery for organ removal such as a hysterectomy is another example of current surgical research.

Curative research can focus on the use of pharmaceuticals such as antibiotics that eliminate disease. Antibiotics are very good at eliminating bacterial disease and one of the few areas where medication alone can cure a disease. A current subject of curative pharmaceutical research is macular degeneration, a vision problem that causes loss of sight in the center of the visual field through destruction of the retina. There are two types of macular degeneration, dry and wet. Dry is the most common form; as of yet there is no cure, only minimal control by vitamins and minerals. However, there is new curative treatment for macular degeneration. Three new drugs, Avastin, Lucentis, and Macugen, are being tested. As of 2010, all were in various stages of clinical testing and have caused reversal of the blindness in the early stages (http://clinicaltrials.gov/ct2/results?cond=%22Macular+Degeneration%22).

control research
Research whose major aim is to control symptoms, not cure the disease or condition. Pain medications control the symptoms of arthritis; they do not cure the underlying disease.

A second type of research is **control research**, designed to reduce the symptoms or severity of the disease. Chemotherapy, heart medications, and thyroid hormone are three examples of controlling diseases. Chemotherapy combined with other treatments may reduce or eliminate the cancer from a body, but often control of the disease process is the major goal. Heart medications control the rate and strength of the heartbeat to improve the person's quality of life, but they do not cure heart disease. Thyroid hormone is given to replace the body's own when the thyroid ceases to function effectively. Although it mimics the original glandular function, it does not cure the processes that destroyed the thyroid or cause it to regenerate. These three treatments are results of research where the goal was to control a process, not cure it. The goal of stem cell and human genome research is to be able to regenerate tissue and make unnecessary the use of thyroid, insulin, antidepressives, and other medications that only control diseases. The ambition is to cure the condition with genetic manipulation.

The third type of research is **prevention research**, which looks for the causes of a condition or disease and then tries to determine how to keep it from happening. Prevention research can focus on any of four phases. In the first phase, it must be determined what diseases and conditions affect the population. Epidemiologists identify and track diseases. This is the primary responsibility of the CDC. In the second phase, the **vector**, or causative agent, for the diseases is identified. Once what causes the disease is known, the vector can be eliminated or controlled. For example, mosquitoes are the vector for malaria, West Nile disease, and many others. If mosquitoes are eradicated, no more malaria. The third phase is to find the predisposing factors that put a person at risk for a disease. These include genetic predispositions (inherited diseases), environmental factors (contaminated water, soil, air), and personal behaviors (e.g., unprotected sex, skydiving, or smoking). The fourth phase is the identification of agents, actions, and behaviors that will most likely prevent the condition. The other three phases have determined that the nicotine and tar in cigarettes cause certain types of lung cancer and predispose the individual to atherosclerosis. The pressing question is how to get people either never to smoke or never to stop smoking. After 25 years of research on this subject, the rate of smoking in the late teens and early 20s has dropped by only a few percentage points. Getting large numbers of people to adopt healthy lifestyles is a major area of preventive research.

prevention research Research whose major aim is to find ways to prevent a disease or condition. For example, preventive research found that diet, exercise, and certain drugs like aspirin may prevent a second heart attack.

vector An organism that transmits disease-causing microbes from infected individuals to other persons or from infected animals to human beings. Fleas were the vectors from rats to people in the great plagues.

Funding and the Grant Process

In the United States, the federal government's expenditures for health care research are about $30.5 billion a year (http://www.nih.gov/about/budget.htm). This does not include the amount spent by state governments in matching grants or state research priorities. Pharmaceutical companies spend approximately the same amount of money in research to generate new drugs each year as the total U.S. government research budget for all types of health care research.

Much more money is spent on the cure and control of disease than on the prevention of disease in the first place. With the ever-increasing cost of health care, this needs to change. Healthy lifestyle behaviors could save billions of dollars each year. It costs much less to give all pregnant women prenatal care than it does to care for one baby with multiple-system problems because the mother did not get prenatal folic acid or had undiagnosed gestational diabetes or toxemia.

Through the Department of Health and Human Services (DHHS), the U.S. government is the largest health research organization in the world. The DHHS oversees 12 different agencies, each of which does some aspect of health care research (see Table 12.2).

When scientists have an idea they wish to investigate, the first step is to apply for a research grant to the appropriate agency. Identifying the appropriate agency is not as easy as it seems. For instance, the National Institutes for Health (NIH) alone has 25 different centers. Each center does both primary research on the area of interest and all of the types of prevention and health outcomes research (see Table 12.3). The NIH

Table 12.2	*Departments of Health and Human Services*

Administration for Children and Families
Administration on Aging
Food and Drug Administration
Health Resources and Services Administration
Centers for Medicare and Medicaid Services
Agency for Healthcare Research and Quality
Indian Health Services
National Institutes of Health
Centers for Disease Control and Prevention
Agency for Toxic Substances and Disease Registry
Substance Abuse and Mental Health Services Administration
Program Support Center

Table 12.3	*National Institutes of Health* (Web sites)

Center of Women's Health	www.4women.gov
National Cancer Institute (NCI)	www.cancer.gov
National Eye Institute (NEI)	www.nei.nih.gov
National Heart, Lung, and Blood Institute (NHLBI)	www.nhlbi.nih.gov
National Human Genome Research Institute (NHGRI)	www.genome.gov
National Institute on Aging (NIA)	www.nia.nih.gov
National Institute on Alcohol Abuse and Alcoholism (NIAAA)	www.niaaa.nih.gov
National Institute of Allergy and Infectious Diseases (NIAID)	www.niaid.nih.gov
National Institute of Arthritis and Musculoskeletal and Skin Diseases (NIAMS)	www.niams.nih.gov
National Institute of Biomedical Imaging and Bioengineering (NIBIB)	www.nibib2.nih.gov
National Institute of Child Health and Human Development (NICHD)	www.nichd.nih.gov
National Institute on Deafness and Other Communication Disorders (NIDCD)	www.nidcd.nih.gov
National Institute of Dental and Craniofacial Research (NIDCR)	www.nidcr.nih.gov
National Institute of Diabetes and Digestive and Kidney Diseases (NIDDK)	www.niddk.nih.gov
National Institute on Drug Abuse (NIDA)	www.nida.nih.gov
National Institute of Environmental Health Sciences (NIEHS)	www.niehs.nih.gov
National Institute of General Medical Sciences (NIGMS)	www.nigms.nih.gov
National Institute of Mental Health (NIMH)	www.nimh.nih.gov
National Center on Minority Health and Health Disparities (NCMHD)	www.ncmhd.nih.gov
National Institute of Neurological Disorders and Stroke (NINDS)	www.ninds.nih.gov
National Institute of Nursing Research (NINR)	www.ninr.nih.gov
National Library of Medicine (NLM)	www.nlm.nih.gov
Warren Grant Magnuson Clinical Center (CC)	www.cc.nih.gov
Center for Information Technology (CIT)	www.cit.nih.gov
National Center for Complementary and Alternative Medicine (NCCAM)	www.nccam.nih.gov
National Center for Research Resources (NCRR)	www.ncrr.nih.gov
John E. Fogarty International Center (FIC)	www.fic.nih.gov
Center for Scientific Review (CSR)	www.csr.nih.gov

controlled a research budget of $30 billion in the fiscal year 2009 (http://www.nih.gov/about/budget.htm).

Located in Bethesda, Maryland, the NIH has about 75 buildings on more than 300 acres. These include a clinical research hospital and research center where patients undergoing clinical trials are cared for by NIH staff nurses, physicians, and other health care providers.

A research scientist or team of researchers decides which of the NIH centers is responsible for the research they are interested in and then applies to that institute. Four times a year, the NIH grant screeners receive 10,000 grant applications to review. The research grants may be as small as $50,000 or as large as many millions depending on what is being researched, how many researchers are involved, and for how long. The standard research grant is for 5 years and can be extended if necessary. Research ideas are funded using a priority system based on the research that identifies the major areas of health care concern in the United States.

For example, a nurse scientist who is interested in the benefits of patient teaching for first-time mothers would apply to the National Institute of Nursing Research (a center of the NIH) for funding for the project. Because there are many requests for grants and few granted, the first step may be to take the NINR research training course. This course takes the new researcher through the steps necessary to write a successful grant. It may take a year to write the grant, then another year to actually get the grant. Then the researcher must report to the NINR each quarter and submit a budget each year. This elaborate process allows the NIH to have a very competitive process for researchers and enough oversight to ensure high-quality research that does not endanger patients or their rights.

An Ounce of Prevention

It has been said that "an apple a day keeps the doctor away." Whether that particular statement is true or not, the focus of prevention is to reduce the amount of health care individuals need.

Prevention research and health goals in the United States are a major focus of both individuals and government agencies. The CDC is the agency charged with tracking health behavior of Americans. But many other agencies and organizations engage in prevention research, tracking, and public service campaigns. The NIH, the Robert Wood Johnson Foundation for health care research, the Susan B. Komen Foundation for breast cancer, and the American Lung and American Cancer Associations are a few of the leading groups interested in disease prevention and research in the United States.

The leading causes of death are tracked, and programs are instituted to help lessen the impact of these diseases. Table 12.4 lists the major causes of death. When age and gender are taken into account, the leading causes of death in subgroups can vary considerably from this list.

Many of these causes of death are linked to certain **risk factors** and thus can be changed by changes in behavior. Risk factors such as smoking, high-fat diet, sedentary lifestyle, high blood pressure, elevated cholesterol, obesity, diabetes, and alcohol abuse are linked to the increased incidence of heart disease, cancer, and stroke. Smoking is implicated in 20 percent of all deaths (Morbidity and Mortality Weekly Report 2008).

risk factors Anything that contributes to a person getting ill. A feature of someone's habits, genetic history, or personal history that increases the probability they will get a particular disease or injury. Smoking is a risk factor for lung cancer.

Table 12.4	*Leading Causes of Death in the United States, 2006*

Deaths and Mortality
- Number of deaths: 2,426,264
- Death rate: 810.4 deaths per 100,000 population
- Life expectancy: 77.7 years
- Infant Mortality rate: 6.69 deaths per 1,000 live births

Number of deaths for leading causes of death:
- Heart disease: 631,636
- Cancer: 559,888
- Stroke (cerebrovascular diseases): 137,119
- Chronic lower respiratory diseases: 124,583
- Accidents (unintentional injuries): 121,599
- Diabetes: 72,449
- Alzheimer's disease: 72,432
- Influenza and Pneumonia: 56,326
- Nephritis, nephrotic syndrome, and nephrosis: 45,344
- Septicemia: 34,234

Source: Deaths: Final Data for 2006, tables B, D, 7, 30 http://www.cdc.gov/nchs/fastats/deaths.htm.

Morbidity and Mortality (Related to Tobacco Use)

Tobacco and Disease

■ Tobacco use causes—

Cancer
Heart disease
Lung diseases (including emphysema, bronchitis, and chronic airway obstruction)

■ Cigarette smoking increases the length of time that people live with a disability by about years.

■ For every person who dies from a smoking-related disease, 20 more people suffer with at least one serious illness from smoking.

Tobacco and Death

Worldwide

Tobacco use causes more than 5 million deaths per year.

Current trends show that tobacco use will cause more than 8 million deaths annually by 2030.

On average, smokers die 13 to 14 years earlier than nonsmokers.

In the United States

Cigarette smoking is the leading preventable cause of death.

Cigarette smoking is responsible for about 1 in 5 deaths annually, or about 443,000 deaths per year.

An estimated 49,000 of tobacco-related deaths are the result of secondhand smoke exposure.

Tobacco-Related Costs and Expenditure in the United States

Costs of Smoking

■ Annually, in the United States, **cigarette smoking** costs more than $193 billion:
$193 billion =
$97 billion in lost productivity
+
$96 billion in health care expenditures

■ Annually, in the United States, **secondhand smoke** costs more than $10 billion in health care expenditures.

State Spending on Tobacco Control

States have billions of dollars available to them—from tobacco excise taxes and tobacco industry legal settlements—for preventing and controlling tobacco use. States currently use a very small percentage of these funds for tobacco control programs:

■ $24.9 billion was available to states in 2007 from tobacco taxes and legal settlements

- States spent less than 3% of the $24.9 billion in 2007 on tobacco control programs
- Investing only 15% (i.e., $3.7 billion) of the $24.9 billion would have funded every state tobacco control program at CDC-recommended levels

Cigarette Industry Spending

The cigarette industry spends billions each year on advertising and promotions:

- $13 billion total spent in 2005 (latest available data)
- $36 million spent a day in 2005 (latest available data)

Tobacco Use in the United States

Numbers of Smokers

Millions of people in the United States smoke cigarettes.

Current* Smokers

19.8% of U.S. adults (43.4 million people 18 years of age and older)

20.0% of high school students

36.4% of American Indian/Alaska Native adults

21.4% of white adults

19.8% of African American adults

13.3% of Hispanic adults

9.6% of Asian American adults (excluding Native Hawaiians and other Pacific Islanders)

*Current smokers are defined as persons who reported smoking at least 100 cigarettes during their lifetime and who, at the time of interview, reported smoking every day or some days.

Starting to Smoke

Thousands of young people and adults begin smoking every day:

- Each day, about 1,000 persons younger than 18 years of age become regular smokers (i.e., begin smoking on a daily basis).
- Each day, approximately 1,800 adults 18 years of age and older become daily smokers (i.e., begin smoking on a daily basis).

Quitting

Many adult smokers want or try to quit smoking:

- Approximately 70% of smokers want to quit completely.
- Approximately 40% of smokers try to quit each year.

Cessation treatments found to be effective include the following:

- Brief clinical interventions
- Counseling
- Over-the-counter and prescription nicotine replacement products (e.g., nicotine gum, inhaler, nasal spray, lozenge, or patch)
- Prescription nonnicotine medications, such as bupropion SR (Zyban®) and varenicline tartrate (Chantix®)

Source: http://www.cdc.gov/Nchs/fastats/smoking.htm.

Healthy People 2020

As you learned at the beginning of this text, according to the CDC's *2002 National Health Survey*, America's health is good overall, but certain areas need improvement. Based on these survey findings, the DHHS released a document called *Healthy People 2020*, which contains two broad health goals. The first goal is to increase the quality and years of healthy life, and the second is to eliminate health disparities. Currently, the CDC is reviewing and updating *Healthy People 2010*, and the new document *Healthy People 2020* is in the final development phase. The new goals have been adopted and are reflected in the tables. **Health-related quality of life (HRQOL)** integrates both physical and mental health dimension so that health is no longer the opposite of disease and death but a concept that stands for well-being (DHHS 2010). *Healthy People 2010* included over 467 objectives designed to obtain health; these are divided into 28 focus areas for national health. The new 2020 goals include 36 areas of

Health-related quality-of-life (HRQOL) The physical and mental well-being of an individual that looks at the quality and quantity of a healthy life in terms of years.

focus. The subjects for prevention campaigns and budget come from these focus areas. The new focus areas are presented in Table 12.5.

The progress made toward these goals was discussed in Chapter 1. Many of the focus areas are influenced by personal behavior patterns. As health care professionals design strategies to improve health, models of behavior such as the Health Promotion Model used in nursing can be helpful. The model has three components: individual characteristics, behavior-specific cognitions and affect, and behavioral outcomes (Pender, Murdaugh, and Parsons 2002). Without understanding the influence of the first two components, the final step of health-promoting behavior is unlikely to occur.

Table 12.5	*Healthy People 2020* **Proposed Focus Areas at a Glance**

Access to Health Services
Adolescent Health
Arthritis, Osteoporosis, and Chronic Back Conditions
Blood Disorders and Blood Safety
Cancer
Chronic Kidney Diseases
Diabetes
Disability and Secondary Conditions
Early and Middle Childhood
Educational and Community-Based Programs
Environmental Health
Family Planning
Food Safety
Genomics
Global Health
Health Communication and Health IT
Healthcare-Associated Infections
Hearing and Other Sensory or Communication Disorders
(Ear, Nose, Throat—Voice, Speech, and Language)
Heart Disease and Stroke
HIV
Immunization and Infectious Diseases
Injury and Violence Prevention
Maternal, Infant, and Child Health
Medical Product Safety
Mental Health and Mental Disorders
Nutrition and Weight Status
Occupational Safety and Health
Older Adults
Oral Health
Physical Activity and Fitness
Public Health Infrastructure
Quality of Life and Well-Being
Respiratory Diseases
Sexually Transmitted Diseases
Social Determinants of Health
Substance Abuse
Tobacco Use
Vision

Source: http://www.healthypeople.gov/hp2020/Objectives/TopicAreas.aspx.

Different strategies are needed at different ages and genders (Haynes, Boese, and Butcher 2004). For children, health promotion should include routine infant screenings, immunizations, instruction to caregivers on accident prevention and proper diet and exercise, and dental care. Adolescents as a group are very healthy, but many unhealthy practices, such as smoking, substance abuse, and unprotected sex, begin at this time. Promotion activities should focus on education.

Health promotion for adult men and women is quite different, primarily because of reproductive health issues. For women, family planning and prenatal care are essential, as are detection and prevention of unique cancers and osteoporosis. Although men are at risk for all the causes of death listed in Table 12.4, prostate cancer applies only to men. Men are also at much higher risk for violence.

The health of older adults is an increasing concern given the overall aging of the population and increased longevity. Poor nutrition and vision and hearing problems are particularly acute in this population. Accident prevention is essential because falls can contribute to a host of other, more severe health problems.

Women's Health

Women's health is one of the areas in which the least progress has been made toward the *Healthy People 2010* goals (National Women's Law Center and the Oregon Health & Science University 2004). The 2004 report singles out access to care as one of the areas that has not improved and indeed has fallen behind the goals set in the *Healthy People 2010*. Only 2 of the 27 benchmarks goals have been reached or are likely to be reached by 2010. In looking at specific goals, the report states,

- In some states, only one in three women have health insurance of any type.
- Only 17 states provide poor women with safe abortion procedures.
- Less than half the states (20) require that private insurers cover contraceptives as they do other drugs.
- Only three states meet the national goal for women getting pap smears.
- Only one state meets the national goal for achieving a low percentage of women who smoke.
- Only 19 states have met the colorectal cancer screening goal.

Because many women and at least one in every four children in the United States live in poverty, access to care will remain a social, political, and health problem for years to come.

We know how to prevent or mitigate many diseases, but we do not know how to ensure that women and men who need basic health care get it. If we cannot meet the first focus on healthy people, it is unlikely that significant gains will be made on the other 27 goals, which all require access to health care to implement.

The current debate on health care offers a unique opportunity to focus on reproductive health. The average woman spends 5 of the 35 years of fertility having children and 30 years trying not to get pregnant. It takes a healthy woman to have a healthy baby. The need for increased access to reproductive health care is demonstrated by the high rate of unintended pregnancies, low birth weight and neurologically impaired babies, increased maternal diabetes and hypertension, increased sexually transmitted diseases (STDs) in all age groups, and inadequate access to breast care and uterine/cervical cancer screening. The United States does not have a seamless continuum of care that addresses pre-conception, pregnancy planning, birth spacing, emergency contraception, post-natal care, and general reproductive health. We also lack a health care delivery system that integrates reproductive health into primary care delivery for either women or men. For many women, primary care in the reproductive years may be delivered by a variety of health care providers-physicians (MD and OD), nurse practitioners, complimentary medicine providers, and both certified and lay mid-wives, which increases the fragmentation of care for women.

The Business Response for Prevention

Corporations and insurance companies are as concerned about improving health as the federal government is. Lost productivity and increasing insurance costs affect businesses directly, with some estimating that preventable health expenditures cost employers an average of $1,685 per employee, a total of $226 billion per year (Clark 2008). This has led businesses and insurance companies to take a proactive role in health education and promotion.

Many employers provide worksite-based programs for health promotion and disease prevention. The data from one survey indicate that 72 percent of companies surveyed provided education on lifestyle behaviors; 52 percent offered wellness programs (Banham 2010).

A review of the workplace research by DHHS indicates improved health for employees and increased productivity and cost savings for the employer as a result of these programs (DHHS 2003). The DHHS study focused on five health issues: overweight and obesity, diabetes, cardiovascular disease, asthma, and tobacco use.

> Overweight and obesity: People who are overweight or obese use more physician and hospital services and pay more for medications, with a total cost to the nation of $69 to $117 billion per year. This figure includes the cost of treating obesity-related disorders such as arthritis, heart disease, type 2 diabetes, hypertension, and stroke. Lost workdays and restricted-activity days cost businesses in the form of health insurance, sick leave, life insurance, and disability insurance.
>
> Diabetes: The American Diabetes Association puts the cost at $132 billion. Data from the CDC indicate 8.3 lost workdays for those with diabetes compared to 1.7 for those without. Virtually all health plans offer disease management programs, which have a big impact, often cutting costs about 20 percent per month.
>
> Cardiovascular disease: Total costs were estimated at $329 billion for 2002.
>
> Asthma: Total costs were estimated at $14 billion in 2001, which includes $4.6 billion related to lost productivity.
>
> Tobacco use: Total costs are estimated at $138 billion. Smokers are more expensive to employers than nonsmokers. Plans to help employees quit smoking cost $0.89 to $4.92 per smoker compared to treating smoking-related illness at $6 to $33 per smoker.

Clearly businesses and their insurance companies have a huge financial incentive to help employees improve their health. The question that isn't clear is which programs return the most benefit for the least cost. Organizations such as the Wellness Council of America (www.welcoa.org) have studied workplace programs for more than 20 years; Welcoa estimates that for every $1 spent on wellness programs, the employer saves $3 in health insurance costs. Employers utilize a combination of incentives to encourage participation. These include monetary incentives to complete health assessments or participate in weight management or tobacco cessation programs, and can also include reduced employee contributions to insurance premiums or merchandise (Wells 2010). Under the 2010 Patient Protection and Affordable Care Act, employers can offer up to 30%–50% reductions in health coverage costs as an incentive (Vesely 2010).

The Individual's Response for Prevention

Americans have more access to health information than ever before. One concern is that those people who need information the most—the poor or uninsured—are also the groups least likely to use the Internet as a health resource. Table 12.6 lists some sources of health information. Under the 2010 Patient Protection and Affordable Care Act, food in vending machines and at chain restaurants will have to post nutritional information beginning in 2011.

Data indicate that physical activity can improve many of the health conditions listed in Table 12.4. According to the 2008 National Health Survey, 32.5 percent of adults regularly engage in physical activity. An increased emphasis on fitness has created an entire industry in the last several decades. Fitness industry revenues total almost $21.6 billion, with a total payroll of $7.1 billion. More than 580,000 people are employed by the industry, at 31,000 businesses (U.S. Census Bureau 2007). Fitness centers are available at work, in hospitals, in hotel/motels, on military bases, at schools, colleges, and universities, at apartment complexes, in addition to commercial health clubs. U.S. health clubs have more than 45.5 million members (http://clubindustry.com).

Without exercise, prevention of obesity is very difficult in a fast-food culture. One lunch at McDonald's gives children or adults more calories than they should have all day and almost all the sodium and fat they should have, leaving very little for the other four recommended meals a day (five small meals are preferable to three large ones). A meal composed of a Quarter Pounder with cheese, fries, and a large Coke has a total of 1,430 calories—over a full day's calorie intake, 99 percent of the daily fat recommendation, and 69 percent of the daily recommended sodium intake (A Full Serving of Nutritional Facts http://www.mcdonalds.com/app_controller.nutrition2004). Nutritional information is available from all fast-food companies, making it is possible to eat selections with a better nutritional profile.

Table 12.6	*Sources of Health Information*
General health information	
National Institutes of Health	http://www.nih.gov/
Medline Plus	medlineplus.gov
Selected topics	
Alzheimer's disease	http://www.nia.nih.gov/alzheimers
American Council on Exercise	www.acefitness.org/default.aspx
Cancer	http://www.cancer.gov/ and www.cancer.net
Children's Health	www.kidshealth.org
Family health	www.familydoctor.org
Food Pyramid	www.mypyramid.gov
Full Serving of Nutritional Facts	http:///www.mcdonalds.com/app_controller.nutrition
MayoClinic	www.mayoclinic.com
McDonalds Nutrition	www.mcdonalds.com/us/en/food/food_quality/nutrition_choices.html
Risk assessment	www.YourDiseaseRisk.wustl.edu
Women's Health	http://health.nih.gov/category/WomensHealth

Prevention alone cannot eradicate disease, but it can reduce the impact of most diseases and make functional, if not clinical, cure a possibility. In conclusion, an apple a day may keep the doctor away, but a good education and income will keep disease at bay.

Summary

Health care research and prevention are two ways to minimize the impact of disease on the population. Research can focus on three goals: cure, control, or prevention. Research scientists work in many settings: universities, companies, not-for-profits, and the government. The federal government is the largest sponsor of health care research. The CDC tracks disease and death rates to help formulate and implement programs to prevent or lessen the impact of disease. Personal behavior patterns, such as nutrition, smoking, exercise, weight control, and regular screening, promote healthy outcomes. Access to care is a major determinant of health; income and education are major predictors of access to health care. Women have less access to health care than men and as a result have lower health status.

Questions for Review

1. Give examples of the three major types of research.
2. Describe the function and scope of the Departments of Health and Human Services.
3. What is the NIH, and what does it do?
4. Describe the process of obtaining a research grant from the NIH.
5. How does the government decide which research projects to fund?
6. How is the flu vaccine determined each year?
7. What is the status of women's health goals for *2010 Healthy People*?
8. What incentives can businesses offer to impact health care?

Questions for Discussion

1. What is your experience with the flu vaccine?
   a. Do you get a yearly flu shot? Why? Why not?
   b. Have you had the flu in the last 5 years?
   c. Survey the class: how many have had the flu? The flu shots? How does that compare to the national average?
2. Using a government Web site, describe the research being done on one of the top 10 causes of death.
3. In your opinion, what method should be used to determine the subjects of health care research? Using your method you've chosen, what types of research would be supported?
4. Describe the steps being taken to reach the goal of one of the foci of *Healthy People 2010.*
5. At your school or place of work, what tools are available to help you take care of yourself?
6. Go to the Web sites of several fast-food companies to access nutritional information. How do your favorites compare?
7. How does your state rank in meeting the Healthy People Goals?
8. How would you determine your own health status using assessment tools on the Web?

Chapter References

AARP Bulletin. 2005. *I Can See Clearly Now* 46 (9): 34–35. Available at AARP www.arp.org/bulletin.

Banhan, R. 2010. The financial virtue of wellness. *Treasury & Risk*, May: 36–39.

Clinical Trials http://clinicaltrials.gov/ct2/results?cond=%22Macular+Degeneration%22 Flu.Gov (www.flu.gov).

Centers for Disease Control and Prevention. 2008. Smoking-Attributable Mortality, Years of Potential Life Lost, and Productivity Losses—United States, 2000–2004. *Morbidity and Mortality Weekly Report* <serial online>. 57(45):1226–1228 <accessed 2009 Mar 31>.

Clark, A. 2008. The new frontier of wellness. *Benefits Quarterly*, Second quarter: 23-28.

DHHS (U.S. Department of Health and Human Services). 2010. *Healthy People 2010*. Washington, DC: U.S. Government Printing Office.

DHHS (U.S. Department of Health and Human Services). 2003. *Prevention makes common "cents."* Washington, DC: U.S. Government Printing Office. Available at www.aspe.hhs.gov/health/prevention/prevention.pdf.

Haynes, L., T. Boese, and H. Butcher. 2004. *Nursing in contemporary society*. Upper Saddle River, NJ: Prentice Hall.

Leavell, H., and E. Clark. 1965. *Preventative medicine for the doctor in his community: An epidemiological approach*. 2nd ed. New York: McGraw-Hill.

McDonalds Nutrition Information (http:///www.mcdonalds.com/app_controller.nutrition).

McGinnis, M., and W. Foege. 1993. Actual cause of death in the United States. *Journal of the American Medical Association* 270: 2208.

National Institute of Allergy and Infectious Disease (http://www.niaid.nih.gov/factsheets/flu.htm).

National Women's Law Center and the Oregon Health & Science University. 2004. *Making the grade on women's health: A national and state-by-state report card*.

Pender, N., C. Murdaugh, and M. Parsons. 2002. *Health promotion in nursing*. 4th ed. Upper Saddle River, NJ: Prentice Hall.

U.S. Census Bureau. *2007 Economic Census, Industry series reports. NAICS 713940*.

Vesely, R. 2010. For good behavior. *Modern Healthcare*, 49:19. Retrieved from MEDLINE.

Wells, S. 2010. Getting paid for staying well. *HR Magazine*, February: 59-60.

For Additional Information

Genetics Home Reference (http://ghr.nlm.nih.gov/).

See any of the Web sites listed in Table 12.6.

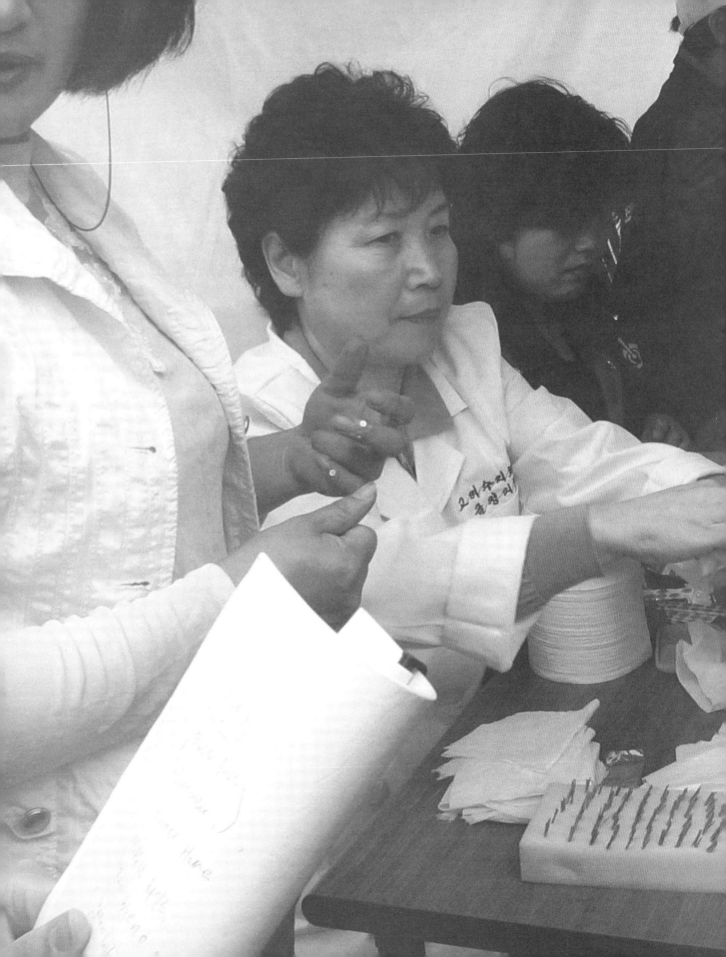

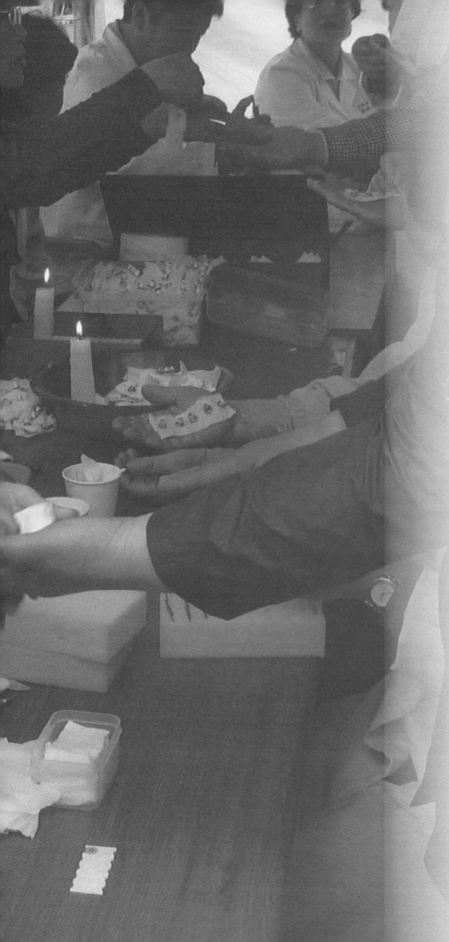

13

Cultural Competency, Health Literacy, and Health Care Ethics

Learning Objectives

After reading this chapter, you should be able to:

1. Define cultural competency.
2. Describe REALM.
3. Explain the ideal of health literacy.
4. Identify the benefits of health and cultural literacy to the country.
5. Assess your own and your family's health literacy.
6. Discuss and give examples of four health literacy strategies.
7. Discuss ethical issues in cultural competency theories.
8. Identify and describe three major ethical theories.
9. Identify four major ethical principles in health care.
10. Discuss the ethical rational for health care reform.

Pima Indians and Diabetes

Sadie is a member of the Pima Indian tribe of the Gila River Indian Community. Her ancestors were among the first people to set foot in the Americas 30,000 years ago. They have lived in the Sonoron Desert near the Gila River in what is now southern Arizona for at least 2,000 years.

What makes the Pima Indian tribe very special in modern medical history is that they have participated in one of the longest-running research projects of the Indian Health Service. For the last 30 years, this tribe has been studied, have taken surveys, and had every aspect of their lives described by researchers. The reason for the interest? Over 50 percent of all adult Pima tribe members have Type II—adult diabetes and at a very young age, usually by 36. In comparison, about 8 percent of the general population in the 20 to 60 age group have Type II diabetes, rising to about 23 percent by age 60. In addition, the tribe's diabetics have a much greater risk of having Kidney Disease of Diabetes Mellitus (KDDM) and kidney failure. The community is the smallest town (population 1,100) in the United States with its own kidney dialysis center.

The sand-colored stucco home where Sadie lives with her husband and three daughters in Gila is neat as a pin. Her household chores are good exercise, she says, to help control her own diabetes. Sadie's mother, who developed diabetes shortly after her daughter was born, died from kidney disease that developed from her long-term diabetes. Her father, a retired heavy equipment operator who had been very active in reservation life, suffered an amputation—a complication of his diabetes—a year ago, after being hospitalized for several long months. "He got a sore on his foot and never got it treated," she explains. Four of her 10 brothers and sisters also have the disease, which runs in families. Although she has seen the worst diabetes can do, Sadie is not giving up. What her father and other family members have gone through makes her want to take care of herself: "I could be in that same situation."

She is also motivated by wanting to see her three daughters, aged 12, 7, and 3, keep their health. All were big babies, and they have remained heavy for their ages. "All of my kids are chubby," she adds. That's common for babies born to mothers who have or are prone to develop diabetes, according to NIH researchers who are studying the disease in the Pima Indians. This mother is trying to teach her daughters to watch what they eat because being overweight increases dramatically the risk of diabetes.

Introduction

The study of ethics and cultural competency in the health care arena originates from the idea that there should be fairness and equality in the delivery of health care benefits. This chapter deals with the institutional issues in health care ethics, rather than the individual case. The same holds true for our discussion of cultural competency: it is not so much being able to talk to a single individual; but to achieve fairness and equality, it is critical to have organizational and institutional tools in place that allow the providers to talk to people at all levels of health literacy.

Culture and Health Care

Variables such as age, gender, ethnicity, and socioeconomic status are strongly related to the level of actual and perceived health within a given population. Culture and cultural values are also related to beliefs about health and illness.

culture An integrated and shared pattern of human behavior.

Although there are different definitions of culture, social scientists agree that **culture** is learned and shared by group members. What you believe, your values, and

Her third-grader, a pretty child with glossy black hair who likes to read when she isn't playing with her cat, already has diabetes. Her mother helps her monitor her blood sugar and is teaching her about choosing healthy foods, although she admits it's hard. When sweets are sometimes given out at school, her daughter gets a toy instead. "I tell her the cookies are gone, but you've still got the toy," her mother says.

Researchers do not yet fully understand why American Indians, and especially the Pima Indians, are more likely to develop diabetes, but one thing is clear—those who are overweight are at high risk. Approximately 95 percent percent of all Pima Indians and 80 percent of all other people with diabetes are overweight (http://diabetes.niddk.nih.gov/dm/pubs/statistics/). Although researchers are still searching for the genes that cause diabetes in many Pima families, they say that cutting fat in the diet and exercising are the best ways yet known to prevent diabetes and modify its long-term effects (http://www.diabetes.niddk.nih.gov/DM/pubs/pima).

"What I really want to do is change the way we eat here," Sadie explains, referring to fried foods and the tacos the family loves. She knows that eating less sugar and fat is important for her family's health. "They say if you bake or broil, it's supposed to be better, and I've been trying to do that lately."

The need to communicate health care information in a culturally effective and caring way to Sadie and the rest of her tribe led to the Indian Health Service health literacy and cultural competency project. This project uses tools designed to improve communication between the health care provider and the tribal member in a respectful and effective way. Since many tribal members are not health literate, have no access to the Internet, and are very wary of abandoning tribal customs and tribal healers, a new approach was needed. The research on cultural competency demonstrated that there were tools that would help Sadie and her family understand and accept the information needed to care for their diabetic family member. REALM (Rapid Estimate of Adult Literacy in Medicine) is one such tool. We will explore others in this chapter.

Sadie's children and grandchildren have a much better chance to live without diabetes through the efforts of the Indian Health Service's Health Literacy and Cultural Competence programs.

Source: Adapted from http://diabetes.niddk.nih.gov/DM/pubs/pima.

---

much of your behavior are culturally determined. Sociologist Robin Williams has identified 12 **core values** of the American culture: individualism, freedom, democracy, equality, achievement and success, efficiency and practicality, progress, science and technology, material comfort, activity and work, humanitarianism, and group superiority (Henslin 2009). Definitions are presented in Table 13.1. However, these values are constantly being changed and challenged as the ethnic landscape and generational adoption of social media and communication evolve.

Often these values come into conflict. For example, Americans value both efficiency and humanitarianism. Therefore, many Americans are dissatisfied with a health care system that treats them efficiently but does not take time to recognize them as individuals. Others view the current system as one that is inherently unjust because the system does not treat people equally. As we will explore women, people of color, and the poor all have issues with health care in the United States.

Of course, in a country as large as the United States there are also subcultures. **Subcultures** are groups that share many of the elements of mainstream culture, but maintain their own distinctive customs, values, norms, and lifestyles. Subcultures can be based on gender, age, ethnicity, religion, sexual preference, and occupation, to name just a few variables. Occupations such as health care and places of employment

Core values Values are shared attitudes and beliefs among group members. Core values are the central values of a culture.

Subculture A group within a main culture that accepts the standards of the main culture, but has distinctive customs and values.

Table 13.1	*Cultural Values in America*
Individualism	Americans believe that individual effort and initiative lead to success. If a person doesn't get ahead, it's his fault.
Freedom	Americans resent any limitation on their personal freedom. Even though Americans are widely aware of the dangers of unhealthy choices such as drinking, smoking, and overeating, they resist any attempt to regulate those behaviors, believing even bad choices to be an individual's right.
Democracy	Americans believe that everyone has the right to express an opinion and that the majority rules.
Equality	Equal opportunity is an ideal of American society.
Achievement and success	Personal achievement is highly valued and is measured by attaining wealth, power, and prestige. For this reason, many people respect physicians.
Efficiency and practicality	Doing things as efficiently as possible and making changes to improve efficiency are considered strengths.
Progress	Americans expect technology to change rapidly.
Science and technology	Americans develop new technology and expect science to control natural forces. If a new disease is identified (e.g., AIDS or SARS), Americans expect scientists to find a cure quickly.
Material comfort	Americans expect to be comfortable. Americans take over-the-counter medications and expect their health care services to be relatively pain free.
Activity and work	Even when not at work, Americans expect people to be "busy." Leisure activities such as sports and exercise are good behaviors.
Humanitarianism	Americans value helpfulness and kindness. They volunteer and contribute to many health-related groups such as the American Cancer Society. In times of mass disasters, they provide aid individually or through the Red Cross and other organizations.
Group superiority	Despite the values of equality and democracy, American have valued some groups more highly than others. In its ugliest form, this value has been expressed as racism.

Source: Henslin 2009.

such as hospitals can be considered as subcultures because they have their own specialized language, customs, and material culture.

Disease and illness occur within a cultural context, even to the extent of defining what is and is not a disease. Some of the aspects of culture that affect health care are identified in Table 13.2.

Table 13.2	*Aspects of Culture That Impact Health Care*	
Language		Beliefs about health and illness
Time orientation		Beliefs about aging
Family practices		Death practices
Childbirth practices		Pain response
Child-rearing practices		Grief response
Food habits		Touch and privacy
Sexuality		

The United States has five ethnic minority groups—Native Americans/Alaskan Native, Hispanics/Latina, Asian, Native Hawaiian, and African American. Data indicate that these cultures have different health outcomes from the dominant white culture. In addition, they have different health practices and access health care differently. A challenge for the health care industry is to ensure that all Americans receive good quality care.

One consequence of culture is that our culture influences the way we see the world. However, as the United States becomes more diverse culturally, it is more common to encounter people of other cultures. As an example of this increasing diversity, in one of my recent classes in Health Care Management, seven different languages were spoken and the students represented four continents. If a person is **ethnocentric**, he or she will evaluate others' customs according to values of his or her own cultural group. This can lead to misperceptions and conflict. Anne Fadiman's account of an epileptic Hmong child's interaction with the U.S. health care system illustrates how vastly different cultures and their perceptions of illness can come into conflict (Fadiman 1997). The U.S. system viewed epilepsy as a disease that needed treatment, whereas the Hmong parents viewed the seizures as evidence of visits by spirits. Ethnocentrism can also affect relations between health care businesses and their employees.

Culture affects how people communicate, understand, and respond to health information. Cultural and linguistic competency of health professionals contributes to health literacy. **Health literacy** is defined as the degree to which individuals have the capacity to obtain, process, and understand basic information and services needed to make appropriate decisions about their health. Culture refers to integrated patterns of human behavior that include the language, thoughts, communications, actions, customs, beliefs, values, and institutions of racial, ethnic, religious, gender, age, or social groups. Competence implies having the capacity to function effectively as an individual and an organization within the context of the cultural beliefs, behaviors, and needs presented by consumers and their communities.

Cultural competence is the ability of health organizations and practitioners to recognize the cultural beliefs, values, attitudes, traditions, language preferences, and health practices of specific cultural groups and to apply that knowledge to produce positive health outcomes. Competency includes communicating in a manner that is linguistically and culturally appropriate. Healthcare professionals have their own culture and language (http://www11.georgetown.edu/research/gucchd/nccc/foundations/frameworks).

Many adopt the "culture of medicine" and the language of their specialty as a result of their training and work environment. This can affect how health professionals communicate with the public. If the patient is health literate, he or she will have the ability to understand health care providers' information such as prescription instructions, disease brochures, and health care instructions. Health literacy is not dependent on the ability to read, but rather to understand what is said to patients regardless of their culture, reading ability, or language (http://www. minorityhealth.hhs.gov).

Ethnocentrism The evaluation of behaviors according to one's own cultural beliefs.

Health literacy The degree to which individuals have the capacity to obtain, process, and understand basic information and services needed to make appropriate decisions about their health.

Cultural competence The ability of health organizations and practitioners to recognize cultural beliefs, values, attitudes, traditions, language preferences, and health practices of specific cultural groups and to apply that knowledge to produce positive health outcomes.

Why Are Cultural Competence and Health Literacy Important?

Cultural competency and health literacy are two of the main ingredients in closing the gap in the disparity of health care services provided to different groups. It's the way patients and health care providers can come together and talk about health concerns so that cultural differences can enhance rather than hinder the conversation. Health care services that are respectful of and responsive to the health beliefs, practices, and cultural and linguistic needs of diverse patients can help bring about positive health outcomes. Research suggests that those who are not health literate experience almost

40 percent more hospitalizations than their health literate counterparts (http://www.ihs.gov/healthcommunications). Culture and language may influence:

- Health, healing, and wellness belief systems
- How illness, disease, and their causes are perceived, both by the patient/consumer and the health care provider
- The behaviors of patients/consumers who are seeking health care and their attitudes toward health care providers.

The increasing population growth of racial and ethnic communities and linguistic groups, each with its own cultural traits and health profiles, presents a challenge to the health care delivery service in this country. It is estimated that over 90 million people in the United States are not health literate. The provider and the patient each bring their individual learned patterns of language and culture to the health care experience, which must be transcended to achieve equal access and quality health care. All groups who are seen as or perceived to be minorities are affected by cultural competency and health literacy issues. In addition to the five major groups listed, women, children, and elders are also affected (http://bioethics.od.nih.gov/culturalcomp.html).

- African Americans
- American Indian/Alaska native
- Asian American
- Hispanic/Latino
- Native Hawaiian
- Women
- Children
- Elders

We measure the degree to which the group is affected by health literacy and cultural issues by looking at the outcomes of specific diseases and health markers as demonstrated by the profile of the Pima Indians. Some of those markers include the level of access to health care, the level of infant and maternal health, and the status of women's health. Other markers include the status of oral health in the population, the number and type of immunizations, and the level of organ donation. The incidence of certain diseases and health issues, such as asthma, cancer, chronic liver, diabetes, hepatitis, HIV/AIDS, obesity, and stroke are also markers.

How Are Health Care Providers Trained in Cultural Competency and Health Literacy?

Thanks to projects like the Indian Health Service's work with the Pima, other Indian tribes, and the work with the Hmong tribes, several tools have been developed to assess and increase cultural competency and health care literacy. One of the most important factors is the ability to use systems already in place in groups to help health providers. In the Pima group, the Healers and Elders were major players in outlining the strategies for intervention in diabetes. Knowing the cultural norms of the tribes, the expectations, fears, and customs allowed researchers to develop tools for health care providers.

Health care providers who are working with specific populations need a good orientation to the customs and beliefs of the group, access to language assistance, and a way to rapidly assess health care literacy and appropriate communication tools. To get someone like Sadie to change her family's diet requires culturally appropriate teaching and communication skills as well as the very practical guides to diet and exercise.

Tools Used to Assess and Improve Health Literacy

It is important to clarify a couple of issues about health literacy. First, health literacy is not the same thing as regular literacy. The health care profession has its own language, medical terminology. For those of you who have taken classes in medical terminology, you know that it takes hard study to learn all the concepts of this language and culture. So it is not surprising that people who have not had this training often find what health care providers say hard to understand. Second, many of the groups are not English language proficient—they come from other countries or parts of this country where English is not the first language. They will need to have language appropriate communication, which does not mean just translating medical terminology into another language.

The Indian Health Service has developed tools to assist the health care provider to assess health literacy in many different populations. A number of cues may be suggestive of low health literacy status. These cues can include:

- Hand brochure to patient upside down and see if he or she correctly aligns the page in order to read it.
- Ask the patient if the print is clear enough to read on the brochure.
- Registration and other forms may be filled out incompletely or incorrectly.
- Patient gives excuses when asked to read something (i.e., forgot reading glasses).
- Patient hands medical brochures/materials to a relative or other person.
- Patient cannot describe how to take medications.

Another tool is the REALM (Rapid Estimate of Adult Literacy in Medicine). This tool asks patients to read and pronounce common medical terms. It has been used to assess health literacy among many different patient populations. A guide to talking with patients provided by the Indian Health Service suggests the following:

How to Talk to Patients of Different Cultures and Languages

When talking to patients about their health care issues, remember that patients may be anxious, worried, distressed, and/or confused. Following are a few tips:

- **Avoid using technical words or jargon.** It may be tough to avoid "physician-speak," but experts say you should assume that all your patients will be confused by most of what you say. If you must use a technical word, define it.
- **Avoid unnecessary details.** Limit the information you cover in order to reduce confusion or information overload. Use simple vocabulary and short sentences. Make no more than two or three key points for each topic.
- **Avoid acronyms.** When you must use an acronym, explain the meaning the first time you use it.

- **Use the "teach-back" method.** Avoid asking patients, "Do you understand?" Most will say they do even when they are confused. Instead say, "I want to make sure I did a good job teaching you. Tell me how you are going to do this when you get home." Research consistently shows that this type of "teach-back" method improves recall and participation in the treatment plan.
- **Use pictures.** Illustrations often convey instructions better than words.
- **Talk to family members.** If you think your patient may have low health literacy, enlist the aid of a family member or friend.

Source: http://www.ihs.gov/healthcommunications/index.cfm?module=dsp_hc_toolkit.

These tools must be used with care and compassion, or they can actually discourage patients from accessing care, much the same way you would be nervous about a quiz (http://www.ihs.gov/healthcommunications).

Ethical Issues in Health Care

The enactment of the Medicare-Medicaid and the End Stage Renal Disease bills in 1965 fundamentally changed the distribution of health care in the United States from a transaction between the health care provider and the patient to an institutional form of government-mediated health care delivery. This made the federal government the largest broker of health care in the world. The enactment of these two bills entitled large specific segments of the population to the social benefits of health care and thus obligated the federal government to provide those benefits in a fair and just manner. So one could argue that the real beginning of health care ethics as a major area of study and policy was in 1965. Coincidentally, this time period was one of great advances in medical technology and drug therapy. We could now keep people alive through the use of ventilators, pacemakers, and modern surgery. So the question became almost immediately—how does society decide who should get these new benefits and who will be left out? These are the major questions of health care ethics.

Because health care concerns human beings' physical and mental well-being, discussions about health care often contain a lot of "shoulds:" "the government should provide basic health care" or "the drug companies should keep drug prices low." In those discussions, a decision about the allocation of scarce resources is based on an ethical viewpoint of how the world should be organized. Health care ethical theories provide a framework to assist patients, health care providers, and policy makers in making these types of decisions.

Ethical issues are those issues in which there are competing values or goods. In an ethical dilemma, there is always more than one answer. This is because both or all the options have some good in them. For example, caring for the elderly is a good. Caring for children is also a good. An ethical dilemma arises when there are insufficient resources to care for both, and choices must be made.

Health care ethics addresses large concepts such as respect for autonomy, nonmaleficency (do no harm), beneficence (do good), justice, veracity (truth telling), privacy, confidentiality, and professional roles. Justice is the major concept used in discussing societal obligations in distributing the health care and will be covered last and in the most detail. The other concepts or principles discussed here are primarily used in the discussion of individual ethical dilemmas and help health care providers and families to talk about ethical decisions they must make on an individual basis.

Autonomy comes from the Greek *auto* (self) and *nomos* (rule)—self rule. Respect for autonomy requires the health care provider to adhere to the patient's decisions. This concept is the basis for our ideas of informed consent, cultural competence, disclosure of risks, and surrogate decision-making. The opposite of autonomy is paternalism—literally the father knows best or in our context of health care—the health care provider knows what is best for the patient.

Nonmaleficency, a technical philosophical term, requires health care providers not to inflict harm intentionally or simply put – at least do no harm. Many bioethical controversies involve the principle of do no harm. Policy makers in states like Oregon had to balance the patient's right of autonomy against the health care providers' mandate to do no harm in the Death With Dignity legislation. Many court cases have revolved around the giving or withholding life-sustaining treatment, again an ethical dilemma involving patient/family wishes and the health care providers' perspective. These are large questions, which involve the patients and their health care providers, but also the public, policy makers, the courts, and legislators.

Beneficence requires us to contribute positively to the welfare of others—do good, not evil. It continues the idea of do no harm into a demand to provide benefits. This principle is expressed when we talk about the government's role in providing public health or when we talk about the need to balance the cost of a program with the benefits it will give to people. The Good Samaritan Rule is a good example of beneficence: you should stop at a wreck and provide first aid if you are able. You are giving a positive benefit to the injured person. Some states have legislated beneficence so that health care providers with basic first aid are required to either stop and help or report injuries. Further legislation has protected the person acting under the Good Samaritan Rule from lawsuits, an expression that the good it does to have people help those who are injured outweighs some legal rights.

Codes of ethics are based on a combination of the concepts just mentioned and the idea that health care professionals are held to a higher ethical standard than nonprofessionals.

These codes of ethics demand a certain standard of behavior if one is to be in good standing with the health care professions. They are universal principles that are required of health care professionals in every aspect of health care from physicians to the scientist and medical records clerk and everyone in between. The major principles involved in professional behavior are veracity (telling the truth) and confidentially. Along with the virtues of compassion, integrity, trustworthiness, and wisdom, these principles guide the health care professional in the care of patients.

Justice and the Health Care System

The principle of justice is probably the most often quoted principle when people talk about health care reform or the government's role in public health. The terms *fairness* and *entitlement* are frequently used in those conversations that discuss allocation of resources. We use theories of justice to help decide how to distribute fairly the benefits of society. These theories were devised because simple ideas of justice do not work well on the macro scale of society. We cannot just divide health care equally among all citizens because some need more and some don't need any at all. So the pie is unequal from the beginning.

There are several major ethical theories used to help health policy makers and governments divide the pie. These include **rights theory, utilitarianism,** and **Kantian** to name a few. Those theories are studied in an ethics, bioethics, or business ethics class in a much greater degree than is possible in this brief overview.

All of these theories have been used to examine the issues of health care in the United States. Policy decisions about health care make trade-offs between three competing "shoulds:"

1. Access: As many people as possible should be able to receive health care services.
2. Quality: The health care services should be of the highest possible quality.
3. Cost: The health care services should not cost too much.

These three policy drivers or shoulds are presented in Figure 13.1. What policy makers usually discover is that they can achieve one or two of these objectives, but that

Rights theory An ethical theory that believes people have certain basic rights as human beings and as citizens.

Utilitarianism An ethical theory that believes resources should be distributed to achieve the maximum benefit.

Kantian theory An ethical theory developed by Immanuel Kant (1724–1804) that says a universal moral law obligates one to treat people as an end in itself.

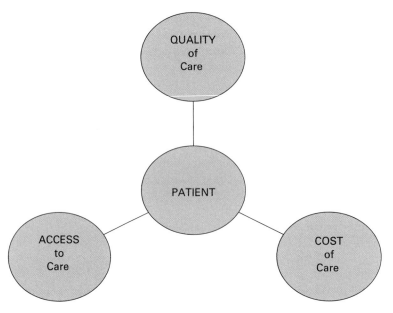

Figure 13.1   Policy Trade-Offs

they cannot simultaneously achieve all three. Ethical theories can provide a rationale and framework for these difficult choices.

In rights theory, health care is viewed as a basic human and citizen right. Currently in the United States, unlike most of the industrialized world, the only people with a right to health care are the 65+ age group. Rights theory and the principle of justice were the primary rationales for the Patient Protection and Affordable Care Act of 2010. The argument was that health care was a right of all citizens, not the few who could pay or belong to special groups, and therefore the government had an obligation to provide basic health care for all. All rights under this theory have a companion obligation.

The utilitarian theory revolves around the idea that health care resources should be allocated where they will do the most good. This would suggest some sort of a rationing of health care so that the most needy would always get health care. John Stuart Mill first introduced this theory in the 19th century. He proposed that moral decisions should be made on the basis of the most good for the most people. In terms of social policy, his theory is a long-term project, not just a simple equation. The health care systems of Britain, Scandinavia, and Canada reflect the Utilitarian idea that health care is a good, and having the most people have access to the system is a societal good that must be shared according to the individuals need for it, regardless of the person's ability to pay. The U.S. system on the other hand is in direct opposition to the Utilitarian belief because access to the societal good of health care is only available to those who have the monetary resources or belong to a very specific group, not according to need.

Kantian theory tells people they ought to treat others as they want to be treated themselves. Furthermore, people should never be treated as a means to an end. In other words, don't use people for your own benefit. This holds true for individuals, corporations, and governments. Research provides a good example of this theory of justice. Research using human subjects should be done in such a way as to protect the subjects from treatment that would not be acceptable to you. This is reflected in the codes of ethics for research (Beauchamp and Childress 2001).

John Rawls and the Theory of Justice

One of the most influential philosophers in the field of health care and the just distribution of societal goods such as health care was John Rawls. His landmark book *A Theory of Justice* was published in 1971. His *justice as fairness* concept has been the basis of policy on a large-scale societal level in such diverse areas as economics, education, and health care ever since. Prior to this work, much of the discussion on health care ethics was centered on the individual patient/provider interaction, not what the government or society as a whole should or should not do.

His theory of justice works so well because it includes basic concepts of social justice, utilitarianism, Kantian theory, and rights theories in one elegant theory. Rawls' theory is based on two principles that then guide moral decision making for society, governments, and individuals when it comes to dividing societal goods such as liberty, opportunity, income, wealth, and the basis of self-respect. The theory also addresses the differences in the natural benefits one is born with, but in no way deserved like health, intelligence, imagination, and position in society at birth. Health care because of its special place in people's lives includes and is influenced by all these goods. The first principle states that each person is to have an equal right to basic liberties compatible with a similar system of liberty for all. In other words, no one has more rights than their neighbor; if one can have health care, all should. The second principle states that the given that there are natural and social inequalities they have to be handled so that they both give the least advantaged as much benefit as is possible. The theory would allow millions to be spent developing a new knee for a basketball star if and only if there was a way to give that same type of knee to a poor child with a congenital defect (a least advantaged person). He further states that all societal benefits must be open to all under the fair equality of opportunity clause. This is the rationale for access to medical school or other public higher education regardless of gender, ethnic background, or other differences for all (Rawls 1971).

This theory of justice works so well because it includes basic concepts of social justice, utilitarianism, Kantian theory, and rights theories in one elegant theory. As we have seen in the recent health care reform debates of 2009/2010, the delivery of health care services is special because it:

- has the overarching goal of reducing pain and suffering
- increases the quality of peoples' lives by prevention of disease and enhancing wellness and fitness
- influences the opportunities a person has in society, and
- has a historical, religious and moral connotation
- is unpredictable and intermittent in its need; it is not usually a continuous life-long need, like food or shelter that is not affected by class or position

This last category of unpredictability is important in a theory of justice trying to account for a large population. There are of course diseases or risks that are greater and that occur more often in one class or position than another. It is, for instance, unlikely that a wealthy person, who was mentally sound, would be the victim of chronic starvation, nor is it likely that a person from the poverty zone in the United States would be made ill by improperly canned French escargot or Russian caviar. However, anyone from any class may develop cancer or pneumonia. These special features of health care complicate any discussion of the delivery system and justice. John Rawls' theory takes into account the need for both equal opportunity, the natural lottery of abilities and talents, the need for a Kantian test of respect for others, and our innate sense that justice and fairness should be the basis for something as important as health care. Under the Rawls' theory of justice in health care, it would not be permissible to deny life and opportunity giving health benefits because someone was a person of color, poor, a woman or child or any other special category, unless that benefit was not available to anyone else.

Women and Health Care Justice

The principles of John Rawls can be used to evaluate the health care system in the United States. In this example of using a moral theory to determine whether a system is fair or just, the case of women and the health care system will be examined. To understand how women are treated in the U.S. health care system, it is necessary to review the model of distribution of health care. In the United States, we have a market model of distribution, perhaps not a perfect model, but it comes closest to describing the system. From a Rawlsian perspective, if health care cannot be distributed in a way that satisfies the two principles of Justice, the distribution method is unjust and should be changed.

Looking at women most easily makes the case for health care reform using a theory of justice. Health care distribution in the United States accounts for about 13 percent of its gross national product or over $8,000 per person (http://www.oecd.org/infobycountry). Yet women, who make up over 50 percent of the population, do not enjoy 50 percent of its benefits (National Women's Law Center 2004). Because women do not enjoy equal access to the opportunities of employment in the health care field (fewer women than men are high-paying providers, administrators, or researchers), they are disadvantaged. They also do not have the financial resources (the median income of women is still less by far than that for men) to compete with males for access to service, access to the benefits of research or treatments. Since a market model distributes health care in the United States by exchanging the benefits of health care for a monetary exchange and women are at an economic disadvantage, women qualify under the theory of justice as least advantaged. The plight of women of color is even more dismal.

Women interact with the health care system at critical points in their lives: when giving birth, at menopause, and in old age. Yet, they are disadvantaged even at these points. A woman having a baby in the United States has less chance of her child living than if she has had the baby in Cuba, which has a universal health care system (http://www.unicef.org/infobycountry/cuba). As she reached menopause in the last four decades, she was given drugs that were known to be dangerous. For example, although the drug manufactures and the FDA knew of the dangers connected to estrogen use, that information was withheld from women from the first studies indicating serious problems in the 1980s to the first black box warning in 2002 for further testing by drug companies (Hulley 2004). But when the drug was used for men for prostate cancer, a very specific warning about its dangers was included (www.ourbodiesourselves.org). This is clearly a case of unequal treatment based on gender and unacceptable under any theory of justice.

Women's issues in old age have very low research priority because they are primarily chronic conditions like heart failure and arthritis. In fact, private foundations are now doing most of the research into breast cancer and arthritis, sponsored mostly by women themselves. However, there is a great deal of government-funded research into disease and conditions of men such as acute heart conditions, prostate cancer, and replacements of knees and hips. Women are consistently treated with disrespect by the health providers and have last place on claims for research money to decrease their morbidity. In addition, the mortality of both mother and infants in the United States is extremely high for an industrialized country—13th in the world. This is not what one would have expected from a just health care system. Indeed, using the Rawlsian theory, it is obvious that the market model of health care is not a just distribution system. It is this conclusion that fuels the continuing call for meaningful health care reform in the United Sates.

Using the Theory of Justice to evaluate other countries is a good way to compare the justice and fairness of systems. The Swedish system, for example, is a wholly nationalized system. Medical, dental, and pharmaceutical needs are met for all citizens by government-sponsored agencies. The basic thrust of the system is to keep people well. As a result, the Swedish people enjoy some of the best health care in the world, their life expectancy is one of the highest (81years), and the maternal and infant mortality is the lowest in the world. In addition, they spend only about one half the money per person–($4,000) on health care as does the United States – ($8,000). The Swedish system does not allow unequal treatment on the basis of wealth or income shares. From a Rawlsian perspective, the Swedish system has several promising features: universal access and equity of care, participation by the public in the allocation of health resources process, regulation of the private sector to insure against vast income disparities, and a philosophy that emphasizes wellness and the dignity of the person. Rawlsian principles would judge it to be more just than the U.S. system on the basis of equity of resource allocation treatment of those who by their health needs would be classed as least advantaged.

This same critique and conclusion could be done with any of the other countries that have health care systems that ensure universal access and care for all citizens that need it. The countries that meet the test of justice and fairness for their health care systems would include Great Britain, France, Germany, Japan, and Canada to name a few (http://www.oecd.org/infobycountry).

Summary

Culture refers to integrated patterns of human behavior that include the language, thoughts, communications, actions, customs, beliefs, values, and institutions of racial, ethnic, religious, gender, age, or social groups. Competence implies having the capacity to function effectively as an individual and an organization within the context of the cultural beliefs, behaviors, and needs presented by consumers and their communities.

Cultural competence is the ability of health organizations and practitioners to recognize the cultural beliefs, values, attitudes, traditions, language preferences, and health practices of specific cultural groups and to apply that knowledge to produce positive health outcomes. Competency includes communicating in a manner that is linguistically and culturally appropriate.

Health literacy is the ability of the individual to understand health care providers' information such as prescription instructions, disease brochures, and health care instructions. Researchers have developed tools for the health professional to use in assessing health literacy and providing linguistically and appropriate patient education materials. Health literacy improves health outcomes.

Health care ethics addresses large concepts such as respect for autonomy, nomaleficency (do no harm), beneficence (do good), justice, veracity (truth telling), privacy, confidentiality, and professional roles. Health care ethics also provides health care professionals with their codes of ethics. These codes demand a certain standard of behavior if one is to be in good standing with the health care professions. There are universal principles including veracity (telling the truth) and confidentially that are the cornerstones of professional behavior and duty to patients. Along with the virtues of compassion, integrity, trustworthiness, and wisdom, these principles guide the health care professional in the care of patients. There are several major ethical theories used to help health policy makers and governments divide the pie. The theory of John Rawls includes basic concepts of social justice, utilitarianism, Kantian, and rights theories. It examines the market model of health care distribution to determine the justice and fairness of our health care system.

Questions for Review

1. What is cultural competency?
2. Why is cultural competency important?
3. Describe health literacy.
4. How is it different from regular literacy and the ability to read?
5. How is health literacy assessed?
6. Define the major health ethics principles.
7. What are the advantages of John Rawls' theory of justice?
8. What are the principles and virtues of professionalism?

Questions for Discussion

1. Refer to the chapter profile. Why was cultural competency and health literacy so important for health care providers in caring for the Pima Indians?
2. Who should be trained in cultural competency and health literacy?
3. How many cultures are represented by the students in your classroom today? Discuss the different health care traditions represented by those cultures.
4. Is cultural competency an ethical question and why?
5. Discus health care reform in terms of ethical theories.
6. Describe a societal ethical dilemma and then apply two different principles of ethics to it and defend your decision in terms of that principle.
7. How do the cultural aspects listed in Table 13.2 impact health care, giving specific examples.

Chapter References

Beauchamp, T. L., and Childress, J. F. 2001. *Principles of Biomedical Ethics.* 5th ed. New York, NY and Oxford, England: Oxford University Press.

Center for Linguistic and Cultural Competency in Health Care, Office of Minority Health (http://www. minorityhealth.hhs.gov).

Culture and Ethnicity in Medicine—Bioethics Resources on the Web—National Institute of Health. (http://bioethics.od.nih.gov/culturalcomp.html).

Fadiman, A. 1997. *The spirit catches you and you fall down: A Hmong girl, her American doctors, and the collision of two cultures.* New York: Farrar, Straus, and Giroux.

Henslin, J. M. 2009. *Sociology: A down-to-earth approach.* 10th ed. Upper Saddle River, NJ: Prentice Hall.

Hulley, S. 2004. The WHI Estrogen-Alone Trial—Do things look any better? *JAMA* 291: 1769–1771.

Indian Health Service Communication Tool Kit (http://www.ihs.gov/healthcommunications/index.cfm?module=dsp_hc_toolkit).

Indian Health Service: White paper on Health Literacy #15A646 – accessed 5/09/2010 (http://www.ihs.gov/healthcommunications).

National diabetes statistics 2007 (http://diabetes.niddk.nih.gov/dm/pubs/statistics/).

National Institute of Diabetes and Digestive and Kidney Diseases (NIDDK). (http://www. diabetes.niddk.nih.gov/DM/pubs/pima).

National Center for Cultural Competence, Georgetown University (http://www11.georgetown. edu/research/gucchd/nccc/foundations/frameworks).

National Women's Law Center and the Oregon Health & Science University. 2004. *Making the grade on women's health: A national and state-by-state report card.*

Organization for Employment, Labour & Social Affairs, OECD Health Data 2009 (http://www. oecd.org/infobycountry).

Our Bodies Ourselves (www.ourbodiesourselves.org/book/menoexcertp.asp?id=58&chaptered=31).

Rawls, J. 1971. *A Theory of Justice.* Cambridge, MA: Harvard University Press.

UNICEF (http://www.unicef.org/infobycountry/cuba).

UNICEF (http://www.unicef.org/infobycountry/usa).

Women's Health Initiative. (www.nhlhi.hih.gov/whi/e-a_advisory.htm).

For Additional Information

Bioethics Resources on the Web http://bioethics.od.nih.gov

Coughllin, S. *Ethical issues in epidemiologic research and public health practice.* Epidemiology and Applied Research Branch, Division of Cancer Prevention and Control, National Center for Chronic Disease Prevention and Health Promotion, Centers for Disease Control and Prevention.Available at http://www.ete-online.com/content/3/1/16.

Drugwatch (www.drugwatch.com/premarian).

Health Care: The White House (http://www.whitehouse.gov/issues/health-care).

HealthReform.gov (http://www.healthreform.gov/).

Hoyert D.L. 2007. Maternal mortality and related concepts. National Center for Health Statistics. *Vital Health Statistics* 3(33).

Obasogle, O. and D. Winickoff. *When is the racial pharmacy bad medicine?* Available at http://www. thehastingscenter.org/Bioethicsforum/.

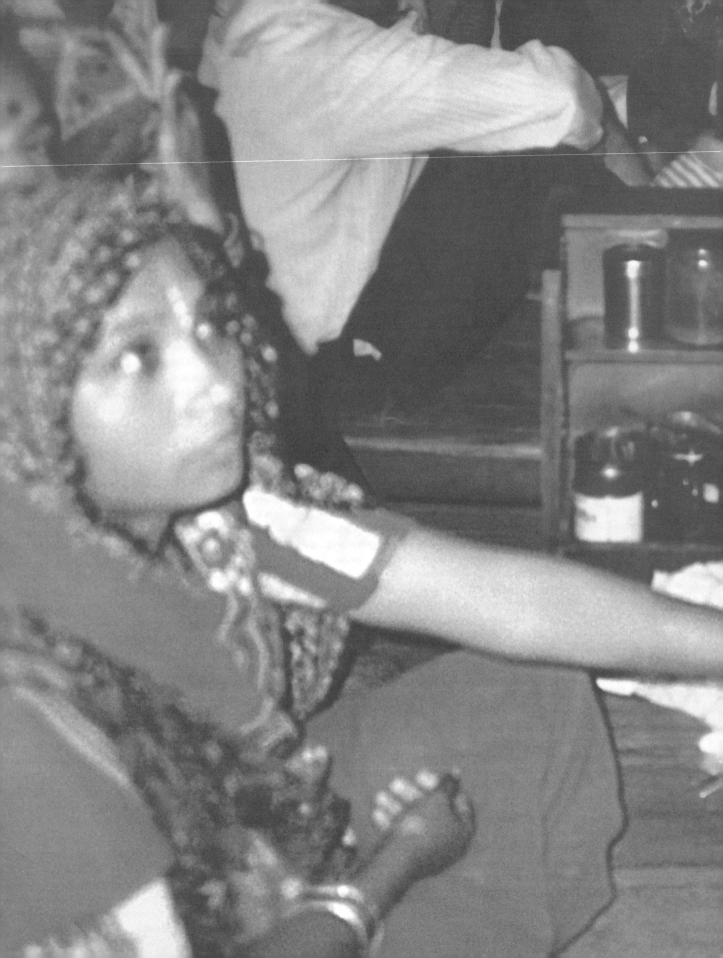

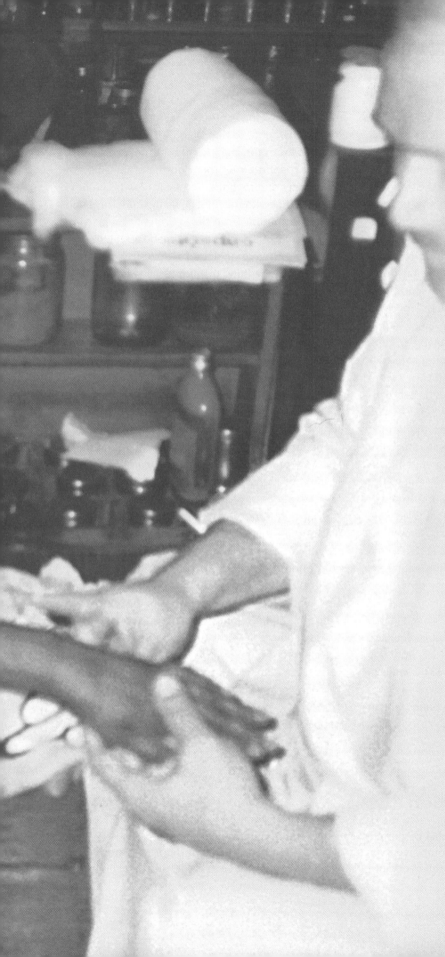

14

International Health Care

Learning Objectives

After reading this chapter, you should be able to:

1. Describe the health care systems of three other countries.
2. Compare the U.S. system to other types of health care systems.
3. Assess health outcomes of health care systems in other countries using health indicators.
4. Plan a trip to a foreign country for a health care need.

Dental Vacation in Mexico

Tom and Becky returned from their Mexican vacation tanned and with wonderful smiles. This was particularly true for Tom. Before he left for Mexico, Tom's smile was literally crooked, since he was missing several teeth from a bicycle accident. His insurance was inadequate to cover the expense of implants, crowns, and bridges. The U.S. dentist had estimated $12,000 dollars above and beyond his insurance. Like most dental policies, there was a yearly cap on expenses that barely covered one crown, let alone a whole mouth restoration. Tom had heard from a friend that he could get good quality dental work done in Mexico for about half what it would be in the United States. Tom's job involved a lot of work with the public, so stringing the work out over 4 years was not a viable option. He and Becky started researching dental care outside the United States. Friends thought they were crazy: after all, wasn't all foreign health care dangerous and prone to complications?

The first thing Tom learned was that many hospitals and clinics in other countries are accredited by the same organization that accredits hospitals here, the Joint Commission. In Mexico, the largest health care provider, Christus Muguerza, has the Joint Commission International Gold Seal of Approval among other certifications. They have hospitals both in Mexico and in eight states in the U.S. Over 28 countries cater to a million patients a year who have health care in a country other than their own (Woodman 2007).

Tom found he could get all the work that he needed done in a dental clinic in Tijuana, Mexico, for roughly half the quoted U.S. price. His implants in the United States would run $2,400–$3,000 apiece; in Tijuana, they were $1,500. His crowns were quoted as $800 to $1,000 in the United States, and in Mexico $375. He could go to Mexico to have his dental work done, take Becky and stay in a four star hotel for 2 weeks, and still save about $3,000. Tom and Becky took the Amtrak train from their home in Portland, Oregon, to San Diego, California, hopped a shuttle from the train station to the border, and the resort shuttle met them on the other sided of the boarder and took them to their resort. The next day, Tom met with the dentist, taking his X-rays and other information from his U.S. dentist with him. The dentist examined Tom and made appointments for the next several days to do the work. Tom reported that the thing that impressed him the most at first was the fact that the dentist gave him his full attention at each appointment—no going from room to room, working on several people at once. He made the crowns himself, fitting them to Tom at each stage, so no need for a long wait between stages. The resort was geared for the medical traveler and provided transportation from the resort to the clinic each day and special foods, and had a pharmacy on site. The dentist gave Tom his cell phone number with instructions to call him if there were any problems. The work was completed with no complications. In Tom's mind, this was the best dental experience of his life.

More and more countries are becoming medical tourism destinations. Medical tourism statistics revealed an anticipated growth of the industry from about $40 billion in 2004 to $100 billion by 2012. It was also estimated that a million and a half Americans sought healthcare outside the United States in 2008. So, pack your bags for a face-lift in Rio de Janeiro, a tummy tuck in Costa Rica, or a hip replacement in Canada.

Sources: Woodman, J. 2007. *Patients beyond borders*. Chapel Hill, NC: Healthy Travel Media: Joint Commission (http://www.medicaltravel.com.mx/certifications); http://www.understanding-medicaltourism.com/medical-tourism-statistics.php.

Introduction

We live in a global community and that community includes health care. This book has up to this point given you a look at the major segments of the U.S. system. This chapter will give an overview of some of the global systems. While all countries have a health care system of some sort, we have chosen only a few below to examine. To compare countries and how well their health care system works, health indicators such as life expectancy, spending on health care, infant and maternal mortality, and the percentage of the citizens covered by the system are used by scientists, researchers, and policy makers.

Both Canada and Mexico are our neighbors, and people travel with relative ease to both countries for business, pleasure, and health care. So, we will explore both those systems. The British system is the oldest National Health care system and a model for many other countries and will be reviewed here. The French and German systems are well-established systems with both strong public and private segments. India is without a doubt the largest system, with a strong traditional medicine and homeopthatic system as well as a flourishing Western-style component. Cuba has a completely nationalized system with one of the best community health systems in the world as well as having doctors and nurses as one of its major exports, a unique concept. Data about these systems are presented in Table 14.1. Keep in mind our own system as you review the global perspective.

Table 14.1	*International Comparison of Selected Health Indicators and Spending*							
	United States	**United Kingdom**	**Mexico**	**Canada**	**Germany**	**France**	**Japan**	**India**
System	Market <65 Single payer >65 Universal veterans	Universal Single payer	3% Market 97 public/ universal	Universal/ Private	Universal Insurance Mandated Private insurance	Universal coverage	Universal coverage	Private Traditional government
Population in millions	307	61	48	30.3	82.1	61.7	128	1.139 billion
Life expectancy	78.1	79	76	80.9	80.0	80.3	82.1	63.7
HC spending as part of GDP	15.3%	8.3%	6%	9.8%	11%	11.1%	8%	5.2%
Per person spending	$8,000	$2,723	$800	$3,643	$2,983	$3.374	$1,927	NA
Infant mortality/ 1,000 births	6.1	4.78	15.3	4.99	3.95	3.31	2.79	49.8
Maternal mortality/ 100,000 live births	11	8.0	60	7.0	4	8	6.0	450
Percentage of citizens covered	82%	100%	100%	100%	100%	100%	100%	NA

Sources: http://data.worldbank.org/indicator/SH.STA.MMRT; http://www.unicef.org/infobycountry/mexico_statistics.html#68; http://www.npr.org; https://www.cia.gov/library/publications/the-world-factbook/rankorder/2091rank.html;.http://www.oecd.org/health/healthataglance.

Health Care Delivery Systems

Single Payer system
The financing of the costs of delivering health care for an entire population through a single insurance pool out of which costs are met. Canada and the United Kingdom are good examples.

The most common system for delivering health care around the globe is what is called a **Single Payer system**. A single payer system is the financing of the costs of delivering universal health care for an entire population through a single insurance pool out of which costs are paid. This is the system those countries with universal access and treatment for all citizens use. All the health care costs are billed to and paid by a single agency within the country, state, or province. Health care providers do not usually bill individual services under this plan, but bill the cost of running the clinic, hospital, or home health unit directly to the government. This system is used in all the Scandinavian countries, Canada, Australia, New Zealand, the United Kingdom, Taiwan, Cuba, and a variation of it in France, Germany, Spain, Italy, and other countries with universal health care as a societal benefit.

The United States and a handful of developing countries use the market economy model to deliver health care. As described in Chapter 2, in a market economy model system, the price and distribution of goods, in this case health care, is determined by supply and demand. It allows the price of health care to increase as demand increases and tends to concentrate service in areas of high population regardless of the need of more rural areas. In addition, if the disease or condition does not generate enough demand, there is little incentive to treat or research the condition. Many countries like Japan use a mixed model in which there is mandatory insurance and the delivery model is a private market model. The market model of health care delivery treats health care like any other product or service, ignoring the very special aspects of health care described in Chapter 13. Generally, we do not choose to have a stroke or break a leg, so there is no freedom of choice involved in our spending of resources. This would seem to invalidate the market model as a sustainable delivery system. Costs rise very rapidly in this system, and there is great disparity between levels of providers with some physicians earning many millions of dollars a year, while nurses and other providers earn a small fraction of that as described in the chapters on health care providers.

The differences in the models of health care delivery are studied by looking at the efficiency and outcomes of the system. We will examine a few below. The U.S. system is not included in this chapter as it has been extensively examined in the previous chapters.

Mexico

Public institutions, state and federal governments, private providers, and private hospitals and clinics provide health care in Mexico. Mexico was in the world spotlight in 2009 during the outbreak of the pandemic H1N1 flu outbreak.

History

The first hospital in Mexico was founded in 1791 by the Bishop of Guadalajara the Hospicio Cabanas. It is not only a functioning hospital today, but is the largest health complex in Central and Latin America and is a World Heritage site. The Mexican Social Security Institute, IMSS (Instituto Mexicano del Seguro Social), was founded in 1943 to provide public health care to all Mexican citizens. In 2003, the Mexican government launched a universal health care plan.

Mexican Health Care Delivery System

The system in Mexico is a three-part system (private, public, and universal) with different levels of care, provider payment, and delivery options depending on the employment status and income of the citizen.

The private system covers roughly 3 percent of the population and caters to the wealthy of the country and the booming medical tourism trade. It is a combination of private insures who facilitate access to state of the art and very high-quality health care and people who are covered by the public system but pay out of pocket for higher-quality services. Non-Mexicans can purchase health care in Mexico by private insurers—both Mexican and American, out-of-pocket payments and other government's national plans (British, Canadian, and French), who reimburse Mexico for their citizens care. The private sector health care is booming in Mexico, partly due to medical tourism. U.S. citizens like Tom flock to Mexico for dental work, cosmetic surgery, cardiac procedures, orthopedic procedures, and ophthalmology procedures. Mexico is also a popular retirement destination for U.S. and Canadian citizens, further increasing the demand for high-quality care. Many Mexican physicians are trained in the U.S. and increasingly U.S. physicians are trained in Mexico.

The public system in Mexico covers wage earners, state employees, and the military. An estimated 50 million workers pay into an insurance plan according to their wages. The IMSS or Mexican Social Security System operates its own clinics and hospitals for insured workers. The quality of these state-run clinics and hospitals varies a good deal. Workers may also opt to use the private system and pay the out-of-pocket expenses. Some 17 million state employees pay into a separate plan administered through the Institute of Security and Social Services, which runs it own clinics and hospitals. The military and employees of the state-owned petroleum company, Pemex, are covered through their own insurance programs. The remaining uninsured Mexicans—about 40 percent of the population—fall under the umbrella of the universal health care plan known as the Popular Health Insurance plan. It was initiated in 2003 with the goal of reducing health care inequities and serving the poorest of citizens. Families pay a premium to join dependent on income (about 20 percent of families pay no premiums) and are required to visit clinics for preventive care (http://content. healthaffairs.org/cgi/content/full/24/6/1467).

Statistics

Universal health in Mexico is credited with an increase in positive health care outcomes in Mexico and reducing catastrophic health cost by as much as 9 percent (*Lancet* 2009). Mexican children now receive the same vaccinations as Canadian children. Malaria and TB cases have dropped (60% and 30%, respectively) since the inception of the plan (E! Science News http://esciencenews.com/sources/science.centric/2009/04/08/).

Mexico spends about $800 or 6 percent of GDP per capita in health care expenditures compared to $8,000 in the United States. Life expectancy in Mexico is 76 years compared with 79 years in the United States.

Canada

The Canadian system for health care delivery can be described as a mixed system, because it is possible to have completely private health care with the patient paying the provider. However, most Canadian health care is provided through the single payer model. Each province in Canada has the constitutional option to opt out of this system, although none have to date. All physician, hospital, pharmaceutical, and clinic fees are set and paid for by the government. A health care provider can not charge more than the government fee, even if the patient is not covered by the public system or is from another country, unless the provider opts out of the system altogether. Other health care expenses such as dentistry and optometry are wholly private sector operations. Each person who enrolls in the program is given a health care card, much like the Medicare card in the United States. All people have the same plan http://www.hc-sc.gc.ca).

In recent years, American citizens have increasingly gone to Canada to purchase prescription drugs and be treated for certain illnesses. U.S. citizens take advantage of the high quality and lower cost of Canadian health care. Canadians also come to the United States for elective surgeries such as hip and heart. Canadians travel to the United States for health care for specialized procedures not available in Canada and in some cases to avoid long waiting times.

History

The early French settlers founded Catholic hospitals in the 1800s. Health care in Canada was private until 1946. At that time, the province of Saskatchewan introduced universal health care coverage. Over the next 10 years, the remaining nine provinces introduced similar coverage. In 1957, the Hospital and Diagnostic Services Act was passed through which the federal government paid 50 percent of costs of the health care programs in all 10 provinces. In 1966, the Medical Care Act was passed that instituted the universal coverage countrywide. The Canada Health Act was passed in 1984 that prohibited extra user fees and extra physician billing fees. The Canadian system, which blends universal health coverage with private sector fee-for-service, is often seen as a model for U.S. health care reform in current and future discussions.

Delivery

The majority of health care in Canada (75%) is funded publicly and delivered privately. The private sector spending is about 30 percent of the total, primarily for services not covered by Canadian Medicare such as dentistry, optometry, some prescription drugs, cosmetic surgery, and for, in some provinces, priority access to health care services. Canadians may also purchase supplementary private health insurance for these services; about 65 percent of the population has this coverage.

The actual delivery of services is the responsibility of the provinces and territories. Although privately funded, most of the services are provided by private enterprises. Most physicians do not receive a salary, but are paid on a fee-for-service basis. They in turn pay their staff, much like private practice physicians in the United States. The role of the federal government is to:

- Provide the funds to deliver the services to the provinces,
- Set and administer the principles of the national health care system,
- Deliver services to specific special groups—veterans, First Nation Peoples, and the Inuit people, and
- Provide public health, health protection programs, and health care research

Both Canadian citizens and health care providers report high approval ratings for this system (Health Canada http://www.hc-sc.gc.ca).

Statistics

In 2005, Canada spent 9.8 percent of GDP on health care, or U.S. $3,463 per capita. Of that, approximately 70 percent was government expenditure, according to the World Health Organization (WHO) (Canada http://www.who.int/countries/can).

India

India has a population of over 1 billion people, with only seven physicians per 10,000 people, according to WHO. India has no central health care system, unlike the other countries we have reviewed. The responsibility for health care is through a system of primary care centers, traditional medicine practitioners, and hospitals. The rural health care system treats less complicated cases and then funnels difficult cases to the urban centers. The system is divided between the modern Western style health care and the traditional systems and homeopathy. Traditional medicine has been practice in India for thousands of years. Traditional systems include Ayureveda, Unani, Siddha, Yoga, naturopathy, and homeopath. These are major delivery systems in India; they treat more people than the modern Western style clinics and hospitals. There are 3,204 traditional hospitals and 725 thousand practitioners in India, according to the Ministry of Health (http://www.india.gov.in/citizen/health/health.php).

The Ayurvedic system is built on the balance in the body of three humors: Vata, Pitta, and Kapha. Health or illness depends on the presence or absence of a balanced state. The diagnosis takes into consideration not only the person's physical state, but also the mental condition, and the person's position in society. The treatments include diet, massage and other bodywork, spiritual guidance, and medicines. People come from all over the world to be treated by the traditional medicine practitioners. Walk into any major U.S. grocery store, and you will find Ayurvedic teas and herbs in the health foods section.

India is also a major medical tourism destination for Western style procedures. India hosts several million foreign visitors seeking high-quality, low-cost health care. Since foreigners pay directly, this form of tourism pumps billions into the Indian economy. Cardiovascular procedures top the list (http://www.indianhealthcare.in).

Summary

Health care in a global community ranges from single-payer systems to traditional medicine systems. Very few systems look like our own system, but our system has aspects of most of the other systems embedded in it. Medical tourism in the past was to a large extent an American experience with people from all over the world coming here for advanced procedures and care. That trend is reversing because of the high cost of American health care and the increasing sophistication of other health care systems. People are going to all corners of the globe for health care from prescription medicines in Canada to heart surgery in India.

To compare countries and how well their health care system works, health indicators such as life expectancy, spending on health care, infant and maternal mortality, and the percentage of the citizens covered by the system are used.

Questions for Review

1. What is a single-payer system?
2. Name two countries with single-payer systems.
3. Compare and contrast the U.S. system with a single payer system.
4. Describe the Canadian health care system.
5. Describe a traditional health care system.
6. Which country spends the most/least on health care?
7. In which country is the risk of dying during childbirth the lowest/highest?
8. In which country do children under the age of one die the most/least?
9. In which country do people live the longest/shortest?
10. What is medical tourism?

Questions for Discussion

1. What type of health care system would you like to live under?
2. Is health care better in the United States? Why or why not? What indicators did you use to define "better"?
3. Should basic indicators of health care be the only measure of a system's success? What other indicators would you use?
4. Would you travel to a foreign country like Tom (see the chapter profile) did for health care to save money?

Chapter References

Department of Health—England (http://www.dh.gov.uk).
Health Canada (http://www.hc-sc.gc.ca).
India Brand Equity Foundation (http://www.ibef.org).
Indian Health Care (http://www.indianhealthcare.in).
Indian Citizen Health (http://www.india.gov.in/citizen/health/health.php).
Joint Commission (http://www.medicaltravel.com.mx/certifications).
National Health Service—England (http://www.nhs.uk).
Organization for Employment, Labour and Social Affairs (http://www.oecd.org/health/healthataglance).
Understanding Medical Tourism (http://www.understanding-medicaltourism.com/medical-tourism-statistics.php).
UNESCO—World Heritage site—Hospitico Cabanas (http://whc.unesco.org/archive/advisory_body_evaluation/815.pd).
Unicef (http://www.unicef.org/infobycountry/).
Unicef—Mexico (http://www.unicef.org/infobycountry/mexico_statistics.html).
Woodman, J. 2007. *Patients beyond borders.* Chapel Hill, NC: Healthy Travel Media.
World Health Organization (http://apps.who.int/whosis/database).
World Health Organization Canada (http://www.who.int/countries/can).

For Additional Information

Organization for Employment, Labour and Social Affairs (http://www.oecd.org/health/healthataglance).
Unicef—Mexico (http://www.unicef.org/infobycountry/).

Glossary

Accounting – The business function that tracks flows of payments in and out of a business.

Activities of daily living – Basic activities such as mobility, eating, toileting, dressing, and bathing.

Actuary – A professional who calculates insurance and annuity risks, premiums, and dividends.

Acute care – Short-term medical care provided to a patient with an immediate need for care.

ADN (associate degree in nursing) – An associate's program typically takes 2 years to complete and is usually offered by a community college.

Advanced practice nurse – A nurse who has obtained a master's degree in a clinical specialty.

Aging in place – A philosophy that allows the aging person or couple to stay in their living situation while growing older with increasing levels of personal and medical assistance as needed. These are adult living communities where the range is from individual homes to a skilled nursing facility in one complex.

Allopathic medicine – A process of treating disease by using standard treatments, such as surgery and drugs.

Alzheimer's disease – A degenerative disorder that affects the brain and causes dementia.

Ambulatory care – Medical care provided in an office setting to a mobile patient.

Antigenic drift – Describes the gradual and continuous changes in the genetic makeup of some viruses such as the Type B flu virus.

Antitrust law – An area of federal law which prohibits monopolization and other activities that lessen competition in the marketplace.

Assessment – The process of determining the health needs of a community.

Assisted living facilities (ALFs) – Homes or apartment-like living spaces that allow for independent activities such as cooking and bathing and also provide care such as medication or treatment delivery; a nonmedical model of chronic care living arrangements.

Assurance – The process of making sure that correct actions are taken to protect community health.

Benefits – The items that are covered under an insurance plan. Also referred to as coverage.

Biochemical – Involving chemical substances present in living organisms, such as dopamine.

Blind random trial – A clinical trial method in which no one knows which drugs the participants are receiving until the trial is finished.

Block grants – A system in which the federal government provides large sums of money to regions and states for projects; started under President Ronald Regan in the 1980s.

Board certification – A physician may become board certified by completing additional years of residency in the specialty and passing an exam.

Board of directors – A group that sets the overall direction for a group or business.

BSN (Bachelor of Science in Nursing) – A bachelor's program usually takes 4 years to complete.

Burden of disease – The cost of a disease in terms of the individual, family, and community disability, including lost work, family relationships, and community participation.

Burnout – A psychological condition in which a person loses the ability to care and becomes apathetic. Stress and overwork are thought to cause burnout.

Business – The activity of providing goods and services to customers for profit.

Business cycle – Regular cycles of decline and growth in an economy over a time period.

Capitation – A payment method under which each patient is entitled to receive a set dollar amount of services in each time period.

Case – A term used in health statistics to refer to each person who has a disease.

Centers for Disease Control and Prevention (CDC) – A group of federal governmental agencies responsible for collecting and interpreting health care statistics.

Centers for Medicare & Medicaid Services (CMS) – The federal agency that administers the Medicare and Medicaid programs; previously known as the Health Care Financing Administration (HCFA).

Certified nurse-midwife (CNM) – An advanced practice nurse who provides prenatal and postpartum care and delivers infants.

Certified registered nurse anesthetist (CRNA) – An advanced practice nurse who specializes in anesthesia.

Chronic condition – An illness or injury lasting more than 90 days; a nonacute illness such as asthma.

Clinical nurse specialist (CNS) – An advanced practice nurse who specializes in a field such as oncology, neonatal care, or mental health.

Clinical trial – The process of testing a new drug, treatment, or medical device on humans in a controlled manner.

CME (continuing medical education) – The state requirement that physicians receive a certain amount of additional training and education to remain licensed.

CNA (Certified Nursing Assistant) – A nurse's aide who has received the credential of CNA.

Cognitive – Relating to the process of thinking or acquiring knowledge. Cognitive diseases disrupt the ability to acquire or remember knowledge.

Communicable disease – A disease that spreads from person to person; another term for infectious disease.

Community hospital – A nonfederal hospital facility that is available to the public.

Compliance program – A program that is implemented in a business to ensure that it stays in compliance with current legislation, especially changes in the Medicare or Medicaid programs.

Computer axial tomography (CT) scan – Machine that visualizes the inside of the human body using a combination of X-ray technology and computerized axial tomography; results are viewed on the computer.

Continuum of care – The philosophy that the health care system should facilitate an individual's care from complete independence to dependence.

Control research – Research whose major aim is to control symptoms, not cure the disease or condition. Pain medications control the symptoms of arthritis; they do not cure the underlying disease.

Coordination of benefits – If a service is covered under more than one policy, then the insurance companies determine which policy pays.

Copayment (coinsurance) – A payment made by the insured at the time services are received.

Core values – Values are shared attitudes and beliefs among group members. Core values are the central values of a culture.

Corporation – A legal form of business ownership that can have many owners. The percentage of the business owned is determined by the number of shares held by the owner, also known as a shareholder.

Cost/benefit analysis – The process of comparing the specific costs of a treatment to the benefits obtained by that treatment.

Counterculture – A group within a main culture that rejects the standards of the main culture.

Cultural relativism – The evaluation of other cultures by their own standards.

Culture – An integrated and shared pattern of human behavior.

Curative medical care – Medical care that helps cure an already ill or infected person.

Curative research – Research whose major aim is to find a cure for a specific disease.

Current procedural terminology (CPT) – A part of the HCPCS used to code procedures and services performed by providers.

Deductible – An amount specified in the insurance policy that must be paid by the insured before the insurance company will pay.

Delivery models – Systems to bring a particular type of care to individuals and groups.

Demand – The amount of a good a buyer is willing to purchase at a given price.

Demographic – The data from human populations that describe vital statistics, size, and distribution.

Diagnostic tests – Tests ordered by a physician to provide information that assists in making a diagnosis.

Diploma program – Hospitals used to provide on-the-job training programs for nurses and award a diploma upon completion. Very few diploma programs still exist.

Disability Adjusted Life Years (DALY) – The number of years a disease reduces the lifespan.

Drug resistant – The term used to describe when a disease or bacteria are not affected or stopped by the use of common antibiotics and other drugs.

Eating disorders – A group of diseases that describes a patient's focus on food, obsessive eating, or not eating, along with faulty perception of body image.

Economic indicators – Key measurements that provide information about the health of the economy.

Electrocautery – The process of destroying tissue by an electrically heated instrument.

Electron beam computer tomography – Uses electron beams instead of X-rays for computerized axial tomography and also viewed on computer. Compared with the traditional CT scan, it does not require the patient to be completely still, is less enclosed, and costs more.

ELSI programs – Programs around the world that study the ethical, legal, and social aspects of the availability of genetic information.

Employee Retirement Income Security Act of 1974 (ERISA) – Federal legislation that mandates how employer-funded benefit plans must be administered.

Enrollees – The employees who sign up for insurance coverage from the employer.

Enrollment period – The time period during which people, usually employees, can sign up for or change their insurance coverage.

Epidemic – A term used to describe a disease that is widespread in a population.

Epidemiology – The study of the nature, cause, control, and determinants of the frequency of disease, disability, and death in human populations. Also the study of the history of a disease and its distribution throughout a society (public health).

Ethnocentrism – The evaluation of behaviors according to one's own cultural beliefs.

Etiology – The study of the causes and origins of disease.

Exclusive Provider Organizations (EPOs) – Delivery networks in which patients must use the services of those providers.

Explanation of benefits (EOB) – A form sent to the patient that explains which claims were paid at what level.

Federal Employees Health Benefits Program (FEHBP) – An employer-sponsored health insurance program available to employees of the federal government.

Fee-for-service – A method of reimbursement that presets the fee that will be paid for the service provided.

For profit – Making a profit is identified as the primary reason for the business to exist.

Fortune Global 500 – The top-earning 500 companies in the United States as listed by *Fortune* magazine.

Foundation – A type of non-profit organization that raises money and then distributes it to other organizations in support of their programs.

Gatekeeping – A process of restricting access to services.

General and family practitioner – Physician who focuses on providing comprehensive health care to patients of all ages.

General hospitals – Hospitals that provide a range of services.

Generic drug – A drug sold or dispensed under a name that is not protected by a trademark, usually a chemical name or description (e.g., acetaminophen instead of Tylenol).

Gene sequencing – The process of determining the individual arrangement of nucleotides that compose a given gene; used extensively in drug research.

Gene therapy – The treatment of disease using normal or altered genes to replace or enhance nonfunctional or missing genes.

Governing board – A group who sets the overall direction for a group or business.

Gross Domestic Product (GDP) – The dollar value of all the final goods and services produced by businesses within a country's borders.

Group practice – A group of several physicians who practice as a group.

Healthcare Common Procedure Coding System (HCPCS) – A classification system used to code and process an insurance claim.

Health information record – Contains the patient's personal, financial, and social data as well as the medical data. The health information record replaces the term *medical record*.

Health Insurance Portability and Accountability Act of 1996 (HIPAA) – A federal law that mandates insurance portability and sets up procedures for electronic data exchange.

Health Maintenance Act of 1973 – Federal legislation that provided incentives for the formation of Health Maintenance Organizations.

Health Maintenance Organization (HMO) – Employer prepays a flat fee to the HMO; employees receive services as they need them.

Health-related quality-of-life (HRQOL) – The physical and mental well-being of an individual that looks at the quality and quantity of a healthy life in terms of years.

Histology – The study of body tissues.

Human Genome Project – An international cooperative scientific project to map the 60,000 human genes that make up the human genetic code.

ICD-9-CM – The abbreviation for the International Classification of Diseases, 9th Revision, Clinical Modification. This classification is used to code office visits to process an insurance claim.

Imaging technology – A broad term referring to the many forms of technology that allow an image of the patient's body to be produced.

Implants – Medical devices that are placed inside the human body for therapeutic purposes, such as an insulin pump or artificial knee joint.

Indemnity – One party is exempted from incurred liabilities by the other party.

Independent practice association (IPA) model – The IPA markets the health plan. Physicians contract with the IPA to treat members of the HMO.

Individual retirement account (IRA) – Individuals may deposit money into an IRA to save for retirement. These accounts have certain tax benefits, and there are penalties for withdrawing the money prior to retirement.

Infectious disease – A disease that can spread from person to person (versus a genetic disease or a disease that is not contagious).

Inflation – An increase in the price level.

Information technology – The business function that manages all the technology used to run the business and collects information for decision making.

Inpatient care – The patient needs care that requires being admitted to the hospital.

Institutional review board (IRB) – The group of people appointed by the government or a university to oversee any research on animals or humans.

Interest – The amount, stated as a percentage, paid to borrow money.

Internal medicine – An area of medicine that focuses on the body's organs, such as the heart, eyes, ears, kidneys, and the digestive, respiratory, and vascular systems.

Investigational new drug (IND) application – The notice to the FDA (Food and Drug Administration) that the drug company intends to begin clinical tests on humans.

Ischemic cardiac diseases – A group of conditions characterized by a decreased blood flow to the heart.

Joint Commission on Accreditation of Healthcare Organizations (JCAHO) – National organization that evaluates and accredits health care organizations.

Kantian theory – An ethical theory developed by Immanuel Kant (1724–1804) that says a universal moral law obligates one to treat people as an end in itself.

Latex allergies – Many medical practitioners and patients are allergic to latex, which is the most commonly found material in gloves used in medical procedures.

Licensed practical nurse (LPN) – A nurse who has completed a state-approved program and passed a national exam. Generally, LPNs are supervised by RNs when providing patient care.

Limited liability partnership – A specific type of partnership arrangement in which a partner's liability is limited to the amount of the capital contribution.

Long-term care – The federal health care definition of long-term care is more than 60 days.

Magnetic resonance imaging (MRI) – Technology that uses electromagnetic radiation to visualize the body's soft tissues, such as the brain and spinal cord.

Major depression – A depression that lasts for a significant period of time or recurs frequently; a medical diagnosis.

Malpractice – The act of providing professional services that are below the standard of quality for that profession.

Managed care – Describes the combination of payments for health care and delivery of services into one system.

Management – The business function of planning, organizing, directing, and controlling the business's resources.

Market economy – An economy in which many sellers compete for customers.

Marketing – The business function that focuses on the exchange process between the business and its customers.

Medicaid – A federal and state program that funds health care primarily on the basis of the recipient's income.

Medical devices – The range of medical technologies that are used for therapeutic purposes, such as cardiac pacemakers and thermometers.

Medical history – The record of a patient's health, physicians' visits, symptoms, prescribed treatments, regular medications, and family medical history.

Medical imaging – Viewing the inside of the human body using a variety of techniques such as X-rays and CT scans.

Medical model – A viewpoint about health that focuses on the diagnosis and treatment of disease.

Medical nutrition therapy – The use of nutrition to support health in a patient.

Medical Power of Attorney – A person appointed by another who can give consent for medical care or can withhold medical care. It is a legal document that empowers the surrogate decision maker in all health care decisions if the patient is unable to make decisions.

Medical Practice Act – State legislation that sets out the requirements for physician licensure in that state.

Medical staff – Responsibility for quality patient care belongs to the physicians who make up the hospital's medical staff.

Medical technology – Therapeutic and diagnostic devices used to prevent, treat, diagnose, and assist patients medically. The X-ray machine is an example of medical technology.

Medicare – A federal program that pays health care costs for the elderly, the permanently disabled, and those with end-stage renal disease.

Medicare Advantage – A revision of the Medicare + Choice offered under Part C of Medicare.

Medicare Part A – This part of the Medicare program pays for inpatient hospital services, critical access to hospitals, and skilled nursing facilities.

Medicare Part B – This part of the Medicare program pays for physician services, outpatient hospital care, and some services and supplies.

Medicare Part C – This part of the Medicare program is an additional insurance plan intended to cover the gaps in Part A and Part B coverage.

Medicare Prescription Drug, Improvement, and Modernization Act of 2003 – The most recent modification of the federal legislation; in particular, it added coverage for prescription drugs.

Mental health – The ability to cope with change, a positive outlook on life, ability to interact in close relationships in a loving and supportive manner, and the general feeling of well-being that can be assessed in the individual.

Minimally invasive surgery – Use of fiberoptics, guided images, microwave, and other technologies to do surgery rather than cutting large sections of tissue.

Mission statement – A short statement that articulates the reason for the organization's existence.

Monitoring – The regular review of disease data to determine changes in disease levels.

Monopoly – An economy with only one seller. The one seller is able to set whatever price it chooses.

Mood – The state of mind experienced at a particular time.

Mood disorder – An altered state of mind, such as the continuous sadness known as depression.

National codes (HCPCS level II codes) – The part of HCPCS used to code procedures and services not found in the CPT.

National Institutes for Health (NIH) – A group of federal governmental agencies responsible for the health of the nation.

Needlestick injuries – Health practitioners can be injured and exposed to disease if they are inadvertently stuck by a needle.

Network HMO – The HMO contracts with at least two group medical practices, described as "in network" to provide services.

New Drug Application (NDA) – The formal request from the FDA to be allowed to market a new drug.

Not-for-profit – The primary reason for the business to exist is some reason other than profit.

Not-for-profit hospitals – The primary purpose of the hospital is something other than profit.

Nurse Practice Act – State legislation that sets out the requirements for nurse licensure in the state.

Nurse practitioner (NP) – Advanced practice nurse who provides basic primary health care.

Nurse's aide – Health care worker who provides the most basic level of patient care, such as feeding and hygiene.

Nurse supervisor – A nursing position with more responsibilities and requiring more experience than a staff nurse.

Nursing home – An old-fashioned word designating a chronic care facility.

Nursing Interventions Classification (NIC) – A list of 542 interventions that are the nursing treatments of choice for each nursing diagnosis.

Nursing Outcomes Classification (NOC) – A list of 385 identified outcomes that are responsive to nursing care.

Nursing process – An organizing framework that provides a systematic method to deliver patient care.

Oligopoly – An economy with only a few sellers.

Osteopathic medicine – A process of treating patients by providing preventive and holistic care.

Outpatient care – Also referred to as ambulatory care. The patient does not require admittance to a hospital.

Outsourcing – The process of buying goods or services from another provider rather than performing them by the business.

Over-the-counter (OTC) – Drugs and medical devices that may be sold without a written health care provider's order. Aspirin and crutches are examples.

Parenteral nutrition – Any method of delivering nutrition that is not by mouth, such as by an intravenous line or by a direct tube into the stomach or intestine.

Parity – Equality; in this context, it means equality of benefits between insurance coverage for mental health and medical coverage.

Partnership – A legal form of business ownership that involves at least two people called *partners*.

Patient advocate – Hospital employee whose role is to take the side of the patient in all discussions and disputes.

Pediatrician – A physician who focuses on providing care to children.

Pharmaceuticals – Bioactive agents in the human body for therapeutic purposes (e.g., antibiotics).

Phlebotomist – A health care professional who collects blood samples.

Policy – The agreement, or contract, that describes all of the terms and conditions of an insurance policy.

Policy development – The process of making a collective decision about what needs to be done to protect the community's health.

Preauthorization – Many insurers require that certain procedures be authorized by the insurer before they are performed. Failure to obtain preauthorization may result in denial of the claim.

Predisposition – In medicine, a susceptibility to a disease or condition because of hereditary or other factors.

Preferred Provider Organization (PPO) – A delivery network that manages and negotiates contracts on behalf of the providers, who provide services at lower cost.

Premium – The price paid by the insured for insurance coverage.

Prepaid group practice model HMO – Physicians are employees of an independent group that contracts with the health plan to provide services.

Prepaid health plan (PHP) – Refers to plans in which fixed payments are made before services are rendered.

Prescription drug – A drug that must have a health care provider's written order (prescription) to be dispensed.

Prevention efforts – Health programs and behaviors that prevent illness from occurring.

Preventive research – Research whose major aim is to find ways to prevent a disease or condition. For example, preventive research found that diet, exercise, and certain drugs like aspirin may prevent a second heart attack.

Primary care – Basic and routine care that can be delivered by a provider in an office or clinic.

Primary care physician – The physician who sees a patient regularly for routine and preventive care.

Primary prevention – Focuses on preventing disease or problems. Seat belts are a primary prevention technique against injuries in a collision.

Privately owned hospitals – Hospitals owned by non-government entities.

Production – The business function that designs and manages the process that manufactures the business's products.

Profit – The amount left when a business subtracts its expenses from its revenues. If the amount is a negative number, it is a loss.

Proprietary – Owned by an individual or group of individuals: a for-profit arrangement.

Prospective payment system (PPS) – A payment system in which the amount of reimbursement is determined prior to the patient receiving services and is based on the patient's classification into a diagnostic-related group (DRG).

Public hospitals – Hospitals owned by the federal, state, or local government.

Quarantine – Forced isolation of a person to prevent a disease from spreading.

Radio frequency ablation (RFA) – Uses microwaves to destroy tissue.

Reciprocity agreement – An agreement between two states in which each accepts the professional licensing requirements of the other.

Recombination – The genetic process of new gene combinations that gives rise to offspring that have a combination of genes different from those of either parent.

Registered nurse (RN) – A nurse who develops and manages a nursing care plan for a patient.

Rehabilitation – Therapy or other help given to a patient to enable the person to live a healthy and productive life.

Research and development (R&D) – The process of examining and bringing a product to market.

Residency – The last stage of physician training. After medical school, the student completes on-the-job training in his or her specialty.

Residential care – A living arrangement in which the person resides or lives full time at a facility.

Rights theory – An ethical theory that believes people have certain basic rights as human beings and as citizens.

Risk factors – Anything that contributes to a person getting ill. A feature of someone's habits, genetic history, or personal history that increases the probability they will get a particular disease or injury. Smoking is a risk factor for lung cancer.

Risk of loss – The probability that the insured-against event will occur.

Risk pooling – The process of combining all the insureds into one group so the group's overall risk of loss is reduced.

Sandwich generation – The generation that is currently working and taking care of children and parents, thus sandwiched between two dependent age groups.

Secondary care – Involves routine hospitalization and surgery on a short-term basis.

Secondary prevention – Focuses on early detection and prevention such as mammograms and breast exams.

Self-insured plan – A plan where an employer pays for employees' health care.

Self-referral arrangements – Health care providers are prohibited under federal law from referring patients to laboratories or other health services in which they have a financial interest.

Sick role – A pattern of behavior that is expected by the culture from a person who is defined as sick.

Single payer system – The financing of the costs of delivering universal health care for an entire population through a single insurance pool out of which costs are met.

Sole proprietorship – A legal form of business ownership that has only one owner.

Solo practice – A self-employed physician who practices alone.

Somatic – Affecting the body separate from the mind. For example, warm baths are a somatic treatment for calming the body.

Spend down – Redistributing assets so that the individual will be Medicaid eligible.

Staff model HMO – Physicians are employees of the HMO and paid a salary.

Staff nurse – An entry-level position for a nurse.

State Board of Nursing – Each state has an agency that oversees the profession and accredits educational programs.

State Children's Health Insurance Program (SCHIP) – A federal program that targets low-income children whose parents do not qualify for Medicaid yet are unable to afford private health insurance.

Strategic planning process – The formal process of setting the direction of an organization.

Subculture – A group within a main culture that accepts the standards of the main culture, but has distinctive customs and values.

Supervised clinical experience – Nursing students obtain hands-on experience with patients as part of their education.

Surgeon – A physician who performs operations.

Surveillance – The continuous search for and documentation of disease in public health.

Sustainable competitive advantage – Anything about a business that allows it to outperform other businesses and maintain its position over time.

SWOT analysis – A method used by businesses to analyze the external environment.

Talk therapy – Psychotherapy invented by Sigmund Freud that involves primarily talking rather than somatic or drug therapy.

Technician – A person who performs the routine tasks in a laboratory setting.

Technologist – A professional who performs testing services. A technologist usually has more training than a technician.

Technology – The application of knowledge based on inventions, innovations, and discoveries in science.

Tertiary care – Complex and specialized care delivered in specific institutional settings, such as burn treatment.

Tertiary prevention – A focus on keeping the disease or condition from deteriorating further (e.g., water exercise for people with joint problems or better insulin compounds and delivery systems for diabetics to prevent further complications).

The insured – The person who will receive benefits under the terms of an insurance policy.

Therapy – Remedial treatment of a disorder.

Third-party administrator (TPA) – A company that manages the paperwork for an employer who establishes a self-insured plan.

TRICARE – A health insurance program offered by the Department of Defense to military personnel.

Unemployment – A lack of jobs in an economy for those willing and able to work.

Usual, customary, and reasonable payment program (UCR) – A method of reimbursing providers by examining what other providers are paid for that service.

Utilitarianism – An ethical theory that believes resources should be distributed to achieve the maximum benefit.

Utilization measures – Measures that indicate whether an organization is being used to its full capacity.

Vector – An organism that transmits disease-causing microbes from infected individuals to other persons or from infected animals to human beings. Fleas were the vectors from rats to people in the great plagues.

Wellness model – A viewpoint about health that focuses on the prevention of disease.

Workers' compensation – A program that provides health care benefits to employees who are injured on the job.

Index